Interventions for Alzheimer's Disease

A Caregiver's Complete Reference

Interventions for Alzheimer's Disease

A Caregiver's Complete Reference

Ruth M. Tappen, Ed.D., R.N., FAAN
Florida Atlantic University

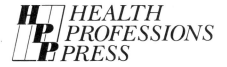

HEALTH
PROFESSIONS
PRESS

Baltimore • London • Toronto • Sydney

Health Professions Press, Inc.
Post Office Box 10624
Baltimore, Maryland 21285-0624

Typeset by PRO-IMAGE Corporation, York, Pennsylvania.
Cover design by James V. McCabe, Four Winds Productions, LLC,
Baltimore, Maryland.
Manufactured in the United States of America by
The Maple Press Company, York, Pennsylvania.

Library of Congress Cataloging-in-Publication Data

Tappen, Ruth M.
    Interventions for Alzheimer's disease : a caregiver's complete reference / Ruth M. Tappen
        p. cm.
    Includes bibliographical references and index.
    ISBN 1-878812-39-4
    1. Alzheimer's disease—Patients—Care. I. Title.
    RC523.T37   1997
    362.1′96831–dc21

                                                                                    97-1680
                                                                                    CIP

British Library Cataloguing in Publication Data are available from the British Library.

Contents

About the Author

Ruth Tappen, Ed.D., R.N., FAAN, is Christine E. Lynn Eminent Scholar and Professor in the College of Nursing at Florida Atlantic University. She holds a doctorate in nursing education from Teachers College, Columbia University, and has completed a postdoctoral fellowship in instrumentation and clinical research at the College of Nursing, University of Arizona.

Her work is concerned primarily with the care of older adults, particularly those with long-term chronic conditions such as Alzheimer's disease and related dementias. Her research has been funded by the Robert Wood Johnson Foundation; the Division of Nursing, Bureau of Health Professions, Department of Health and Human Services; and the National Institute for Nursing Research, National Institutes of Health.

Dr. Tappen is the author of numerous articles on practice, administration, and education related to older adults, and has presented a number of papers on her research, both nationally and internationally. She is also the author of the textbook *Nursing Leadership and Management: Concepts and Practice*, now in its third edition.

Dr. Tappen is a Fellow of the American Academy of Nursing and served as an Ombudsman for the District X Long Term Care Ombudsman Council, Broward County, Florida. She is also adjunct nurse researcher and associate of the Geriatric Research Education and Clinical Center (GRECC) of the Veterans Administration Medical Center, Miami.

Theris Touhy, M.S.N., A.R.N.P., C.S. (author of Chapter 12), is a nurse practitioner and clinical nurse specialist in gerontological nursing. She is a Visiting Assistant Professor in the College of Nursing, Florida Atlantic University, and Clinical Nurse Specialist, Extended Care Program, Veterans Affairs Medical Center, West Palm Beach.

Ms. Touhy is the author of several articles and chapters on the creation of a caring-based curriculum, interventions in long-term care, and the use of story in becoming acquainted with older people. She has held leadership positions in several long-term care facilities and is a frequent presenter on clinical and nursing issues related to the care of older adults.

Preface

This book is written for professionals who find themselves responsible for the planning, administration, or provision of services for the increasing number of older people with Alzheimer's disease and the related dementing diseases. It provides a background for understanding the disease itself and suggests a wide range of potentially effective interventions for people in the early, middle, and late stages of Alzheimer's disease. Most important, this information is provided within a framework of care and concern for the person with the disease and an emphasis on honoring the person's rights to respect, privacy, and preservation of dignity.

It was not all that long ago that people would say, "My mother has Alzheimer's, but thank God, she has no idea what's happening to her anymore." Although the person's level of awareness and the degree of comprehension of what is happening diminish as the disease progresses, these abilities do not disintegrate entirely. Thus, it is no longer possible to console ourselves with myths. People with Alzheimer's disease and related dementias do feel the pain and the frustrations that accompany their losses. They experience the same emotions as do people without cognitive impairment: fear, anger, love, and joy. Which of these emotions predominates can be affected to a great extent by the kind of help that is offered to people with dementia and the manner in which it is offered. It is hoped that this book will contribute to the humanizing of the care of people at all stages of this terrible disease.

He who has a why to live can bear with almost any how.

Friedrich Nietzche

Understanding Alzheimer's Disease

Chapter 1

Course of
Alzheimer's Disease

[Y]ou feel the loss over and over till you think you might go mad. You are literally watching someone's mind die. . . . Alzheimer's drags it out to the limits of human endurance. . .

H. Anifantakis (1991)

For many people, receiving a diagnosis of Alzheimer's disease may be more frightening than receiving a diagnosis of cancer. Cancer is clearly physical; a tumor can be visualized, and even leukemic cells can be pictured. The disease can be understood in terms of cell growth that has gotten out of control. Fighting cancer is a matter of finding the right combination of drugs, surgery, radiation, and determination to survive.

Alzheimer's disease, by contrast, has been described as a "mind-robbing, body sparing" condition (Whitehouse, Lerner, & Hedera, 1993, p. 603). It is a failure of one of the most mysterious organs of the human body, the brain. Attempts to describe the function of the brain become mired in explanations of electrochemical transmissions and neural networks that never quite seem to provide an understanding of what thinking is or what can interfere with it. It is probably safe to say that thinking about how one thinks is something most people rarely do. Even more problematic is thinking about how another person is having difficulty thinking. Yet this is exactly what must be done to understand Alzheimer's disease and related dementias.

ALZHEIMER'S DISEASE–DELIRIUM–DEMENTIA

Alzheimer's disease, delirium, and dementia once were lumped together under the term *senility*. The most dangerous aspect of this overgeneralization was its consequences for diagnosis and treatment: Delirium may be reversible, whereas the dementias generally are not. Severe depression may also mimic dementia and may be difficult to distinguish from dementia without a comprehensive health history, extensive neuropsychological testing, and treatment with medication and psychotherapy.

Delirium

Delirium is a temporary condition that may be mistaken for dementia. The person with delirium may be either overactive (*hyper*active) or underactive (*hypo*active) (Lee & Loring, 1993). The hyperactive person may actually appear to be psychotic: restless, excitable, hallucinatory, incoherent, and disoriented (not knowing where he or she is or what day it is). The hypoactive person may seem dazed, listless, lethargic, slow to respond, and unable to understand what is happening.

Delirium is usually the result of an underlying physical problem. It occurs more often in very old ("old-old," people over age 80) people because their nervous systems are more vulnerable than are the nervous systems of younger people, who generally have more physical reserves. Medically prescribed drugs are one of the most common causes of delirium in older people. Other common causes include oxygen deficiency, dehydration, hypo- or hyperthermia (too low or too high a body temperature), and hypo- or hyperglycemia (blood sugar that is too low or too high). Remembering how it feels to have a high temperature with the flu is one way to understand some of the sensations of a hyperactive delirium. Even one's sense of time is changed by the high temperature: Time seems to move more slowly as the body's metabolic rate is increased by a high temperature.

If delirium is recognized early enough and treated adequately, it is usually reversible. When it is not correctly diagnosed and treated, the affected person may be mistakenly diagnosed as having dementia, and even placed in a nursing facility and maintained on the very same drug that caused the delirium. Fortunately, most medical personnel are now aware of this potential danger.

Dementia

In contrast to that of delirium, the onset of dementia is almost always slow and insidious, rather than sudden. In fact, it is often difficult to pinpoint the onset of a dementia. A slow, steady decline is typical. A notable exception is the vascular dementias, which are known for their stepwise course and fluctuation in severity (see Chapter 3). A person with vascular dementia may seem lucid one day and unable to carry on a conversation the next day.

Dementia is the general term used for diseases, including Alzheimer's disease, that are characterized by progressive cognitive impairment and the emotional and behavioral problems that result from the cognitive decline (Sungaila & Crockett, 1993). They are both progressive and degenerative in nature, as opposed to the reversible nature of delirium. The DSM-IV definition of dementia specifies impairment in ability to learn new material, remember previously learned material, or both and at least one of the following: aphasia, apraxia, agnosia, or disturbance in executive functioning (American Psychiatric Association, 1994). The term *aphasia* refers to difficulty in expression and comprehension of written or spoken language. *Apraxia* is difficulty carrying out purposeful movements. *Agnosia* is difficulty interpreting sensory stimuli (Kolb & Wishaw, 1990). *Executive functioning* is the ability to direct one's own behavior; impairment is demonstrated by behaviors such as carelessness, impulsivity, excitability, lack of motivation, and inability to plan and carry out purposeful behavior (Lezak, 1983). These impairments must be sufficient to interfere with an individual's occupational or social functioning and represent a decline from previously higher levels of function.

A number of different chronic degenerative dementias exist, including the vascular dementias, alcohol-related dementia (Korsakoff's syndrome), the dementia of Parkinson's disease, Lewy's bodies, Pick's disease, normal-pressure hydrocephalus, and Alzheimer's disease. The differences among the most common of these dementias are explained further in Chapter 3.

Alzheimer's disease is the most common type of dementia of the middle and later years of life. It was named after Alois Alzheimer, who first related it to the plaques and tangles that characterize the disease neurologically. The name was first applied only to early-onset dementia but has since been extended to include later-onset dementia as well because both types of dementia are now thought to be the same disease process. Unlike Parkinson's disease or Korsakoff's syndrome, Alzheimer's disease is not linked to another disease process. For this reason, it is often called primary degenerative dementia of the Alzheimer's type. Primary degenerative dementia of the Alzheimer's type is characterized by the cognitive deficits and interference with function described previously as well as the following criteria designed to distinguish it from other dementias (American Psychiatric Association, 1994):

- A gradual and continuing cognitive decline
- Lack of evidence that the decline is the result of other neurological problems such as stroke, Parkinson's disease, Huntington's chorea, or the effects of substance abuse
- Cognitive deficits do not occur only during delirium
- Cognitive deficits are not the result of depression or other psychiatric problems

ONSET AND TIME FRAME

Although each one is different, family members' stories of how they first discovered that their loved one had Alzheimer's disease or another kind of dementia often reveal similar patterns.

> My father-in-law was an avid reader. We exchanged books for years. When he was hospitalized, I noticed that he was not making any progress in his new book. He was on page 3 for a week. Later we found out that he had vascular dementia.

> My mother was a bookkeeper. She was always so proud of her attention to detail. Then she started complaining about the bank—how they were giving her so much trouble. They kept calling her, she said, and were really rude to her. We discovered that her checking account was overdrawn for the first time in her life. She had been writing huge checks to all kinds of charities that we had never heard of before. None of the bills were paid. We had to take over her finances after that. We found out that she had Alzheimer's disease.

> He was outside with the children. Suddenly they were calling me, "Grandpa fell!" He'd never done that before. He said he tripped over an uneven spot in the sidewalk and that he would fix it for us before someone really got hurt. It happened a few more times before we finally realized that something was wrong and insisted that he see a doctor. By then he was forgetting things, too. Sometimes he was as sharp as a tack and then he would be real hazy, real uncertain about what he was saying or doing. He was finally diagnosed as having a vascular dementia.

> My wife was in her early 50s. She had always been a very active, very intelligent woman. She could speak three languages fluently and read two others. When she began having trouble remembering things, she signed up for a memory-improving course at the community college. She took [classes] for a year but the problem got worse. Now she can't speak but she does know who I am. It

was when we moved from Princeton to New Brunswick that I realized how bad it was. She couldn't find our own apartment, couldn't get back from the store, couldn't find our mailbox downstairs. They used to call what she has presenile dementia but the doctor said it was just early-onset Alzheimer's disease. She is still a beautiful woman.

In each of these stories the disease had been present for some time before the family member realized that something was wrong. Although each one discovered it in a different way, their sorrow is evident in the way they describe how intelligent, active, or responsible their loved one had been up to that time. In each story the loss is substantial and will increase as the disease progresses.

An interesting study of 100 people whose Alzheimer's disease was confirmed at autopsy gives us an idea of the time frame of the disease (Kukull et al., 1994). For the average person, the presence of Alzheimer's disease is diagnosed 32 months after symptoms are first noticed. This hypothetical "average person" was placed in an institution 25 months after that and died 44 months later. People under age 65 at the time of diagnosis were not placed in a long-term care facility as soon and usually lived longer than the average of 8.4 years after onset of symptoms. Heart disease, stroke, cancer, and other common causes of death among older people are predominant causes of death in people in the earlier stages of Alzheimer's disease. Reduced ability to recognize and report symptoms may contribute to delay in treatment and should be of concern to caregivers. In the severe stage, pneumonia and Alzheimer's disease are most often listed as the causes of death (Kukull et al., 1994).

STAGES

The various stages through which Alzheimer's disease progresses can be described in several different ways. The easiest to remember are those that use three stages describing the mild, moderate, and severe forms of the disease. Benson (1989) enumerated these three stages as follows:

Stage I: 1–3 years
Memory: New learning and remote recall impaired
Visuospatial: Mild disorientation in unfamiliar surroundings
Language: Word-finding difficulty, poor word list generation
Motor: Normal
Electroencephalogram (EEG):   Normal
Computed tomography (CT):   Normal

Stage II: 2–10 years
Memory: Recent and remote recall impaired further
Visuospatial: Disorientation
Language: Speech fluent but aphasic
Motor: Restlessness evident
EEG: Slowing of background rhythm
CT: Mild ventricular dilation and sulcal (i.e., groove, furrow of the brain) enlargement

Stage III: 8–12 years
Memory, Visuospatial, and Language: Severely deteriorated
Motor: Limb rigidity and flexion posture common
EEG: Diffusely slow
CT: Ventricular dilation, sulcal enlargement

This brief outline presents a picture of the gradual but unrelenting deterioration that occurs with Alzheimer's disease.

Probably the best-known set of stages describing the deterioration of function experienced by the person with Alzheimer's disease is the more detailed FAST (Functional Assessment Staging), developed by Reisberg and associates (Sclan & Reisberg, 1992) (see Table 1.1). An earlier version of the FAST was called the Global Deterioration Scale. The FAST predicts the order in which the functional decline occurs and can be used to track the progression of the disease in an individual.

Some controversy has arisen over the accuracy of these stages, especially over the degree to which most people with Alzheimer's disease actually display this progression of symptoms. Nevertheless, the stages are a useful summary of the changes that occur in Alzheimer's disease and can be helpful in classifying individuals with the disease.

The FAST has seven stages. Two of the stages have substages as well, allowing ranking of an individual on 1 of 16 sequential functional levels from "normal" (no objective or subjective decrease in function) to "severe" (profound decrease in function; outside support essential).

The FAST distinguishes between the fully functional older adult and the older adult who complains of some problems with remembering important things but has no observable deficit. These are Stages 1 and 2 on the FAST. It is important to note that the boundary between normal aging changes and dementia is not sharp and clear (Oxman & Baynes, 1994). In fact, the minor problems of Reisberg and co-workers' Stage 2 are more likely to be *age-associated memory impairment* (AAMI) than Alzheimer's disease.

Table 1.1. Functional Assessment Staging (FAST) in normal aging and in Alzheimer's disease (AD)

FAST stage	Characteristics
1	*No objective or subjective functional decrement*
2	*Subjective functional decrement, but no objective evidence of decreased performance in complex occupational or social activities*
3	*Objective functional decrement of sufficient severity to interfere with complex occupational and social tasks*
4	*Deficient performance in the complex tasks of daily life* (e.g., planning dinner for guest, handling finances)
5	*Deficient performance in basic tasks of daily life, such as choosing proper clothing*
6	*Decreased ability to dress, bathe, and toilet independently*
6a	*Difficulty putting clothes on properly*
6b	*Unable to bathe properly; may develop fear of bathing*
6c	*Inability to handle mechanics of toileting* (e.g., forgets to flush, does not wipe properly)
6d	*Urinary incontinence*
6e	*Fecal incontinence*
7	*Loss of speech, locomotion, and consciousness*
7a	*Ability to speak limited (1 to 5 words a day)*
7b	*All intelligible vocabulary lost*
7c	*Nonambulatory*
7d	*Unable to sit up independently*
7e	*Unable to smile*
7f	*Unable to hold up head*

From Reisberg, B. (1988). Functional Assessment Staging (FAST). *Psychopharmacology Bulletin, 24,* 653–659; reprinted by permission.

AAMI is a benign forgetfulness that does not worsen in the malignant manner that the dementias do. A Finnish study found that 42% of men and 36% of women age 60–78 have AAMI (Koivisto et al., 1995). The important point is that most forgetfulness is not the beginning of Alzheimer's disease, although what it is exactly and even whether it is entirely a subjective feeling or a biologically determined decline in function, are still a matter of some controversy (Larrabee & McEntee, 1995). On some occasions older people need to be reassured that AAMI is benign.

The person at Stage 3 on the FAST experiences some difficulty remembering important events such as appointments. Everyday items (e.g., keys, glasses, wallets) are frequently misplaced and increasingly difficult to find. The person may become lost in unfamiliar places and experience anxiety or mild panic before becoming reoriented. These problems are often the beginning of a dementia but may be the result of some other cause, including a physical illness such as pneumonia that has reduced the oxygen supply in the blood and consequently compromised brain function, or a drug that has a toxic effect on the brain. Some people at this stage seem to become concerned about their problems (e.g., the woman in her early 50s described by her husband in the last vignette). Others seem to ignore them or simply ascribe them to the effects of old age.

An individual whose difficulties have progressed beyond the third stage on the FAST is often distressed by what is happening. Some try to hide their increasing disability and are quite successful at it for a considerable length of time, particularly if they are not too greatly challenged—by a demanding job, for example. At this stage, co-workers, family members, and friends notice the changes, if they have not done so already. A person in this fourth stage, called *mild Alzheimer's disease*, has trouble balancing a checkbook, planning a dinner, traveling alone, or maintaining any kind of employment. If the person is still working, the problems become very apparent at this stage. Other responsibilities, such as maintaining a household or baby-sitting grandchildren, also become too difficult to perform alone. The following is a description of the progression to Stage 4 by a family member:

> About 9 years ago, my wife began to display difficulty remembering things. She didn't say much about it, but everything took so much longer for her to do. For example, she was a Sunday school teacher and her Sunday school preparation would stretch out and out and out. She would take more time but she appeared to be less and less effective with the children.
>
> The interesting thing was that she thought she was doing very well. But the children recognized the difference and responded by running off, not showing up, and so forth. (Tappen, 1990)

The husband describes what happened as his wife entered the fifth stage on the FAST:

> She didn't want any help. She didn't even want me to know what was going on. She began to fall apart in the way she dressed. For example, she was always after me to buy her pantyhose. She was always out of pantyhose and blaming it on the cats. In truth, she was putting more and more pairs of pantyhose on at one time. The same thing happened with bras: She began putting on more and more bras. It also showed up in feeding the cats. She would forget that she had fed the cats and she would feed the cats again and again. There would be cat dishes all over the place. (Tappen, 1990)

At FAST Stage 5, or *moderate Alzheimer's disease*, simple tasks become increasingly difficult. The affected person begins to experience difficulty choosing clothes, doing the housework, or driving a car. The following is another example from a family member:

> It was 4 years ago that I noticed my husband was not taking messages on the telephone properly. He was saying somebody called, but he wouldn't get the name or number. He'd always done it before. Actually, he wasn't doing much of anything. He'd always been working with his books before. He's a writer and a teacher. He would just sit there and look at it, doing nothing, not even turning a page, but I thought he was tired or something.
>
> Then, when I went into the hospital, he did not come to see me or anything because he had forgotten how to get on the bus. I realized when I got home that he couldn't do a thing. He couldn't even fix a piece of bread for me. He did not know where the bread was. He had done these little things for me before but now he couldn't do anything. (Tappen, 1990)

When the disease becomes *moderately severe* (Stages 6a–6e), the person begins to need help putting on clothes correctly, not just choosing them. This is followed by a need for help with bathing, toileting, and staying continent (i.e., not having accidents) of urine and stool, in that order. The individual at this stage frequently needs help.

The person with *severe Alzheimer's disease* (Stages 7a–7f) speaks very little, only a few words or phrases a day. This already-limited vocabulary finally shrinks to just a word or two, although vocalizations (i.e., nonword sounds) may continue and may be loud at times. After this point, the individual gradually loses his or her ability to walk, to sit up, to smile, and, eventually, even to hold the head up (Sclan & Reisberg, 1992).

COGNITIVE CHANGES

A number of important cognitive functions are affected by Alzheimer's disease and related dementias. Cognitive functions, as opposed to the motor and sensory functions of the brain, are "the sum of the brain's power to acquire, process, integrate, store and retrieve information" (Oxman & Baynes, 1994, p. 6).

Changes in Memory

Decline in memory function is the core symptom of Alzheimer's disease. However, memory is not a unitary phenomenon. Different types of memory are affected in different ways by the disease.

Short- and Long-Term Memory   One important distinction among different types of memory is the length of time information is retained. *Immediate* memory is retained for a matter of seconds. This is also called primary memory. *Short-term*, or secondary, memory is retained for a matter of minutes rather than seconds. *Long-term*, or tertiary, memory is remote memory that may be measured in days or years (Squire, 1987).

Immediate and short-term memory are impaired in the earlier stages of Alzheimer's disease. In testing situations, people with Alzheimer's disease have difficulty repeating a series of numbers (e.g., a telephone number) back to an examiner or recalling a list of objects (e.g., a shopping list) a few minutes later. Later in the disease, memory of the past, both historical (e.g., who was president at a given time) and personal, is also impaired (Oxman & Baynes, 1994), probably as a result of difficulty in retrieving these "old" memories (Kopelman, 1992).

Declarative and Procedural Memory   A second important classification of memory focuses on the type of information remembered rather than the length of time it is retained. Squire's (1987) model is relatively easy to understand (see Figure 1.1). In Squire's model memory is divided into declarative and procedural categories. Shepherd (1988) describes procedural memory as "knowing how" and declarative memory as "knowing that" (p. 610).

Procedural memory refers to what the individual can remember how to do—that is, general skills, procedures, and rules (cognitive operations) such as writing, typing, solving rule-based puzzles, or riding a bicycle (Moscovitch, 1992). It is more automatic and less conscious than declarative memory. Procedural memories are not usually classified as immediate, short-term, or long-term. Procedural memory is believed to be spared until the late stages of Alzheimer's disease (Eslinger & Damasio, 1985), which has important implications for selecting interventions (see Chapters 5 and 7). Operant conditioning (i.e., using rewards to reinforce desired behavior) is considered to be a type of procedural memory. It has been found to be useful in assisting people with Alzheimer's disease to regain basic skills and control some behaviors.

Declarative memory refers to memory of facts and events. This type of memory is divided further into *episodic* and *semantic* memory. Episodic memory involves remembering specific events, or episodes, in one's life. Unlike semantic memories, episodic memories are linked to specific times and places. Semantic memory, in contrast, is knowledge unrelated to a specific event; facts, concepts, and vocabulary are components of semantic memory. For example, the multiplication table, once memorized, becomes a part of semantic memory. Recalling a particularly agonizing session spent memorizing the multiplication tables before a test, however, would be a function of episodic memory.

Declarative memories may be held for a fleeting moment for immediate recall, retained for a few minutes, or stored in long-term memory. These are the memories most profoundly affected by Alzheimer's disease. It is believed that acquisition and storage of information may be most affected in Alzheimer's disease whereas retrieval of stored information may be most affected in Huntington's and Parkinson's dementias (Pillon, Deweer, Agid, & Dubois, 1993). This, too, has implications for the way programs to help people use their remaining abilities are designed (see Chapters 5 and 7).

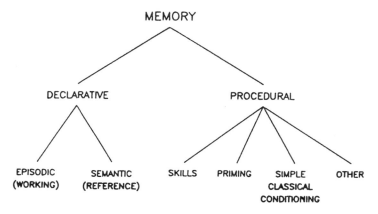

Figure 1.1. Procedural and declarative memory. (From PROCEDURAL AND DECLARATIVE MEMORY by LR Squire. Copyright [c] 1987 BY LR SQUIRE. Used by permission of Oxford University Press, Inc.

Changes in the Use of Language

Communication deficits increase dramatically as Alzheimer's disease progresses. In the early stages of the disease the problem is mild, even subtle (Bayles & Kaszniak, 1987). The individual experiences difficulty finding the right word and remembering people's names, a disorder called *anomia*. To compensate, the individual talks around the missing word, a process called *circumlocution*.

> An older couple are outside, planting their spring garden. The husband has mild Alzheimer's disease.
>
> HUSBAND: Would you hand me that . . . uh . . . that . . . thing over there?
>
> WIFE: What thing over here?
>
> HUSBAND: The handle. That thing there with the handle.
>
> WIFE: Do you mean the rake?
>
> HUSBAND: Yes.

At this stage communication difficulties reflect slower processing of information, reduced attention, and memory problems, particularly word-finding problems. Longer pauses, use of indefinite words (e.g., "that *thing* over *there*"), and circumlocutions are common. If tested, the person with mild dementia may have difficulty with a task such as naming other objects that belong in the same category as a given object (Bayles, Tomoeda, & Trosset, 1992) but will otherwise perform quite well.

On the positive side, much ability remains. The person has no trouble speaking per se; that is, the motor aspects of communication, which can be affected by other diseases, apparently are not affected at all. Speech is clear, fluent, and grammatically correct (at least as correct as it ever was). The total number of words used in a specific task such as describing a picture is the same as that used by older people without cognitive impairment. The description itself, however, is less concise, contains less information, and uses more incomplete phrases and more repetition of ideas than the descriptions produced by people of the same age with no cognitive impairment (Tomoeda & Bayles, 1993; To-:noeda, Bayles, Trosset, & Warren, 1991).

As Alzheimer's disease progresses, communication difficulties become more apparent (Kertesz, 1994). Sentences are more frequently left unfinished and become increasingly vague. More phrases are left incomplete. The total number of words used in a task such as describing a picture diminishes significantly, and the information given is diminished (Tomoeda et al., 1991). In fact, a person at this stage participating in an object-naming test may be able to provide less than 10% of the names he or she could have supplied at the mild stage (Bayles et al., 1992). The anomia continues and intensifies. Substitutions are more common: An umbrella may be called a rain hat, a tree may be called a plant.

Even when cognition is moderately impaired, the person with Alzheimer's disease can read printed material aloud quite well, but may not be able to explain what he or she just read. Writing tasks are more difficult for people with vascular dementias than for those with Alzheimer's disease because of the motor skills involved.

Speech is still quite fluent and grammatical: tenses are correct, negatives are used where needed, words are clearly articulated, subjects and verbs are used correctly. Speech may ramble, however, and become rather difficult to follow as references become increasingly indefinite.

> A father and son are sitting and talking with a visitor in the lounge of a small nursing facility.

FATHER: That man couldn't get the work done. There was never time. He would just work but the doors didn't close. He could do it. All the time, the doors were open. He did work though.

SON TO VISITOR: I think he's talking about the poultry farm he and my mother used to have. They had a handyman who was very slow. My father liked him but could never get him to finish a job.

Well into the course of the disease, people will make great efforts to avoid exposing the extent of their deficits.

When asked to spell *world* backward, Cora began with "d . . . l . . ." but could not finish. Then, when the examiner asked her to count backward from 100 by 7s, Cora tilted her head, looked at the examiner, and, in a querulous tone, asked, "Why should I do *your* homework?"

Up to this point in the disease course the individual with Alzheimer's disease has been able to communicate his or her needs and concerns, even if with some difficulty. In the most severe stage, however, communication can become a great frustration for caregiver and care receiver alike. (*Note*: The use of some specific strategies to facilitate communication can reduce some of this frustration, and may even help a person maintain the ability to communicate longer.) Typically, verbal communication diminishes to a few words or phrases, many of which are just "Yes," "No," or "Get out of here!" When very frustrated or upset, the increasingly inarticulate person may simply scream. Vocalizations—the "ah's" and "mm-hmmm's" that everyone uses at times—may become the only verbal communication still used. Nonverbal communication may continue: pushing people away; reaching out for a desired dessert or for a hug; kicking the care provider to ward off unwanted assistance.

Is it accurate to call this communication problem aphasia? The answer is no if the term *aphasia* is used to refer to a problem caused by a specific focal lesion (one that is localized within a defined area of the brain), such as that which occurs in strokes. However, if the symptoms, rather than the underlying cause, are what is meant by "aphasia," then the communication deficits of Alzheimer's disease can be described in terms of the various types of aphasias (Kertesz, 1994).

Additional Cognitive Changes

Memory deficits, especially deficits in episodic memory, usually appear first in Alzheimer's disease. These are generally followed by deficits in abstract reasoning, attention, language, and visuospatial perception, in that order (Zec, 1993).

Abstract Reasoning   Abstraction is often the second cognitive function to demonstrate evidence of decline in the early stages of Alzheimer's disease. On testing, the person with Alzheimer's disease is able to understand common proverbs, such as "a rolling stone gathers no moss," but cannot explain them satisfactorily. In Pick's disease abstraction is actually more impaired than is memory (Oxman & Baynes, 1994).

Mathematical skills (e.g., addition, subtraction) are also affected early in the disease, as evidenced by the common problem with balancing a checkbook. It is thought that problem solving is also affected, although the research on changes in this cognitive function is still relatively limited.

Attention   It is impossible to pay attention to every one of the millions of bits of information coming into the brain through its sensory ports (e.g., eyes, ears, nose) at any given time. Therefore, it is necessary to filter this information and to select only the information that requires attention. The person with mild dementia shows little change in the ability to attend to a task, including being able to shift attention from one task to another. For example, on testing, the task of crossing out all 8s on a page full of numbers is relatively easy at this stage. However, when the person reaches the moderate stage of Alzheimer's disease, this task and others like it become more difficult. Attempts to attend to two different tasks at once usually end in failure. This fact is useful to know when helping a person with advanced Alzheimer's disease try to regain some independence in activities of daily living: doing one task at a time is more likely to be successful.

Visuospatial Abilities   Visuospatial difficulty is also minimal in the early stages of Alzheimer's disease but becomes evident in the middle stages and eventually becomes severe. Many of the examples are well known. Getting lost and driving or walking around for hours before finding the way home is often the first evidence of visuospatial problems. Later, the individual may even have difficulty finding his or her way around at home. Finding the toilet in time to avoid incontinence is a common problem in the later stages. Finally, failing to recognize a familiar face causes great distress to the unrecognized family member or friend and is frequently remarked on if it occurs. In the sixth stage, moderately severe Alzheimer's disease, some individuals may not recognize their face in a mirror, which is probably part of a more generalized visuospatial deficit in face recognition (Biringer & Anderson, 1992).

Cognitive Slowing   Slowing, a generalized reduction in the speed with which a cognitive function is carried out, occurs in all older people. In Alzheimer's disease, however, the reduction is greater and increases with the progression of the disease.

Awareness of Deficits   Awareness of the extent or effects of the deficits is said to be limited. It is believed that people with Alzheimer's disease underestimate the severity of their deficits or fail to ascribe a problem that occurs to their deficits. For example, it is not uncommon for a person with Alzheimer's disease to accuse someone else of having stolen a misplaced watch or ring. It is also not uncommon for a person with the disease to believe that his or her spouse is having an affair based on the slimmest of evidence, such as arriving home a little late or admitting a repair person into the home. Risky behavior may also result from underestimation of impairment. A common example is refusal to give up driving a car (Zec, 1993). Yet, conversations with individuals in the middle and late stages of Alzheimer's disease indicate that they *are* aware of their not-knowing. "I don't know, I don't know, I don't know" is not an uncommon response to questions. Some ascribe their not-knowing to medications, others to being "crazy"; most have no explanation, but can identify a change from their previous levels of cognitive ability. Only a few individuals give excuses or attribute their problems to others (Tappen, Williams-Burgess, Fishman, & Touhy, 1997).

NEUROLOGICAL CHANGES

It is generally believed that motor areas (those that regulate physical activity) and sensory areas (e.g., vision, hearing) of the brain are spared until late in the disease. However,

there are some neurological changes that eventually affect the person's physical movement and interpretation of sensory input.

Olfaction, the sense of smell, is impaired to some degree in about half of all people
over age 80. In people with Alzheimer's disease this proportion increases to 90% (Oxman
& Baynes, 1994). These facts are important to know for two reasons: The first is the
sense of smell is protective; for example, it alerts people to the presence of smoke and
to the possibility of spoilage in food. A second reason is that interesting scents (e.g.,
lemon, pine) have been used in some recreational activities in Alzheimer's groups. If the
statistics are correct, many participants will have trouble identifying the scent as a result
of reduced olfaction.

Increased muscle tone has been found in the extremities of people with Alzheimer's
disease, particularly in severe Alzheimer's disease. It has also been observed that people
with Alzheimer's disease do not swing their arms as freely as others do when they walk
and that they shuffle when they walk. Their steps may be uneven in length and they
may take longer than the average length of time to turn around and walk in the other
direction (Funkenstein et al., 1993). They do not, however, seem to have less strength
than do other older people. All of these changes may eventually interfere with walking,
an important source of exercise for older people.

Diminished spontaneous movement of both the face and the extremities has also
been noted. This may contribute to others' impression of apathy or depression in the
individual.

Alternating hand movements are clearly impaired in people with Alzheimer's disease, who find it difficult, for example, to open and close their hands (make a fist) and
perform other hand movements (e.g., finger tapping) (Funkenstein et al., 1993). This
impairment may affect their ability to participate in games and crafts requiring similar
movements.

REFERENCES

American Psychiatric Association. (1994). *Diagnostic and statistical manual of mental disorders
    (DSM-IV)* (4th ed.). Washington, DC: American Psychiatric Press.
Anifantakis, H. (1991). *The diminished mind: One family's extraordinary battle with Alzheimer's.*
    Blue Ridge Summit, PA: TAB Books (McGraw-Hill).
Bayles, K.A., & Kaszniak, A.W. (1987). *Communication and cognition in normal aging and de-
    mentia.* San Diego: College-Hill Press/Little, Brown.
Bayles, K.A., Tomoeda, C.K., & Trosset, M.W. (1992). Relation of linguistic communication abil-
    ities of Alzheimer's patients to stage of disease. *Brain and Language, 42,* 454–472.
Benson, F. (1989). The Anglo-American view. In T. Hovaguimian, S. Henderson, Z. Khachaturian,
    & J. Orley (Eds.), *Classification and diagnosis of Alzheimer disease: An international perspec-
    tive.* Toronto: Hans Huber.
Biringer, F., & Anderson, J.R. (1992). Self-recognition in Alzheimer's disease: A mirror and video
    study. *Journal of Gerontology: Psychological Sciences, 47*(6), 385–388.
Eslinger, P.J., & Damasio, A.R. (1985). Alzheimer's disease spares motor learning. *Society for
    Neurosciences Abstracts, 11,* 459.
Funkenstein, H.H., Albert, M.S., Cook, N.R., West, C.G., Scherr, P.A., Chown, M.J., Pegrim, D.,
    & Evans, D.A. (1993). Extrapyramidal signs and other neurologic findings in clinically diagnosed
    Alzheimer's disease. *Archives of Neurology, 50*(1), 51–56.

Kertesz, A. (1994). Language deterioration in dementia. In V.O.B. Emery & T.E. Oxman (Eds.), *Dementia: Presentation, differential diagnosis, and nosology* (pp. 123–138). Baltimore: The Johns Hopkins University Press.

Koivisto, K., Reinikainen, K.J., Hanninen, T., Vanhanen, M., Helkala, E.L., Mykkanen, L., Laakso, M., Pyorala, K., & Riekkinen, P.J. (1995). Prevalence of age-associated memory impairment in a randomly selected population from eastern Finland. *Neurology, 45,* 741–747.

Kolb, B., & Wishaw, I.Q. (1990). *Fundamentals of human neuropsychology.* New York: W.H. Freeman.

Kopelman, M.D. (1992). The "new" and "old": Components of anterograde and retrograde memory loss in Korsakoff and Alzheimer patients. In L.R. Squire & N. Bulters (Eds.), *Neuropsychology of memory* (pp. 130–146). New York: Guilford Press.

Kukull, W.A., Brenner, D.E., Speck, C.E., Nocklin, D., Bowen, J., McCormick, W., Teri, L., Pfanschmidt, M.L., & Larson, E.B. (1994). Causes of death associated with Alzheimer's disease: Variation by level of cognitive impairment before death. *Journal of the American Geriatrics Society, 42,* 723–726.

Larrabee, G.J., & McEntee, W.J. (1995). Age-associated memory impairment: Sorting out the controversies. *Neurology, 45,* 611–614.

Lee, G.P., & Loring, D.W. (1993). Acute confusional states in toxic and metabolic disorders. In R.W. Parks, R.F. Zec, & R. F. Wilson (Eds.), *Neuropsychology of Alzheimer's disease and other dementias.* New York: Oxford University Press.

Lezak, M.D. (1983). *Neuropsychological assessment* (2nd ed.). New York: Oxford University Press.

Moscovitch, M. (1992). A neuropsychological model of memory and consciousness. In L.R. Squire & N. Bulters (Eds.), *Neuropsychology of memory* (pp. 5–22). New York: Guilford Press.

Oxman, T.E., & Baynes, K. (1994). Boundaries between normal aging and dementia. In V.O.B. Emery & T.E. Oxman (Eds.), *Dementia: Presentation, differential diagnosis, and nosology* (pp. 3–18). Baltimore: The Johns Hopkins University Press.

Pillon, B., Deweer, B., Agid, Y., & Dubois, B. (1993). Explicit memory in Alzheimer's, Huntington's, and Parkinson's diseases. *Archives of Neurology, 50*(4), 364–379.

Sclan, S.G., & Reisberg, B. (1992). Functional Assessment Staging (FAST) in Alzheimer's disease: Reliability, validity and ordinality. *International Psychogeriatrics, 4*(Suppl. 1), 55–69.

Shepherd, G.M. (1988). *Neurobiology.* New York: Oxford University Press.

Squire, L.R. (1987). *Memory and brain.* New York: Oxford University Press.

Sungaila, P., & Crockett, D.J. (1993). Dementia and the frontal lobes. In R.W. Parks, R.F. Zec, & R.F. Wilson (Eds.), *Neuropsychology of Alzheimer's disease and other dementias.* New York: Oxford University Press.

Tappen, R.M. (1990). *The challenge of caregiving: Caring for a family member with Alzheimer's disease* [Videotape]. Coral Gables, FL: University of Miami.

Tappen, R.M., Williams-Burgess, C., Fishman, S., & Touhy, T. (1997). *Persistence of self in advanced Alzheimer's disease.* Manuscript submitted for publication.

Tomoeda, C.K., & Bayles, K.A. (1993). Longitudinal effects of Alzheimer's disease on discourse production. *Alzheimer's Disease and Associated Disorders, 7*(4), 223–226.

Tomoeda, C.K., Bayles, K.A., Trosset, M.W., & Warren, D.K. (1991). *Cross-sectional and longitudinal analysis of Alzheimer's disease effects on oral discourse in a picture description task.* Unpublished report, University of Arizona, Tucson.

Whitehouse, P.J., Lerner, A., & Hedera, P.C. (1993). Dementia. In K.M. Heilman & E. Valenstein (Eds.), *Clinical neuropsychology.* New York: Oxford University Press.

Zec, R.F. (1993). Neuropsychological functioning in Alzheimer's disease. In R.W. Parks, R.F. Zec, & R.F. Wilson (Eds.), *Neuropsychology of Alzheimer's disease and other dementias.* New York: Oxford University Press.

Chapter 2

Pathological Changes

The brain is a mass of cranial nerve tissue, most of it in mint condition.

Robert Half (1993)

Our understanding of what occurs within the brain has advanced rapidly since the 1970s. Before that time, the brain was essentially a "black box" so far as our understanding of what occurred within it was concerned. Information went into the black box, was operated on in some way, and came out, but what went on within the black box either was a matter of conjecture or was ignored altogether (Bloom & Lazerson, 1988). Research has provided us with some answers to the question of what happens within the black box, but there is still a great deal left to learn about the brain and its function. Much also remains unknown about the relationship between the physical damage done to the brain in Alzheimer's disease and the widespread effect of this damage on virtually every aspect of life for a person with Alzheimer's disease.

This chapter briefly considers the complex structure and functions of the brain. Then changes that occur with Alzheimer's disease are described, first at the macrolevel of the brain as a whole, including its component parts, and then at the micro-, or cellular, level of the neuron (nerve cell). In the final section the most commonly proffered theories on the causation of Alzheimer's disease are examined.

THE HUMAN BRAIN

Structure

Many people have likened the outline of the brain to a closed fist (the thumb represents the temporal lobes, the wrist represents the brain stem). To others, the outer aspect of the brain appears to be a mass of congealed spaghetti or pale worms. Whichever comparison one prefers, this outer surface provides few clues to either the complexity or the functions of the human brain.

Anatomists divide the central nervous system into three main parts: forebrain, brain stem, and spinal cord. The *forebrain*, which is of most interest in relation to Alzheimer's disease, consists of the *endbrain* (neocortex, basal ganglia, limbic system, olfactory bulbs, and lateral ventricles) and *between brain* (thalamus, hypothalamus, pineal body, and third ventricle) (Kolb & Wishaw, 1990) (see Figure 2.1).

The neocortex is the largest and most prominent part of the brain. A fissure runs down the center of the neocortex from front to back, dividing it into the left and right hemispheres. The hemispheres can be divided into the frontal, parietal, occipital, and temporal lobes (Figure 2.2). Within these lobes are important smaller structures and regions, some of which are affected by Alzheimer's disease.

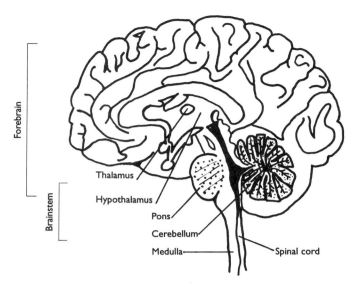

Figure 2.1. The central nervous system: forebrain, brainstem, and spinal cord. (Adapted from Bloom & Lazerson, 1988.)

Function

The brain is the most complex of all organs in the human body. It is estimated that the average adult brain houses somewhere between 10 and 16 billion neurons. Even more incredible is the estimated number of synapses (potential connections between the neurons). If the average number of synapses per neuron is approximately 200 and the average number of neurons is 13 billion, this would yield a total of 2.6 trillion possible synapses (Pechura & Martin, 1991).

Capacity   Of interest to most nonscientists is the brain's enormous capacity for work, including storing and retrieving information (memory). Trehub (1991) offers some interesting estimates based on an average life span of 80 years. Young children probably learn something new every minute that they are awake. (Learning is not limited to the classroom, nor is it limited to reading, writing, and arithmetic. Any new piece of information, from the aroma of freshly cut grass to noticing a new crack in the tile, is learning in the broad sense of the word.) Older people, having learned a great deal already, probably learn something new only every 2 minutes of their waking hours (16 hours a day on average). Given these estimates, an 80-year-old person would have learned a total of 14,016,000 pieces of information in a lifetime, requiring 28,032,000 pairs of neurons to store all of these memories.

Because the storage of most information probably requires a more complicated neuronal circuit than the simple pair of neurons used for this calculation, Trehub multiplied this total by a factor of 10 to get a requirement of 280,320,000 neurons needed to store a lifetime of accumulated information. Even this larger number constitutes only 2% of the total number of neurons in the neocortex, leaving approximately 12 billion for all of the other processes for which the brain is responsible.

Processes   The processes for which the brain is responsible are amazingly varied and complex. These processes can be categorized as primarily sensory, primarily motor, or primarily coordinative. The latter category includes learning and memory (see Table 2.1).

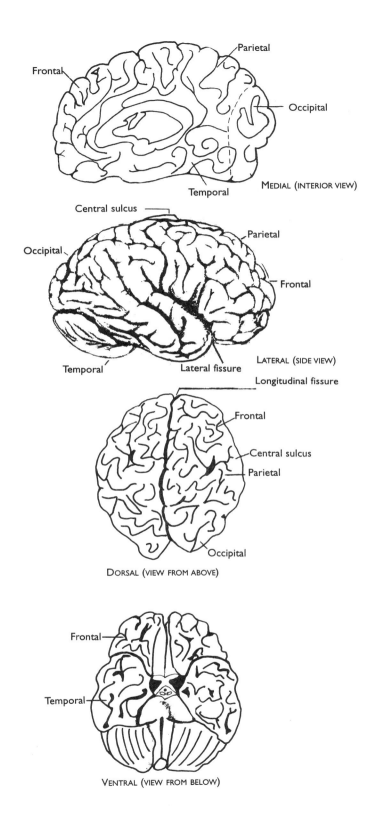

Figure 2.2. Topographical markers and location of the lobes of the neocortex. (Adapted from: FUN-DAMENTALS OF HUMAN NEUROPSYCHOLOGY 3/E by Kolb and Wishaw © 1995 by W.H. Freeman and Company. Used with permission.)

Table 2.1.   Functions of the brain

Sensory	Motor	Coordinative
		Central systems
Taste	Muscle response	Brain–body
Smell	Voluntary	Autonomic (e.g., heart rate)
	Involuntary	Neuroendocrine (e.g., growth hormone)
Hearing		Neuroimmune (e.g., steroidal effect on immunity)
	Glandular response	
Vision	Cilia movement	
Balance		Within-brain
Muscular		Diffuse and specific neurotransmitter systems
		(e.g., dopamine)
Somatosensory		
Chemical		Distributed systems
		Biorhythms
		Behavior (e.g., emotion, learning)

Data from Shepherd, G.M. (1988). *Neurobiology*. New York: Oxford University Press.

The *sensory* processes involve the conversion (transduction) of different stimuli into electrochemical signals by the sensory receptor cells. Sensory modalities include taste, smell, hearing, vision, balance, muscular (e.g., muscle tension, joint position), somatosensory (e.g., touch, pressure, temperature), and chemical (e.g., oxygen level, glucose level, presence of toxins) (Shepherd, 1988).

The *motor* processes involve governance of the responses to the stimuli detected by the sensory processes. The various actions of these responding (effector) organs include muscle responses, either voluntary (e.g., running away) or involuntary (e.g., a startle reaction); glandular responses (e.g., sweating, digestion); and the movement of the cilia that line many organs (Shepherd, 1988).

The *coordinative or central system* processes are higher-level processes that involve mediation of the interactions of various lower-level functions so that they form a coherent response. The central system processes that mediate brain–body interactions include the autonomic nervous system (e.g., increases in heart rate or blood pressure), neuroendocrine system (e.g., the action of the hypothalamic–pituitary system on growth hormones), and neuroimmune system (e.g., the effect of increased corticosteroids on immunity).

Those central system processes that mediate within-brain processes include diffuse and specific neurotransmitter systems and the complicated distributed systems underlying whole-organism behaviors. Neurotransmitters are chemical substances released at the axonal end of the neuron (the projection that sends transmissions) to carry a message across the synapse, or gap between two neurons. The signals are detected by the dendrite of another neuron (the projection that receives such transmissions), providing the chemical link or communication between neurons (Kolb & Wishaw, 1990). Millions of these signals flash through the brain every moment (National Institute on Aging [NIA], 1995, p. 4). The *diffuse transmitters* seem to be more involved in adjusting the excitability of other neurons than in transmitting specific information. In contrast, the *specific transmitters* usually exert a more local effect. For example, dopamine is concentrated in an area called the substantia nigra. Degeneration of these cells and the resulting loss of dopamine synapses is thought to be responsible for the development of Parkinson's dis-

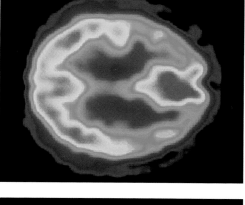
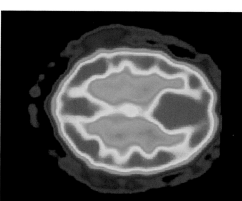

Plate 1. Left) In an individual without cognitive impairment, the red and orange areas of the positron emission tomograph (PET) demonstrate normal glucose metabolism. Right) In an individual with probable Alzheimer's disease, the blue and green areas of the PET scan indicate decreased glucose uptake in the parietal region (see also Figure 2.2). (From Roses, A.D. [1995]. Apolipoprotein E and Alzheimer's disease. *Science and Medicine*, 2[5], 16–25; reprinted with permission. PET scans courtesy of Drs. Gary W. Small and Michael Phelps, University of California, Los Angeles.)

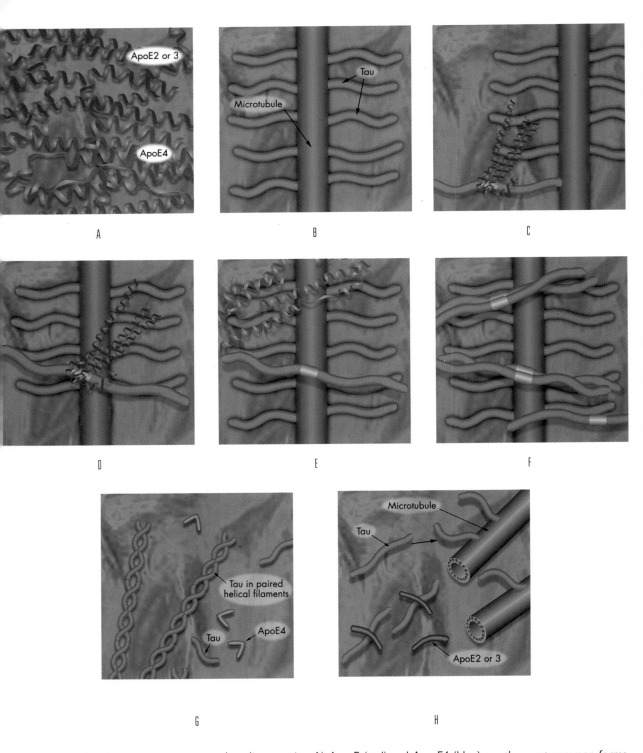

Plate 2. Interaction between tau protein and apolipoprotein. A) Apo E (red) and Apo E4 (blue) are the most common forms of Apo E. B) The microtubule (teal), an important conduit within the neuron, is supported by tau proteins (green). C) Apo E2 or E3 protects the area where tau binds to the microtubule. D) Apo E2 or E3 binds successfully to tau. E) Apo E4 protein does not bind successfully to tau. F) Without the protection of Apo E2 or E3, tau binds to tau and eventually forms tangles. G) Tangles form in the presence of Apo E4. H) The protective effect of Apo E2 or E3 is evident. (Panels A–F adapted from the video "Waves of Stone," produced by Vision Associates, Inc., New York, NY; panels G and H adapted from the *Journal of NIH Research* 1996 calendar.)

ease. A precursor of dopamine, L-dopa is used to treat Parkinson's disease (Shepherd, 1988).

The *distributed systems,* coordinated within various regions of the brain, govern the body's biorhythms and a person's behavior, including feeding, mating, learning and memory, and emotion. These higher-level central system processes are the ones affected most by Alzheimer's disease.

CHANGES ASSOCIATED WITH ALZHEIMER'S DISEASE

Macrolevel Changes

Most of the damage done by Alzheimer's disease is concentrated in areas of the brain that are responsible for memory, language, reasoning, and judgment. The neocortex can lose as much as one third of its volume in Alzheimer's disease (Plate 1; Kolb & Wishaw, 1990). This shrinkage begins long before clinical symptoms of Alzheimer's disease are evident and may be detected by computed tomography (CT) scan or magnetic resonance imaging (MRI) (discussed in Chapter 3) (Roses, 1995). The ventricles (fluid-filled spaces within the brain) are enlarged, as are the clefts (sulci) between the looping ridges (gyri) that are a distinguishing feature of the brain. Neuronal loss is not distributed evenly throughout the neocortex in Alzheimer's disease. The visual (occipital) and sensorimotor areas are relatively spared until late in the disease, as are the frontal lobes for the most part. The greatest change is found in the parietal tertiary areas, the inferior temporal lobes, and the limbic system (see Figure 2.3). The limbic system, including the hippocampus and amygdala, is especially affected by the disease. In particular, the entorhinal area, which is a major relay station between the hippocampus and the neocortex, is damaged. Because the hippocampus is considered vital to the storage of information (research indicates that severe memory loss follows damage to the hippocampus), the disconnection caused by entorhinal damage is believed to be responsible for the early and continuing difficulties with memory found in people with Alzheimer's disease (Braak & Braak, 1994; Kolb & Wishaw, 1990).

Microlevel Changes

Most people are aware of the curious fact that a loss of neurons as the brain ages is a normally occurring event (Gatz, Lowe, Berg, Mortimer, & Pederson, 1994). Another curious fact is that the brains of many apparently cognitively intact older people are found at autopsy to contain some of the plaques and tangles considered to be the hallmarks of Alzheimer's disease. Dr. Alan Roses, a well-respected scientist, hypothesized that everyone would eventually develop Alzheimer's disease if we all lived to 140 years of age (Roses, 1995). Thus, is it possible that Alzheimer's disease is simply the aging process gone awry? If so, why does it go awry and what can we do to prevent this?

It is not possible to answer these questions definitively, but there are many promising hypotheses about the cause of Alzheimer's disease. Before examining these hypotheses, it is important to consider what is known about the cellular level changes associated with Alzheimer's disease. The damage that occurs in Alzheimer's disease at the cellular level affects the metabolism of neurons, repair, and cleanup that maintains cell functioning and communication between the neurons (NIA, 1995).

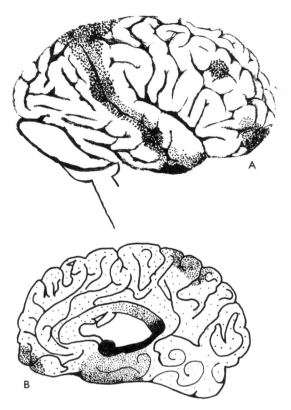

Figure 2.3. Distribution and severity of degeneration in Alzheimer's disease: side (A) and internal (B) views. Darker areas represent more pronounced degeneration. (Adapted from: FUNDAMENTALS OF HUMAN NEUROPSYCHOLOGY 3/E by Kolb and Wishaw © 1995 by W.H. Freeman and Company. Used with permission.)

Structural Changes in Neurons   The reduction in the volume of the cerebral cortex that occurs with Alzheimer's disease may be the result of shrinking rather than complete disappearance of neurons (Finch, 1994; Kolb & Wishaw, 1990). These nerve cells lose most of their dendrites and change in shape from triangular to pear-like (Figure 2.4). Clearly, communication between these neurons is severely impaired when the cells and their dendrites are damaged in this manner (Berg & Morris, 1990). It is important to note that these neuronal changes do not occur in healthy older people.

Plaques and Tangles   Within the cells of the cortex and hippocampus, bundles of thread-like fibrils called *paired helical filaments* or *neurofibrillary tangles* have been found on postmortem examination of the brains of people with Alzheimer's disease. It has been suggested that these tangles are composed of normal substances of the cell that have been altered in some way, because similar tangles can be produced in animals by injecting aluminum salts (Berg & Morris, 1990).

The primary fibrous component of these tangles is abnormally phosphorylated tau, a protein found in the cytoplasm (inside the neuron) (Roses, 1995). In healthy neurons tau forms the crosspieces of tiny tubules that guide nutrients into the far ends of the neurons' axons (Plate 2). In neurons affected by Alzheimer's disease the tau is twisted

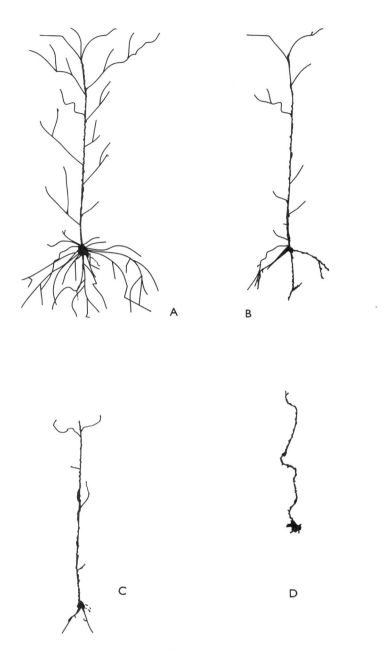

Figure 2.4. Degeneration of a cortical neuron as Alzheimer's disease advances. A, Normal adult pattern; B, early stages; C, advanced stage; D, terminal stage. (Adapted from: FUNDAMENTALS OF HUMAN NEUROPSYCHOLOGY 3/E by Kolb and Wishaw © 1995 by W.H. Freeman and Company. Used with permission.)

into paired helical filaments that no longer support the tubules, allowing them to collapse and subsequently impair the ability of that neuron to communicate with other neurons (NIA, 1995). It has been suggested that one form of apolipoprotein (apo E2) contributes to the stabilization of these tubules but that another form, apo E4, does not (Roses, 1995;

Plate 2). (The potential role of apolipoprotein E in the development of Alzheimer's disease is examined later in this chapter.) Tangles are also found in the brain tissue of people with other forms of dementia, Down syndrome, and Parkinson's disease (Kolb & Wishaw, 1990).

In the tissues that surround and nourish the nerve cells in the brains of people with Alzheimer's disease *neuritic plaques* consisting of a core of *amyloid protein* surrounded by degenerative cell fragments (such as axon terminals) are found. Amyloid protein has also been found in the walls of the delicate cerebral blood vessels that supply the brain with vital oxygen and glucose (Berg & Morris, 1990; Pollen, 1993). Research studies have shown a relationship between the concentration of these plaques and the amount of cognitive impairment that the individual had at the time of death (Blessed, Tomlinson, & Roth, 1968; Kolb & Wishaw, 1990).

These plaques and tangles were first described in 1907 by Alois Alzheimer, for whom the disease is named. Alzheimer described the symptoms of a 51-year-old woman who had severe memory and language problems. With regard to her memory, he wrote, "When the doctor showed her some objects, she first gave the right name for each, but immediately afterward she had already forgotten everything." Her language skills were similarly affected: "She often used confused phrases, single paraphrasic expressions (milkjug instead of cup), sometimes she would stop talking completely" (Pollen, 1993, p. 24). During Alzheimer's lifetime, the presenile (early-onset) dementia that this woman had was considered a different and rarer form of dementia than was the senile (late-onset) variety. An autopsy was performed after this woman died. Her brain had visibly atrophied (shrunk). Microscopic examination revealed the plaques and tangles that have come to be considered the hallmarks of the disease. Alzheimer's description of the tangles, translated from the German, is a vivid one:

> [I]nside an apparently normal-looking cell, one or more single fibers could be observed that became prominent through their striking thickness and specific impregnability. At a more advanced stage, many fibrils arranged in parallel showed the same changes. Then they accumulated forming dense bundles . . . Eventually the nucleus and cytoplasm disappeared, and only a tangled bundle of fibrils indicated the site where once the neuron had been located. (Pollen, 1993, p. 25)

The tangle-filled neurons eventually die (Braak & Braak, 1994). In their place are left "ghost" tangles that stain only faintly compared with the original tangle. These remnants of destroyed neurons are eventually degraded by astrocytes (star-shaped cells) and finally disappear as well.

It is important to note that both plaques and tangles do appear in the brain tissues of cognitively intact older people. It is not their presence alone but their high concentration that is considered evidence of the existence of Alzheimer's disease when the person exhibits the clinical signs of the disease as well (Albert & Moss, 1988).

Neurotransmitters   A significant decrease in the levels of several neurotransmitters is also associated with Alzheimer's disease. Most attention has been focused on changes in the level of acetylcholine, a neurotransmitter strongly associated with memory functions (NIA, 1993). Some studies have shown as much as a 50% decrease in acetylcholine levels in Alzheimer's disease. Other important neurotransmitters whose levels decline in

Alzheimer's disease are dopamine and serotonin, which fall by as much as 50%, and norepinephrine, which falls by as much as 25% (Kolb & Wishaw, 1990).

The combination of neurotransmitter deficiencies, especially that of acetylcholine and serotonin, may be even more significant than the loss of just one neurotransmitter. Animal research has shown that, when both of these neurotransmitters are absent, rats produce an electroencephalograph (which records the electrical activity of the brain) pattern that resembles the pattern for sleep and that they have difficulty learning (Vanderwolf, 1987). If something similar happens in people with Alzheimer's disease, they may experience a "sleeping" neocortex that produces the symptoms of the later stages of the disease (Kolb & Wishaw, 1990, p. 829).

Blood Flow and Glucose Metabolism   Much of the early research on Alzheimer's disease focused on changes in the blood supply to the brain. Many lay people still believe that Alzheimer's disease is primarily the result of a reduction in the flow of blood to the brain caused either by arteriosclerosis or small strokes (see the examination of vascular dementia in Chapter 3).

Brain tissue is sensitive to any decline in oxygen or glucose, those vital substances carried to the brain via the bloodstream. Research indicates that both consumption of oxygen and glucose is less efficient in people with Alzheimer's disease than in unimpaired older people, who experience much more modest declines and are able to compensate for them (Finch, 1994; Kolb & Wishaw, 1990; Metter, 1988). These changes in Alzheimer's disease are considered an effect rather than a cause of the disease.

Staging the Changes

Braak and Braak (1994) have suggested a series of six stages that link the macro- and microlevel changes in the brain with the clinical symptoms of Alzheimer's disease. In defining these stages they used the presence of tangles and neuropil threads, rather than the plaques or other indicators of Alzheimer's disease, as their guide to the advance of the disease.

In the first and second *transentorhinal* stages certain layers of the transentorhinal and entorhinal regions are affected. This stage is the preclinical stage of Alzheimer's disease, in which the individual shows no overt signs of cognitive decline. The third and fourth *limbic* stages are the early stages of clinical Alzheimer's disease, in which mild cognitive changes are apparent. The transentorhinal area becomes severely affected in the third stage. Mild changes occur in the hippocampus, amygdala, basal nuclei, and other structures of the limbic system. Marked involvement of the amygdala, forebrain nuclei, and temporal regions characterize the fourth stage. From Stages 1 to 4, only a small percentage of the total pool of neurons is affected by the disease.

In the final *isocortical* stages the disease spreads outward through the cortex and subcortical areas, affecting increasingly greater portions of the brain. In the fifth stage the entorhinal layers, thalamic nuclei, and related areas are described as "infested" with tangles and related degenerative substances (Braak & Braak, 1994, p. 604). The association areas of the neocortex are now involved, although the motor and sensory areas are only mildly involved. These association areas are important linkages between different cortical and subcortical areas, so higher coordinative brain functions become affected as well.

In the sixth and final stage the entorhinal region is described as denuded of nerve cells, with ghost tangles left to indicate the neurons' former presence. The sensory and motor areas are involved, although the density of degenerative substances is still relatively low in the primary motor areas. The individual now has full-blown Alzheimer's disease (Braak & Braak, 1994).

POSSIBLE CAUSES OF ALZHEIMER'S DISEASE

The search for a cause of Alzheimer's disease has been long and difficult. A continuing controversy rages over which changes are indicators of the cause of the disease and which ones are effects, or outcomes, of the disease (Pollen, 1993). Genetic research may provide the clues that will lead to a comprehensive understanding of how and why Alzheimer's disease occurs in some people but not in others and where attempts to prevent and treat the disease can be focused.

Some general ideas about causation are fairly well established. For example, there are several inherited (familial) forms of the disease, which have been the focus of much research in the 1990s. Like cancer and some other diseases, Alzheimer's disease appears to be a heterogeneous group of dementing diseases that can differ in terms of the age at onset, appearance of symptoms, and severity of the disease (Hooper, 1992). In fact, Alzheimer's disease may not even be solely a disease of the brain, because some of the substances associated with the disease (particularly the amyloid protein) are found in other parts of the body, including the skin (Pollen, 1993).

As with heart disease, there may also be a number of factors that predispose people to Alzheimer's disease in later life. Just as coronary artery disease is affected both by genetic factors that influence the metabolism of cholesterol and by environmental factors such as dietary intake and smoking, it may be that Alzheimer's disease results from some of the changes that accompany aging, such as less blood flow to the brain, as well as from changes in cell metabolism, an increased concentration of calcium ions, and abnormal processing of cell membrane proteins, including the amyloid precursor (Hooper, 1992; Wisniewski, Wegiel, Morys, & Bobinski, 1994).

The information about the causes of Alzheimer's disease comes from a wide variety of sources: large epidemiological studies, highly sophisticated studies of brain function, animal research, and molecular studies of human tissues. New research findings could challenge any or all of these general ideas and the more specific theories that follow in this section.

Incidence and Prevalence

It is estimated that somewhere between 3 and 4 million Americans have Alzheimer's disease or a related dementia. The percentage rises rapidly with increasing age. Information collected about the participants in the Framingham series of studies (relatively strict criteria were used to determine the presence of Alzheimer's disease) shows that the following percentages present with a moderate to severe form of Alzheimer's disease (Bachman et al., 1992):

- 0.4% of people ages 60–64
- 0.9% of people ages 65–69
- 1.8% of people ages 70–74
- 3.6% of people ages 75–79
- 10.57% of people ages 80–84
- 38.6% of people ages 90–95

Above age 75, more women than men present with the disease. However, when the *incidence* (i.e., the number of new cases) was analyzed, it was found that virtually the same number of men and women develop the disease (the statistics were skewed because women live longer than men) (Bachman et al., 1993).

Risk Factors

A number of studies have examined various risk factors associated with Alzheimer's disease. When considering the results of this type of research it is important to remember that such studies do not reveal causes but relationships between factors such as age, education, and various health-related behaviors such as smoking, job-related exposure to toxins, or over- or undereating. For example, although *age* is certainly related to the development of Alzheimer's disease and a person's risk of developing Alzheimer's disease increases steadily with age, age alone is no longer considered the cause of the disease.

Education is an interesting example of the many risk factors that have been related to Alzheimer's disease. Alzheimer's disease has been fairly consistently shown to occur at a higher rate in people with lower educational (<8 years of schooling) and occupational levels. Why is this so? An intriguing explanation is that education itself may have a direct effect on the brain, causing the development of an increased number of synapses that later become a protective reserve against cognitive losses (NIA, 1995). People with Alzheimer's disease with higher levels of education have been found to have a greater degree of physical deterioration in the brain at the same level of symptomatology as people with less education, suggesting that they may cope more effectively for a longer period of time with the effects of the disease (NIA, 1993).

Another possible risk factor is *smoking*. Smokers have been found to have a lower prevalence of Alzheimer's disease than do nonsmokers. This curious finding could be related to the effect on the cholinergic system (producer of acetylcholine) and its nicotinic receptors (Advisory Panel on Alzheimer's Disease, 1993; Taylor & Brown, 1994).

The role of *aluminum* in Alzheimer's disease has been debated since the 1980s. A buildup of aluminum in the brain has been related to the presence of Alzheimer's disease. This relationship has not been considered sufficient reason to advise people to stop using aluminum cookware, although some have done so as a precautionary measure; research indicates that aluminum in cookware is not transferred into food (NIA, 1995).

A number of other factors have been related to the occurrence of Alzheimer's disease. For example, a decline in estrogen levels may increase vulnerability to the disease in postmenopausal women (NIA, 1993), and the use of estrogen replacement therapy may delay the onset of the disease. Estrogen replacement therapy may also enhance the effect of tacrine in the treatment of Alzheimer's disease (Schneider, Farlow, Henderson, & Pogoda, 1996). Head injury at a younger age may predispose people to the disease, as may exposure to various toxic substances. Other neurological diseases, such as Down syndrome and Parkinson's disease, have been related to a higher incidence of Alzheimer's disease (Advisory Panel, 1993; NIA, 1992).

Infectious Agents

No infectious cause for Alzheimer's disease has been found, although some rare forms of chronic progressive dementias can be transmitted from one host to another. For example, kuru is spread through ritual cannibalism in New Guinea. Creutzfeldt-Jakob disease is also infectious (Office of Technology Assessment, 1987). Scrapie is a "slow virus" disease of sheep and goats of interest to researchers because it leaves amyloid fibrils similar to those of Alzheimer's disease in the animals' brains (NIA, 1992). All of these diseases are caused by unconventional viruses that appear to be infectious amyloid proteins (Gajdusek, 1994).

Cholinergic Defect Hypothesis

The theory that Alzheimer's disease results primarily from a defect in the cholinergic system has received considerable support. Drugs that inhibit the cholinergic system, such as scopolamine, can produce memory problems in both humans and primates; drugs that enhance acetylcholine improve memory. Supporters of this theory suggest that depletion of acetylcholine occurs before cell death (Nakamura, 1990). Development of the drug tacrine (see Chapter 8) for treatment of Alzheimer's disease is based on the cholinergic defect hypothesis. Tacrine inhibits an enzyme that breaks down acetylcholine, thus increasing the amount available to the neurons that require it (NIA, 1993). The role of the neurotransmitter acetylcholine has been mentioned several times in this chapter.

In spite of these promising developments the acetylcholine hypothesis is subject to considerable competition from the amyloid theory. Supporters of the amyloid theory point out that, in the cases of familial Alzheimer's disease that have been studied, mutations have been found in the gene coding for the amyloid precursor protein (APP) but not for acetylcholine (Hardy, 1993).

Synaptic Loss

The loss of synapses has been found to be more strongly correlated with the degree of dementia as determined by neuropsychological testing than with the number of plaques or tangles found in the same brain tissue (Terry et al., 1991). Failure of a growth factor may be responsible for the loss of synapses, but there are several other plausible mechanisms as well.

Supporters of the synaptic loss theory contend that the plaques and tangles are important markers of Alzheimer's disease but not the primary contributors to the development of the disease (NIA, 1992). Supporters of the amyloid theory respond that the amyloid deposits occur *before* the loss of synapses and are, therefore, the primary contributors to the development of the disease (Hooper, 1992).

Genetics

Epidemiologic studies have consistently found that a family history of dementia is a risk factor for the development of Alzheimer's disease (Gatz et al., 1994). When combined with the presence of the gene product apo E4 (apo E is the protein, *APOE* is the gene), the risk is significant (Duara et al., 1996). Many experts on Alzheimer's disease continue to speak of two forms of the disease, the *familial*, which is hereditary in some families, and the *sporadic*, or nonfamilial, which is not transmitted by heredity but occurs sporadically in the general population.

Some of the support for the idea that Alzheimer's disease is heterogeneous comes from discoveries of defects on three different chromosomes in different familial groups. The first defect was found in a gene on chromosome 21 that governs the β-APP. This defect was related to a small proportion of families with the familial form of the disease whose members developed Alzheimer's disease in their 50s. The second defect, found in the presenilin-1 gene on chromosome 14, and presenilin-2 on chromosome 1, was related to early onset of Alzheimer's disease in people in their 30s and 40s. The gene for the enzyme AACT (α_1-antichymotrypsin), found in some plaques and tangles, is found on chromosome 14 (Pollen, 1993). AACT probably affects amyloid fibril deposition (Wisniewski et al., 1994). The third discovery was of a relationship between a defect on the *APOE* gene (which encodes the protein that transports cholesterol within the body) on chromosome 19 and late-onset Alzheimer's disease (Hardy, 1993). Apolipoprotein E tends to bind to β-amyloid. This gene may affect development before age 70. Another gene on chromosome 12 may contribute to the risk of developing later-onset Alzheimer's disease (Stephenson, 1997).

A number of families in which Alzheimer's disease appears in a greater than normal proportion of their members generation after generation were studied to find these gene defects. In several mountain villages outside Medellin, Colombia, live members of a large family with an inherited form of Alzheimer's disease. Researchers have traced familial transmission of the disease back to the 1700s in this family. In this autosomal dominant form of the disease, if one parent has Alzheimer's disease, the children have a 50% chance of developing it. The disease appears as soon as the early 30s in some individuals and the 50s in others. As many as 9 or 10 siblings in some of the larger branches of the family have developed Alzheimer's disease. The researchers noted that in Colombia there seems to be less stigma attached to development of the disease and that, because there are no nursing facilities, the families provide care throughout the course of the disease with much tenderness, caring, and interaction with other family members (Kosik, 1997). Many of the affected family members complained of severe headaches before the onset of dementia. Other than this and the early onset, the progression of the disease is similar to that of sporadic Alzheimer's disease (Lopera et al., 1997). Members of such families may be encountered in clinical practice, as in the following:

> A social worker was interviewing the sister of a man applying for admission to an Alzheimer's special care unit. The woman told the social worker, "My older sister and younger brother already show signs of the same problem. My sister is really bad, my younger brother is just beginning to show it, and his wife is really worried about it."

In some cases half or more of the members of a given family are affected by the disease eventually. In some forms of familial Alzheimer's disease the disease appears as early as the third or fourth decade of life (Pollen, 1993).

For people facing such a difficult situation, fear of the disease may become almost incapacitating. Major life decisions, including whether to marry or to have children, are affected by the possibility of developing Alzheimer's disease. If the particular gene responsible for transmission within the family is known, genetic testing can provide an accuracy of prediction for development of the disease of 90% or better. For many people having this information is preferable to living with uncertainty (Pollen, 1993), but others may not want to know as long as there is no way to prevent or cure the disease. Fear of the stigma associated with the disease and the social consequences (including difficulty obtaining health insurance) of a positive test are reasons for recommending anonymous testing and the provision of genetic counseling for those who choose to be tested. Although testing for the three early-onset forms may have some value, testing for risk of later-onset Alzheimer's disease may not be clinically helpful (Post et al., 1997).

Amyloid Cascade Hypothesis

One of the interesting aspects of the genetic discoveries just described is that each contributes in some way to the amyloid cascade hypothesis. Although still an incomplete explanation, this hypothesis is probably the predominant theory of causation (Selkoe, 1994).

In brief, the deposition of amyloid in the plaques and tangles that are considered the primary markers of Alzheimer's disease is believed to be triggered by mutations in the gene that encodes the APP or by binding to the E4 form of apo E. The presence of β-amyloid is considered toxic to the cell (Yankner, Duffy, & Kirschner, 1990). Some consider it a by-product of the brain's attempt to defend itself against or compensate for neuron damage, a type of chronic inflammatory process (Selkoe, 1994). Whatever its purpose, the presence of β-amyloid results in the formation of the plaques and tangles and eventually leads to the destruction of the neuron (Hardy, 1993, 1994). This sequence of events is shown in Figure 2.5.

Role of *APOE4*

Apolipoprotein E is a protein involved in triglyceride metabolism and levels of cholesterol throughout the body. It has been shown to play a role in the repair, growth, and maintenance of myelin and axonal membranes in the nervous system, including the brain (Blass & Poirier, 1996). Most important to the development of Alzheimer's disease is that the *APOE* gene has been associated with the most common form of Alzheimer's disease, the late-onset type that affects 98% of people who develop the disease. This gene has several different variants: *APOE2*, *APOE3*, and *APOE4*. Every human being inherits one variant from each parent; two may be the same (e.g., *APOE3/3*) or there may be a combination such as *APOE3/4*. *APOE2/2* is rare. The most interesting comparison is the age at onset of Alzheimer's disease in people with the *APOE2/3* combination versus those with the *APOE4/4* combination. For people with the *APOE2/3* combination, who comprise 11% of the U.S. population, the average age at onset of Alzheimer's disease is 90. For those with the *APOE4/4* combination, the average age is the early to mid-70s (Roses, 1995).

In other words, *APOE2* appears to have a beneficial effect (delaying onset), whereas *APOE4* has a negative effect (hastening onset). The goal in finding a treatment based on the role of *APOE4* is to either mimic the effect of the beneficial gene (*APOE2*) or stop the effect of the negative gene (*APOE4*). Roses (1995) explains further:

> [I]f a safe medication that mimics the function of apoE2 in the brain can be found, the age of onset curves of individuals without an APOE 2 allele [pair of *APOE* genes] may be made to resemble the best curve. If the average age of onset for the whole population could be switched to greater than 90 years of age, Alzheimer's disease would again become a rare problem. (p. 20)

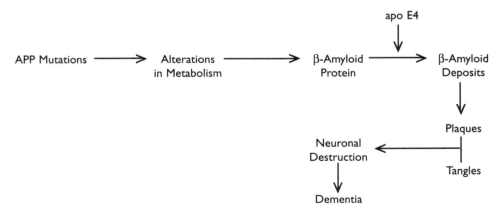

Figure 2.5. Amyloid cascade hypothesis. (Adapted from Hardy, 1993.)

A test for the *APOE* gene is commercially available. However, Mayeux and Schupf (1995) argue that, because the presence of *APOE4* is neither necessary nor sufficient to cause Alzheimer's disease and because neither preventive nor treatment measures are available to respond to the presence of the *APOE4* gene, widespread use of the test would be premature. They also suggest that, when it is appropriate to make these tests generally available, it will be necessary to provide pretest and posttest counseling for everyone who is tested to explore the personal meaning and consequences of the test results.

. . .

Given the variety of factors that appear to contribute to the occurrence of Alzheimer's disease, Blass and Poirier (1996) suggest that it may be the *convergence* of factors that leads to the disease, especially late-onset Alzheimer's disease. They conclude that Alzheimer's disease is probably a syndrome rather than a discrete (i.e., single) disease.

REFERENCES

Advisory Panel on Alzheimer's Disease. (1993). *Fourth report of the Advisory Panel on Alzheimer's Disease, 1992* (NIH Publication No. 93-3520). Washington, DC: Author.

Albert, M.S., & Moss, M.B. (Eds.). (1988). *Geriatric neuropsychology.* New York: Guilford Press.

Bachman, D.L., Wolf, P.A., Linn, R., Knoefal, J.E., Cobb, J., Belanger, A., D'Agostino, R.B., & White, L.R. (1992). Prevalence of dementia and probable senile dementia of the Alzheimer's type in the Framingham study. *Neurology, 42*(1), 115–119.

Bachman, D.L., Wolf, P.A., Linn, R., Knoefal, J.E., Cobb, J., Belanger, A., White, R.B., & D'Agostino, R.B. (1993). Incidence of dementia and probable Alzheimer's disease in a general population: The Framingham study. *Neurology, 43,* 515–519.

Berg, L., & Morris, J.C. (1990). Aging and dementia. In A.L. Pearlman & R.C. Collins (Eds.), *Neurobiology of disease.* New York: Oxford University Press.

Blass, J.P., & Poirier, J. (1996). Pathophysiology of the Alzheimer syndrome. In S. Gauthier (Ed.), *Clinical diagnosis and management of Alzheimer's disease.* Boston: Butterworth-Heinemann.

Blessed, G., Tomlinson, B.E., & Roth, M. (1968). The association between quantitative measures of dementia and of senile change in the cerebral gray matter of elderly subjects. *British Journal of Psychiatry, 114,* 797–811.

Bloom, F.E., & Lazerson, A. (1988). *Brain, mind and behavior.* New York: W.H. Freeman.

Braak, H., & Braak, E. (1994). Pathology of Alzheimer's disease. In D.B. Calne (Ed.), *Neurodegenerative disease.* Philadelphia: W.B. Saunders.

Duara, R., Barker, M.S., Lopez-Alberole, R., Loewenstein, D.A., Grau, L.B., Gilchrist, D., Sevush, S., & Hyslop, S.A. (1996). Alzheimer's disease: Interaction of apolipoprotein E genotype, family history of dementia, gender, education, ethnicity, and age of onset. *Neurology, 46,* 1575–1579.

Finch, C.E. (1994). Biochemistry of aging in the mammalian brain. In G.J. Siegel, B.W. Agranoff, R.W. Albers, & P.B. Molinoff (Eds.), *Basic neurochemistry.* New York: Raven Press.

Gajdusek, D.C. (1994). Infectious and noninfectious amyloidoses of the brain: Systemic amyloidotic neurodegeneration of Creutzfeldt-Jakob disease and aging brain and Alzheimer's disease. In D.B. Calne (Ed.), *Neurodegenerative diseases.* Philadelphia: W.B. Saunders.

Gatz, M., Lowe, B., Berg, S., Mortimer, J., & Pederson, N. (1994). Dementia: Not just a search for the gene. *Gerontologist, 34*(2), 251–255.

Half, R. (1993). Thoughts on the business of life. *Forbes, 152*(12), 216.

Hardy, J. (1993). Genetic mistakes point the way for Alzheimer's disease. *Journal of NIH Research, 5*(11), 46–48.

Hardy, J. (1994). Alzheimer's disease: Clinical molecular genetics. *Clinics in Geriatric Medicine,* *10*(2), 239–247.

Hooper, C. (1992). Encircling a mechanism in Alzheimer's disease. *Journal of NIH Research, 4*(12), 48–54.

Kolb, B., & Wishaw, I.Q. (1990). *Fundamentals of human neuropsychology.* New York: W.H. Freeman.

Kolb, B., & Wishaw, I.Q. (1995). *Fundamentals of human neuropsychology.* (3rd ed.). New York: W.H. Freeman.

Kosik, K.S. (1997). *The Alzheimer gene: One family's burden.* Paper presented at the 3rd Annual Alzheimer's Disease Educational Conference, Alzheimer's Association of Greater Palm Beach, West Palm Beach, Florida.

Lopera, F., Ardilla, A., Martinez, A., Madrigal, L., Arango-Viana, J.C., Lemere, C.A., Arango-Lasparilla, J.D., Hincapié, L., Arcos-Burgos, M., Ossa, J.E., Behrens, I.M., Norton, J., Lendon, C., Goate, A.M., Ruiz-Linares, A., Rosselli, M., & Kosik, K.S. (1997). Clinical features of early-onset Alzheimer disease in a large kindred with an E280A presenilin-1 mutation. *Journal of the American Medical Association, 277*(10), 793–799.

Mayeux, R., & Schupf, N. (1995). Apolipoprotein E and Alzheimer's disease: The implications of progress in molecular medicine. *American Journal of Public Health, 85,* 1280–1284.

Metter, E.J. (1988). Positron emission tomography and cerebral blood flow studies. In M.S. Albert & M.B. Moss (Eds.), *Geriatric neuropsychology* (pp. 228–261). New York: Guilford Press.

Nakamura, S. (1990). Quantitative and qualitative changes of neurotransmitters in Alzheimer's disease. In T. Nagatsu (Ed.), *Senile neurodegeneration and neurotransmitters.* Amsterdam: Elsevier.

National Institute on Aging. (1992). *Progress report on Alzheimer's disease 1992.* (NIH Publication No. 92-3409). Washington, DC: Author.

National Institute on Aging. (1993). *Progress report on Alzheimer's disease 1993.* (NIH Publication No. 93-3409). Bethesda, MD: Author.

National Institute on Aging. (1995). *Progress report on Alzheimer's disease 1995* (NIH Publication No. 95-3994). Bethesda, MD: Author.

Office of Technology Assessment. (1987). *Losing a million minds: Confronting the tragedy of Alzheimer's disease and other dementias.* Washington, DC: Author.

Pechura, C.M., & Martin, J. (1991). *Mapping the brain and its functions: Integrating enabling technologies into neuroscience research.* Washington, DC: National Academy Press.

Pollen, D.A. (1993). *Hannah's heirs: The quest for the genetic origins of Alzheimer's disease.* New York: Oxford University Press.

Post, S.G., Whitehead, P.J., Binstock, R.H., Bird, T., Eckert, S.L., Farrer, L.A., Fleck, L.M., Gaines, A.D., Juengst, E.T., Karlinsky, H., Miles, S., Murray, T.H., Quaid, K.A., Relkin, N.R., Roses, A.D., St. George-Hyslop, P.H., Sachs, G.A., Steinbock, B., Truschke, E.F., & Zinn, A.B. (1997). The clinical introduction of genetic testing for Alzheimer disease. *Journal of the American Medical Association, 277*(10), 832–836.

Roses, A.D. (1995). Apolipoprotein E and Alzheimer's disease. *Science and Medicine, 2*(5), 16–25.

Schneider, L.S., Farlow, M.R., Henderson, V.W., & Pogoda, J.M. (1996). Effects of estrogen replacement therapy on response to tacrine in patients with Alzheimer's disease. *Neurology, 46,* 1580–1584.

Selkoe, D.J. (1994). Biochemistry of Alzheimer's disease. In G.J. Siegel, B.W. Agranoff, R.W. Albers, & P.B. Molinoff (Eds.), *Basic neurochemistry.* New York: Raven Press.

Shepherd, G.M. (1988). *Neurobiology.* New York: Oxford University Press.

Stephenson, J. (1997). Researchers find evidence of a new gene for late-onset Alzheimer disease. *Journal of the American Medical Association, 277*(10), 775.

Taylor, P., & Brown, J.H. (1994). Acetylcholine. In G.J. Siegel, B.W. Agranoff, R.W. Albers, & P.B. Molinoff (Eds.), *Basic neurochemistry.* New York: Raven Press.

Terry, R.D., Masliah, E., Salmon, D.P., Butters, N., DeTeresa, R., Hill, R., Hansen, L.A., & Catzman, R. (1991). Physical basis of cognitive alterations in Alzheimer's disease: Synapse loss is the major correlate of cognitive impairment. *Annals of Neurology, 30*(4), 572–580.

Trehub, A. (1991). *The cognitive brain.* Cambridge, MA: MIT Press.

Vanderwolf, C.H. (1987). Near-total loss of "learning" and "memory" as a result of combined cholinergic and serotonergic blockade in the rat. *Behavioral Brain Research, 23,* 43–57. (Quoted in Kolb, B., & Wishaw, I.Q. (1990). *Fundamentals of human neuropsychology.* New York: W.H. Freeman.)

Wisniewski, H.M., Wegiel, J., Morys, J., & Bobinski, M. (1994). Alzheimer dementia neuropathology. In V.O.B. Emery & T.E. Oxman (Eds.), *Dementia presentations, differential diagnosis, and nosology* (pp. 79–94). Baltimore: The Johns Hopkins University Press.

Yankner, B.A., Duffy, L.K., & Kirschner, D.A. (1990). Neurotrophic and neurotoxic effects of amyloid B protein: Reversal by tachykinin neuropeptides. *Science, 250,* 279–281.

Chapter 3

Clinical Evaluation

In those few minutes I saw him deteriorate in a way I had never seen in any of my previous clinical experience. He went from a cautious but confident patient to a man shocked by the realization that he could not remember or think about some relatively simple questions that he seemed to know that he should be able to answer. . . . [T]he look on his face was one of shocked discovery.

J.T. Tapp (1989, p.12)

A major frustration for professionals, patients, and patients' families is that there is no definitive test for diagnosing Alzheimer's disease. In fact, the closest we can come to a diagnosis in 1997 is a clinician's decision that a person *probably* has Alzheimer's disease because other possible causes of his or her intellectual decline have been eliminated from consideration. The diagnosis of Alzheimer's disease still cannot be confirmed until an autopsy is performed postmortem (after the person dies). However, the accuracy of clinical diagnosis has improved considerably, and most clinicians are relatively confident of their decision when they conclude that a person has Alzheimer's disease.

The process of establishing the presence of Alzheimer's disease presents a number of challenges: eliminating other causes of intellectual decline, distinguishing Alzheimer's disease from other types of dementia, and helping the patient and his or her family cope with the realization that Alzheimer's disease is probably the cause of the problem.

ESTABLISHMENT OF THE PROBABILITY OF ALZHEIMER'S DISEASE

The first signs of Alzheimer's disease are subtle ones that can be mistaken for the effects of fatigue, anxiety, or overwork. Eventually, however, a critical event brings the person to the physician's office: overdrawing the checking account, being brought home by the police after getting lost, changing behavior or mood, even exhibiting an unrelated illness. Some people are shocked by the diagnosis, whereas others have suspected it for some time. All who are diagnosed as having Alzheimer's disease or who have a loved one who receives this diagnosis are in need of accurate, up-to-date information about the disease and professional guidance in managing the care of the person with the disease. The Alzheimer's Association (1996) suggests that people with dementia and their families need answers to the following questions after a diagnosis is made:

- What does the diagnosis mean?
- What symptoms can be anticipated next?
- How will these symptoms change over time?
- What kind of care is needed now? In the future?
- What kind of treatment is available? How effective is it?
- Is participation in a research study possible? What are the risks?
- What services and resources are available? How are they accessed? (p. 10)

Most primary care physicians once simply ascribed memory loss to old age, or diagnosed the problem as "senility" and declared that there was nothing that could be done about it. Their best advice would be "You'll just have to live with it." This is no longer the case. Most primary care physicians and nurse practitioners are alert to the signs of Alzheimer's disease, sympathetic to the shock experienced by the patient and family on learning the diagnosis, and aware of the various treatments and community resources available to them.

This increased awareness is true of the public as well. Most people have at least heard the term *Alzheimer's disease*, although some mistake it for "old timer's disease." Most recognize the seriousness of the diagnosis, and few are nonchalant about it. Probably the greatest change that has occurred with increasing public awareness is that people are inclined to seek assistance, such as confirmation of the diagnosis, more information about the disease, and help in managing the consequences of the disease.

The most commonly used diagnostic guidelines and the use of interviews, observation, and testing in determining whether an individual has Alzheimer's disease are explicated in the following sections.

DIAGNOSTIC GUIDELINES

In 1984 the National Institute of Neurological and Communicative Disorders and Stroke and the Alzheimer's Disease and Related Disorders Association (NINCDS-ADRDA) formed a work group to develop a set of guidelines for the diagnosis of Alzheimer's disease. Because the diagnosis requires considerable clinical judgment, the group defined two levels of certainty regarding the diagnosis: *possible* Alzheimer's disease, if there are atypical features or other problems that could be responsible for the dementia, and *probable* Alzheimer's disease, if there are no other apparent problems that could be responsible for the symptoms and the symptoms fit the typical picture (McKhann et al., 1984). A summary of the criteria may be found in Table 3.1. When the accuracy of clinical diagnoses is compared with pathological evaluations done on autopsy, from 68% to 100% of the clinical diagnoses are confirmed by the autopsy results. Usually, the accuracy rate is considerably higher for probable rather than possible Alzheimer's disease. In an analysis of cases in which an incorrect diagnosis of Alzheimer's disease had been made (Klatka, Schiffer, Powers, & Kazee, 1996), five clues that the problem may not be Alzheimer's disease were noted:

1. Signs of Parkinson's disease, especially tremors at rest and cogwheel rigidity (rigidity that occurs in bursts, like the ratchets of a cogwheel)
2. Absence of language dysfunction, especially in moderate to severe stages
3. Absence of visuospatial impairment, such as difficulty copying complex designs or picture identification
4. Evidence of marked early personality change
5. Focal neurological signs

Only the latter feature, focal neurological signs, is included as an exclusionary feature in the most widely used guidelines for diagnosing Alzheimer's disease clinically (Table 3.1) (Klatka et al., 1996).

A different set of guidelines may be found in the *Diagnostic and Statistical Manual of Mental Disorders (DSM-IV)* (American Psychiatric Association, 1994), which defines various psychiatric disorders. For example, dementia is defined as a decline in memory from previously higher levels that is sufficient to impair occupational or social function

Table 3.1.   NINCDS–ADRDA criteria

Criteria for probable Alzheimer's disease
Dementia established by clinical examination and documented by the Mini-Mental State Exam or
   similar test
Deficits in two or more areas of cognition
Progressive worsening of memory and other functions
No disturbance of consciousness
Onset between age 40 and 90, most after age 65
Absence of systematic disorders or other brain diseases that account for the progressive deficits
   in memory and cognition

Eliminate from consideration if evidence of
Sudden onset
Focal neurological signs (e.g., hemiparesis, incoordination early in illness)
Seizures or gait disturbances at onset or very early stage

Additional supportive evidence
Impaired activities of daily living
Normal lumbar puncture
Normal or nonspecific change in electroencephalogram
Cerebral atrophy on computed tomography
Family history of similar disorders

Features consistent with Alzheimer's disease
Progressive deterioration of specific cognitive functions (aphasia, agnosia)
Plateaus in course of illness
Associated symptoms of depression, incontinence, catastrophic outbursts, sexual disorders, weight
   loss
Motor disorders in advanced stages, seizures

Adapted from McKhann et al. (1984).

and includes one of the following as well: aphasia, apraxia, agnosia, or disturbed executive function. Dementia of the Alzheimer's type is a dementia as defined by NINCDS-ADRDA that is characterized by gradual onset and continuing cognitive decline that is not accounted for by other central nervous system disease, delirium, or depression.

Many of the diagnostic terms used in relation to Alzheimer's disease have different meanings for professionals from different disciplines. For example, depression, delirium, and dementia are considered separate diagnostic entities in the psychiatric literature. Dementia includes both intellectual and functional deficits. Neurologists, however, look at dementia not as a diagnosis but a syndrome characterized by deterioration of intellectual ability (Maletta, 1990). Still other health care professionals, such as nurses, may prefer to use the term *cognitive impairment* rather than to use a medical diagnosis to refer to the decline in intellectual ability.

DIAGNOSTIC TECHNIQUES

The diagnostic techniques employed in clinical evaluation of a person with Alzheimer's disease or related dementias are interview and observation, cognitive testing, and imaging technologies. The Agency for Health Care Policy and Research (AHCPR) clinical practice guidelines for initial assessment of Alzheimer's disease (Costa et al., 1996) emphasize the importance of using a combination of sources, rather than a single source (e.g., MMSE; see pp. 42–43), in assessing an individual.

Interview and Observation

An interview can provide some clues indicating the presence of dementia. Report of memory problems from the patient or family, a change or incongruity in appearance or behavior, and a pattern of deflecting difficult questions or decisions to someone else are frequently noted during an interview (Drachman, Friedland, Larson & Williams, 1991).

Prior to the mid-1990s many physicians used a rule of thumb that if a person reported memory loss, he or she did not have dementia. This rule was based on the idea that people with Alzheimer's disease had little or no insight into the level of their own cognitive disabilities (Drachman et al., 1991). Clinical experience since then suggests that this rule is not necessarily true. Little correlation exists between an older person's self-report and memory problems found during objective testing (Duara, 1994). Some individuals report more memory loss than is found on testing, others less. Family members' reports, in contrast, are usually supported by objective cognitive testing when they state that there is no problem. They also have been found to be relatively accurate when they report that there is a problem (Koss, Patterson, Ownby, Stuckey, & Whitehouse, 1993).

Some family members find it easy to describe in detail the changes that they have observed, whereas others need some prompting to elaborate on what they have noticed. The following questions, derived from the Riege Short-Memory Questionnaire (1982), can be used to elicit the necessary information from family members:

- Can your family member give someone directions to your home?
- Can your family member remember what he or she did last Sunday?
- Does your family member usually remember where he or she parked the car?
- When your family member leaves the store, can he or she remember how much change he or she received?
- If you asked your family member to get you five items at the grocery store, could he or she do that and not forget any item? (Koss et al., 1993)

These questions can be reworded to ask the patient for the same information, such as, "Do you have trouble remembering where you parked the car?" or "Do you remember what you did last Sunday?" AHCPR clinical practice guidelines for initial assessment of Alzheimer's disease (Costa et al., 1996) recommend use of the Functional Activities Questionnaire (FAQ; Pfeffer et al., 1982), which uses a similar approach (Table 3.2).

It is important to progress beyond the superficial, routine questions of most interviews (e.g., "How are you?"; "What do you think of this weather?") because these queries can be answered virtually automatically. Instead, the person can be asked to describe a typical day or his or her home situation in order to ascertain the ability to provide specific information, deal with abstraction, and remember details of recent events. The list of symptoms in Table 3.3 may also be helpful in querying for information.

Some family members will discuss such problems openly in the presence of the person suspected of having Alzheimer's disease or a related dementia. Others, however, are reluctant to do this for fear of embarrassing or frightening the person or because it provokes an angry denial (often resulting from embarrassment or fear). In either case it may be necessary to speak with the patient and family separately because either or both may prefer a private interview initially. In the long run, however, open communication about the problem is preferred and should be encouraged.

In addition to asking questions for the purpose of ruling out other causes of the memory loss and taking a careful history of the memory loss itself, a history of similar memory problems in the same and preceding generations should be elicited. Familial and

Table 3.2. Functional Activities Questionnaire (FAQ)

The FAQ measures an older adult's functional abilities based on information gathered from loved ones, caregivers, and the like. These individuals rate the older person on his or her performance of 10 complex, higher-order activities.

Performance levels are rated from 0 to 3 (normal–dependent), as follows:

0	Normal
1	Has difficulty, but can do without assistance
2	Needs assistance
3	Dependent

Additional response options are scored as follows:

0	Didn't do the activity, but could do now
1	Didn't do the activity and would have difficulty now

ACTIVITIES

1. Writing checks; paying bills; balancing a checkbook
2. Assembling tax records or business affairs
3. Shopping for clothes or groceries without assistance
4. Participating in a game; working on a hobby
5. Preparing a full meal
6. Heating water; making coffee
7. Keeping track of current events
8. Concentrating on, understanding, and discussing a TV show or magazine article
9. Driving; calling for a taxicab
10. Remembering family birthdays or to take medications

To arrive at the total score, individual scores should be added. Total score can range from 0 to 30; the higher the score, the poorer the functional ability of the older adult, and vice versa. AHCPR recommends a cutpoint of 9, which indicates that the older adult is dependent in 3 or more activities.

From Costa, P.T., Williams, T.F., Somerfield, M., et al. (1996). *Recognition and initial assessment of Alzheimer's disease and related dementias*, no. 19. AHCPR Publication No. 97-0703. Rockville, MD: U.S. Department of Health and Human Services, Public Health Service, Agency for Health Care Policy and Research.

nonfamilial types of Alzheimer's disease are usually identified on the basis of family history but may be identified by laboratory tests as well in the future. The distinction between these types is important to members of the individual's family, particularly to younger generations making decisions about marriage and childbearing (Pollen, 1993).

Observation of the individual who may have Alzheimer's disease is also helpful in establishing a diagnosis. For example, uncombed hair, a misbuttoned shirt or sweater, or mismatched clothes would be incongruous on a person who usually dressed well (Drachman et al., 1991). People with Alzheimer's disease often avoid exposing their disability by evading or talking around a subject (*circumlocution*). A common response to a question that the person cannot answer would be, "Oh, that's easy, everyone knows that," or "Why do you want to know that?" If family members are present, the person will often turn to them to supply the answer, which family members often do unconsciously. Taken on an individual basis none of these signs means that the person has dementia.

Table 3.3. Symptoms that may indicate the presence of dementia

Does the older adult experience difficulty with any of the following activities?[a]

_____ *Learning and retaining new information.* Is the person more repetitive? Does the person have difficulty remembering recent conversations, events, appointments, and the like? Does the person misplace objects frequently?

_____ *Handling complex tasks.* Does the person have difficulty following a complex train of thought or performing tasks that require many steps (e.g., cooking)?

_____ *Reasoning ability.* Is the person unable to create a logical plan to solve problems at work or at home? Does the person demonstrate uncharacteristic disregard for proper public or social behavior?

_____ *Maintaining spatial ability and orientation.* Does the person have difficulty driving, organizing, or finding his or her way around familiar places?

_____ *Using language.* Does the person have difficulty finding the right words to express him- or herself meaningfully? Can the person understand conversations and contribute to them?

_____ *Maintaining usual behaviors.* Does the person appear more passive and less responsive than usual? Is the person more irritable than usual? Is the person more suspicious than usual? Does the person misinterpret visual or auditory stimuli? Is the person suddenly dressing haphazardly or failing to dress?

From Costa, P.T., Williams, T.F., Somerfield, M., et al. (1996). *Recognition and initial assessment of Alzheimer's disease and related dementias*, no. 19. AHCPR Publication No. 97-0703. Rockville, MD: U.S. Department of Health and Human Services, Public Health Service, Agency for Health Care Policy and Research.

[a]Positive findings (indicated by check mark or X in the space provided) in any of these areas generally indicate the need for further assessment for the presence of dementia.

However, if the signs are part of a larger pattern reflecting a decline in intellectual ability, they are sufficient indications for further evaluation and testing.

Cognitive Testing

The best known and probably most widely used general test of cognitive function is the Mini-Mental State Examination (MMSE; see Figure 3.1) (Folstein, Folstein, & McHugh, 1975). Known more familiarly as the "Mini-Mental" or the "Folstein," the MMSE is a brief test of orientation, immediate and delayed recall, calculation, concentration, language, and praxis (action). Scores range from 0 (no items answered correctly) to 30 (all items answered correctly). A score of less than 21 may be considered indicative of dementia. The Blessed Information-Memory-Concentration test, the Blessed Orientation-Memory-Concentration test, or the Short Test of Mental Status may also be used (Costa et al., 1996).

A full battery of cognitive tests has far more depth and breadth. The Consortium to Establish a Registry for Alzheimer's Disease (CERAD) recommends a comprehensive battery of clinical and neuropsychological tests for people with Alzheimer's disease (Morris et al., 1989; Welsh et al., 1994). The clinical assessment portion of the CERAD battery includes the following components:

• Semistructured interview with patient and significant other
• Physical examination
• Neurological and laboratory examination

- Drug inventory
- Depression scale
- General health history
- Blessed Dementia Scale (Blessed, Tomlinson, & Roth, 1968)
- Clinical Dementia Rating Scale (Berg, 1988)

The neuropsychological assessment portion of the battery includes measures of the primary areas of cognition affected by Alzheimer's disease, such as memory, language, praxis, and general intellectual status. The tests suggested include the following:

- Verbal Fluency—Animal Naming Test (naming as many animals as possible in 1 minute)
- Modified Boston Naming Test (naming objects presented one at a time as line drawings; Goodglass & Kaplan, 1983)
- MMSE
- Constructional Praxis (reproducing four line drawings of figures of increasing complexity, e.g., circle, diamond, intersecting rectangles, cube)
- Word List Recall
- Word List Recognition

This battery takes about 20–30 minutes to administer. Apraxia, impairment in skilled motor activities, may be tested in the following ways:

- Pantomime—"Show me how you would use a _____."
- Imitation of pantomime—"Watch how I use a _____; then you do it."
- Use of an actual object—"Here is a _____. Show me how you would use it."
- Imitation of examiner using an object
- Identification of the correct pantomime performed by examiner (Mohr, Willmer, & Mendis, in press, in Dastoor & Mohr, 1996)

Interpretation of the results of these and similar tests must be made in light of other information about the person. For example, an individual with hearing or vision impairments clearly would be at a disadvantage in responding to this test. People who have had strokes and have residual aphasia may know the correct answer to a question but be unable to communicate it to the examiner. For these and similar reasons, scores on such tests must be interpreted cautiously.

Imaging Technologies

We have come a long way from the original flat, two-dimensional X ray that first allowed a look inside the human body without performing surgery. The imaging technologies (see following) provide information about the structure and function of the healthy brain and what can go awry when the brain has a disease. None of these technologies offers a certain diagnosis of Alzheimer's disease, but they do assist in the elimination of other causes of dementia (e.g., tumors, subdural hematomas) and promise an objective source of information about the presence of dementing disease and the effectiveness of treatment in the future (Fontaine & Nordberg, 1996; National Institute on Aging [NIA], 1995).

Computed Tomography   The use of computers has contributed a great deal to the advances in imaging techniques. The well-known computed tomography scan (CT, CAT scan) uses narrow X-ray beams to examine the brain from various angles. These cross-sectional images are used to create a computer-generated three-dimensional picture from

Instructions for Administration of Mini-Mental State Examination

Orientation

(1) Ask the patient for the date. Then ask specific questions (e.g., "Can you also tell me what season it is?"). 1 point for each correct answer. (2) Ask the patient "Can you tell me the name of this hospital?" (town, county, etc.). 1 point for each correct answer.

Registration

Ask the patient if you may test his or her memory. Then say the names of 3 unrelated objects, clearly and slowly, about 1 second for each. After you have said all 3, ask him to repeat them. This first repetition determines the score (0–3) but keep saying them until he or she can repeat all 3, up to 6 trials. If the patient does not eventually learn all 3, recall (below) cannot be tested meaningfully.

Attention and Calculation

Ask the patient to begin with 100 and count backwards by 7. Stop after 5 subtractions (e.g., 93, 86, 79, 72, 65). Score the total number of correct answers. If the patient cannot or will not perform this task, ask him or her to spell the word "world" backwards. The score is the number of letters in the correct order (e.g., dlrow = 5, dlorw = 3).

Recall

Ask the patient if he or she can recall the 3 words you previously asked him or her to remember. Score 0–3.

Language

Naming: Show the patient a watch and ask him or her what it is. Show the patient a pencil and ask him or her what it is. Score 0–2.

Repetition: Ask the patient to repeat the sentence after you. Allow only one trial. Score 0 or 1.

3-Stage command: Give the patient a blank piece of paper and repeat the command. Score 1 point for each part correctly executed.

Reading: On a blank piece of paper print the sentence CLOSE YOUR EYES in easy-to-read capital letters. Ask the patient to read the sentence and do what it says. If the patient does close his or her eyes, score only 1 point.

Writing: Give the patient a blank piece of paper and ask him or her to write a sentence. Don't provide the sentence yourself; the sentence should be a complete one.

Copying: Ask the patient to copy the design. The patient must copy all the angles and 2 must intersect to score 1 point.

Sensory Level

Estimate the patient's sensory level along a continuum from left (ALERT) to right (COMA).

(continued)

Figure 3.1. The Mini-Mental State Examination. (Adapted from Folstein, M.F., Folstein, S., & McHugh, P.R. [1975]).

SUBJECT NAME: _____   ID#: _____

TEST POINT: _____   TESTING DATE: _____   EXAMINER: _____

MINI-MENTAL STATE EXAMINATION

MAX SCORE	ACTUAL SCORE	
		ORIENTATION
5	_____	What is the (year) (season) (date) (day) (month)?
5	_____	Name the (state) (county) (town) (hospital) (floor) we are in/on.
		REGISTRATION
3	_____	Name 3 objects: (apple) (table) (penny) [1 second to say each]. Ask the patient all 3 after you have said them. Give 1 point for each correct answer. Then repeat them until he or she learns all three. (Count trials and record.)
		Trials _____
		ATTENTION AND CALCULATION
5	_____	Serial 7's. Begin with 100 and count backwards by 7. 1 point for each correct. Stop after 5 answers. Alternatively spell "world" backwards.
		RECALL
3	_____	Ask for the 3 objects repeated above. 1 point for each correct answer.
		LANGUAGE
9	_____	Show a watch and pencil and ask the patient to name them. (2 points)
	_____	Repeat the following: "No 'ifs,' 'ands,' or 'buts.' " (1 point)
	_____	Follow a 3-stage command: "Take a paper in your right hand, fold it in half, and put it on the floor." (3 points)
		Read and obey the following:
	_____	Close your eyes (1 point)
	_____	Write a sentence (1 point)
	_____	Copy the design (1 point)
30	_____	**TOTAL SCORE**

Assess patient's level of consciousness along a continuum:

_____

ALERT   DROWSY   STUPOR   COMA

Figure 3.1. (*continued*)

which a number of problems can be identified, such as atrophy, tumors, edema, and infarction in the brain (Kee, 1983).

Magnetic Resonance Imaging   Magnetic resonance imaging (MRI) uses external magnetic fields to produce more precise (higher resolution) three-dimensional views of the brain without the radiation exposure of the CT scan (Souder, Saykin, & Alair, 1995).

Far more subtle changes can be detected with MRI than with CT scans. Advances will make this possible even at the molecular level (Giacometti, Davis, Alazrake & Malko, 1994; Pechura & Martin, 1991). MRI picks up much smaller infarcts than can CT and may confirm the presence of vascular involvement in a dementia (Whitehouse, Lerner, & Hedera, 1993). Both CT and MRI can be used to rule out normal-pressure hydro-cephalus, subdural hematomas, and tumors (Drachman et al., 1991). Absence of any cerebrovascular lesions on CT or MRI is considered good evidence against vascular in-volvement (Drachman, 1993).

Positron Emission Tomography   The use of CT and MRI provides information about the *structure* of the brain. Positron emission tomography (PET) provides information about the cellular *function* of the brain. Utilizing short-lived radioactive markers to tag selected molecules injected into the bloodstream, a PET scan can trace the volume and flow of blood through the brain and the level of consumption of oxygen and glucose and of action of neurotransmitters (Fontaine & Nordberg, 1996).

Decreased blood flow, glucose uptake, or both in a particular area is indicative of inactivity or inhibition, both of which are problematic to the individual (Pechura & Martin, 1991). Although both oxygen and glucose consumption decrease with age, the decline is exaggerated when diseases such as Alzheimer's disease are present. Also, be-cause differences in function across the various sectors of the brain can be identified with PET, this approach may be useful in early stages of the disease, when clinical manifes-tations do not indicate the type of dementia that is developing (Fontaine & Nordberg, 1996).

Single-Photon Emission Computed Tomography   Single-photon emission com-puted tomography (SPECT) is a further enhancement of imaging technology that pro-duces even better spatial resolution (Baron & Marchal, 1992). Different patterns of uptake of radioactive markers on SPECT images are indicative of different types of dementias. For example, in a study comparing SPECT results with clinical diagnoses and autopsy results, the posterior temporal and parietal lobes on both sides showed decreases in uptake in individuals with Alzheimer's disease and Parkinsonian dementia, as would be expected. Those who had frontotemporal dementia had a different pattern focused in the frontal lobes. An irregular or mottled pattern was found in people with Jakob-Creutzfeldt de-mentia, and focal (localized) areas of decreased uptake were found in people with ischemic (insufficient blood supply) lesions (Read et al., 1995). Using SPECT, one finds an increase in cerebral blood flow in the frontal cortex while taking verbal memory tests in unim-paired controls but not in people with Alzheimer's disease (Fontaine & Nordberg, 1996).

Magnetic Resonance Spectroscopy   Using magnetic resonance spectroscopy (MRSI), we can detect abnormal concentrations of important chemicals without using the radio-active markers as in the PET and SPECT technologies (NIA, 1995), because the resonance frequency of various chemicals differ. For example, the hydrogen in water can be distin-guished from the hydrogen in lipids on the basis of slight differences in frequency. In the brain, concentrations of such important chemicals as choline can be analyzed with this noninvasive procedure (Giacometti et al., 1994).

Electroencephalogram   Some useful information also can be obtained through the use of electroencephalography. The electrical activity of the brain can be recorded by an electroencephalogram (EEG). The EEG is particularly useful in evaluating seizures and is also useful in identifying Jakob-Creutzfeldt dementia, a disease that can be transmitted to other people through corneal transplants or contaminated brain electrodes (Berkow & Fletcher, 1992; Drachman et al., 1991). The magnetic fields generated by brain activity also can be measured by an EEG (Pechura & Martin, 1991).

Test Administration   When using imaging techniques in the diagnosis of Alzheimer's disease, the equipment used may be problematic. The PET and MRI scanners often have been likened to a washer or dryer in a giant laundromat. The patient must lie completely still with his or her head within a doughnut-shaped scanner for as long as 30 minutes. Although the scan is not painful, it can be uncomfortable, especially for people with claustrophobia. People with Alzheimer's disease who find it difficult to remain still or who are easily frightened by new surroundings may need special advance preparation (e.g., procedures explained) before these tests are performed. New "open" designs of MRI scanners also may be useful.

DIFFERENTIATION OF ALZHEIMER'S DISEASE FROM OTHER DEMENTIAS

Probably the most compelling reason to attempt to differentiate Alzheimer's disease from other types of dementia is the possibility of finding a different type of chronic or reversible dementia, one for which certain precautions must be taken or for which some specific treatment is available.

Vascular Dementia

Second only to Alzheimer's disease in frequency, vascular dementia is less well defined as a clinical entity. Although the occurrence of strokes does not necessarily lead to lasting cognitive impairment, it is thought that some chronic progressive dementias are the result of multiple cerebral infarctions (areas of necrosis in the brain caused by insufficient blood supply). Vascular dementia has been associated with large vessel occlusion, localized ischemic damage, small vessel disease, and global brain ischemia resulting from inadequate perfusion. Clinically, vascular dementia has a more abrupt onset than does Alzheimer's disease, and the decline progresses in a stepwise rather than steady and gradual fashion. Early gait disturbance, unsteadiness and falls, urinary incontinence, and emotional incontinence (instability) are more common in vascular dementia. Psychomotor retardation (slowing), perseveration (repetitiveness), and mood changes are also found. Focal (localized) neurological signs and symptoms are associated with vascular, not Alzheimer's-type, dementia (Morris, 1994). When these focal signs and symptoms are absent, or when CT or MRI do not indicate the presence of cerebrovascular lesions, or both, vascular dementia is unlikely (Roman et al., 1993).

In 1975 Hachinski and colleagues developed a set of criteria for use in distinguishing vascular (multi-infarct) dementias from dementias of the Alzheimer's type (see Figure 3.2). Although relatively useful in distinguishing pure Alzheimer's disease from pure vascular dementia, the Hachinski criteria provide less guidance when dementia and stroke coexist (Roman et al., 1993).

Normal-Pressure Hydrocephalus

A relatively unusual form of dementia, normal-pressure hydrocephalus is a condition in which the ventricles of the brain are dilated but the cerebrospinal fluid pressure remains at normal levels (Berkow & Fletcher, 1992). Clinically, the person is cognitively impaired, incontinent of urine, and experiences gait and balance disturbance. This problem is treated

PATIENT NAME: _____   ROOM #: _____

PHYSICIAN: _____   DATE: _____

ISCHEMIC SCORE

FEATURE	SCORE
Abrupt onset	2
Stepwise deterioration	1
Fluctuating course	2
Nighttime confusion	1
Relative preservation of personality	1
Depression	1
Somatic complaints	1
Emotional incontinence	1
Hypertension	1
Stroke and associated atherosclerosis	2
Focal neurological signs and symptoms	2
TOTAL	

INTERPRETATION

7 or above indicates multi-infarct dementia

4 or below indicates primary degenerative dementia

Figure 3.2. Criteria distinguishing vascular dementia and Alzheimer's-type dementia. (Adapted from Hachinski, V.C., Iliff, L.D., Zilhka, E., DuBoulay, M.B., McAllister, V.L., Marchall, J., Russell, R.W.R., & Simon, L. [1975]. Cerebral blood flow in dementia. *Archives of Neurology, 32*, 632–637; reprinted by permission.)

surgically: The excess fluid is shunted away from the brain into a major vessel. Unfortunately, normal-pressure hydrocephalus is difficult to diagnose, even with imaging techniques, and it is difficult to predict which patients will benefit from the shunting procedure, which has a high complication rate (Clarfield, 1994).

Reversible Dementias

The terms *acute confusional state, delirium,* and *reversible dementia* are often used interchangeably to describe an individual experiencing an acute episode of impaired cognition related to hypoxia, drug toxicity, or other insults to the brain. If prolonged, the condition can become chronic and the damage permanent. Reversible dementia also can be used to refer to an individual whose cognitive ability has been diminished as a result of a potentially treatable underlying emotional or physiological process: fluid and electrolyte abnormalities, hypoglycemia, thyroid disorders, subdural hematoma, brain tumor, or nutritional deficiency. The most common of these processes are overmedication and depression (Morris, 1994). These chronic insults to the brain may be superimposed over existing Alzheimer's disease or vascular dementia, exacerbating the cognitive deficits.

A complete history and physical examination, including drug inventory and blood tests, may be necessary to eliminate the possibility of reversible dementia. Comprehensive blood chemistry, blood count, urinalysis, and chest films (to detect problems contributing to hypoxemia) are often ordered to assess the patient.

Depression

Distinguishing depression from dementia requires a different approach. Intellectual performance is affected by both depression and dementia. To complicate matters further, many individuals in the early stages of Alzheimer's disease are also clinically depressed. A research study comparing four groups of people—those with very mild Alzheimer's disease, major depression, both Alzheimer's disease and depression, and healthy people—found that several neuropsychological tests may be helpful in distinguishing Alzheimer's disease from depression (des Rosiers, Hodges & Berrios, 1995). The Kendrick's Object Learning Test, in which patients are shown cards with pictures of multiple household objects for 30 seconds and then asked to recall them, and tests of ability to retain information over the short term (30 minutes) seemed to differentiate these conditions better than did tests using immediate recall. It also has been noted frequently that, because depression is treatable, it is preferable to err on the side of treating it rather than not if it is suspected.

· · ·

Now that awareness of Alzheimer's disease has increased to the point that it is difficult to find an adult who has never heard of it, the danger of Alzheimer's disease being overlooked or neglected is being replaced by the danger of assuming that any progressive dementing process must be Alzheimer's disease. The danger, of course, is that a potentially reversible problem such as depression or vascular insufficiency may progress untreated because the individual is assumed to have Alzheimer's disease, leaving irreversible damage or loss, and even unnecessary placement in a long-term care facility, in its wake. To prevent these potentially disastrous consequences, accurate diagnosis by an expert in the fields of geriatrics, neurology, or neuropsychiatry is an essential first step in the care of an individual who may have Alzheimer's disease.

REFERENCES

Alzheimer's Association. (1996). *Steps to getting a diagnosis: Finding out if it's Alzheimer's disease*. Chicago: Author.

American Psychiatric Association. (1994). *Diagnostic and statistical manual of mental disorders (DSM-IV)* (4th ed.). Washington, DC: American Psychiatric Press.

Baron, J.C., & Marchal, G. (1992). Cerebral and cardiovascular aging and brain energy metabolism: Studies with positron-emission tomography in man. *Presse Medicale, 21*(26), 1231–1237.

Berg, L. (1988). Clinical dementia rating (CDR). *Psychopharmacology Bulletin, 24*, 637–639.

Berkow, R., & Fletcher, A.J. (1992). *The Merck manual*. Rahway, NJ: Merck Research Laboratories.

Blessed, G., Tomlinson, B.E., & Roth, M. (1968). The association between quantitative measures of dementia and senile change in the cerebral gray matter of elderly subjects. *British Journal of Psychiatry, 114,* 797–811.

Clarfield, A.M. (1994). Reversible dementias from gross structural lesions. In V.O.B. Emery & T.E. Oxman (Eds.), *Dementia: Presentations, differential diagnosis, and nosology* (pp. 64–76). Baltimore: The Johns Hopkins University Press.

Costa, P.T., Williams, T.F., Somerfield, M., et al. (1996). *Recognition and initial assessment of Alzheimer's disease and related dementias,* no. 19. AHCPR Publication No. 97-0703. Rockville, MD: U.S. Department of Health and Human Services, Public Health Service, Agency for Health Care Policy and Research.

Dastoor, D., & Mohr, E. (1996). Neuropsychological assessment. In S. Gauthier (Ed.), *Clinical diagnosis and management of Alzheimer's disease* (pp. 71–81). Boston: Butterworth-Heinemann.

des Rosiers, G., Hodges, J.R., & Berrios, G. (1995). The neuropsychological differentiation of patients with very mild Alzheimer's disease and/or major depression. *Journal of the American Geriatrics Society, 43,* 1256–1263.

Drachman, D.A. (1993). New criteria for the diagnosis of vascular dementia: Do we know enough yet? *Neurology, 43,* 243–245.

Drachman, D.A., Friedland, R.P., Larson, E.B., & Williams, M.E. (1991). Making sure it's really Alzheimer's. *Patient Care, 25*(18), 13–43.

Duara, R. (1994). *Advances in diagnosis of Alzheimer's disease and related disorders.* Paper presented at Advances in Geriatrics VI, Miami, FL.

Folstein, M.F., Folstein, S.E., & McHugh, P.R. (1975). Mini-Mental State Exam: A practical method for grading the cognitive state of patients for the clinician. *Journal of Psychiatric Research, 120,* 189–198.

Fontaine, S., & Nordberg, A. (1996). Brain imaging. In S. Gauthier (Ed.), *Clinical diagnosis and management of Alzheimer's disease* (pp. 83–105). Boston: Butterworth-Heinemann.

Giacometti, A.R., Davis, P.C., Alazrake, N.P., & Malko, J.A. (1994). Anatomic and physiologic imaging of Alzheimer's disease. *Clinics in Geriatric Medicine, 10*(2), 277–298.

Goodglass, H., & Kaplan, E.C. (1983). *The assessment of aphasia and related disorders.* Philadelphia: Lea & Febiger.

Hachinski, V.V, Iliff, L.D., Zilhka, E., DuBoulay, M.B., McAllister, V.L., Marchall, J., Russell, R.W.R., & Simon, L. (1975). Cerebral blood flow in dementia. *Archives of Neurology, 32,* 632–637.

Kee, J.L. (1983). *Laboratory and diagnostic tests with nursing implications.* Norwalk, CT: Appleton-Century-Crofts.

Klatka, L.A., Schiffer, R.B., Powers, J.M., & Kazee, A.M. (1996). Incorrect diagnosis of Alzheimer's disease. *Archives of Neurology, 53,* 35–42.

Koss, E., Patterson, M.B., Ownby, R., Stuckey, J.C., & Whitehouse, P. (1993). Memory evaluation in Alzheimer's disease: Caregivers' appraisals and objective testing. *Archives of Neurology, 50*(1), 92–97.

Maletta, G.J. (1990). The concept of "reversible" dementia: How nonreliable terminology may impair effective treatment. *Journal of the American Geriatrics Society, 38*(2), 136–140.

McKhann, G., Drachman, D., Folstein, M., Katzman, R., Price, D., & Stadlan, E.M. (1984). Clinical diagnosis of Alzheimer's disease: Report of the NINCDS-ADRDA Work Group under the auspices of Department of Health and Human Services Task Force on Alzheimer's Disease. *Neurology, 34,* 939–944.

Morris, J.C. (1994). Differential diagnosis of Alzheimer's disease. *Clinics in Geriatric Medicine, 10,* 257–276.

Morris, J.C., Heyman, A., & Mohs, R.C. (1989). The Consortium to Establish a Registry for Alzheimer's Disease (CERAD). I: Clinical and neuropsychological assessment of Alzheimer's disease. *Neurology, 39,* 1159–1165.

National Institute on Aging. (1995). *Progress report on Alzheimer's disease 1995* (NIH Publication No. 95-3994). Washington, DC: Author.

Pechura, C.M., & Martin, J.B. (1991). *Mapping the brain and its functions: Integrating enabling technologies into neuroscience research.* Washington, DC: National Academy Press.

Pfeffer, R.I., Kurosaki, T.T., Harrah, C.H., et al. (1982). Measurement of functional activities of older adults in the community. *Journal of Gerontology, 37*, 323–329.

Pollen, D.A. (1993). *Hannah's heirs: The quest for the genetic origins of Alzheimer's disease.* New York: Oxford University Press.

Read, S.L., Miller, B.L., Mena, I., Kim, R., Itabashi, H., & Darby, A. (1995). SPECT in dementia: Clinical and pathological correlation. *Journal of the American Geriatrics Society, 43*, 1243–1247.

Riege, W.H. (1982). Self-report and tests of memory in aging. *Clinical Gerontologist, 1*, 23–36.

Roman, G.C., Tatemichi, T.K., Erkinjuntti, T., Cummings, J.L., Masdeu, J.C., Garcia, J.H., Amaducci, L., Orgogozo, J.M., Brun, A., Hofman, A., et al. (1993). Vascular dementia: Diagnostic criteria for research studies. Report of the NINDS-AIREN International Workshop. *Neurology, 43*(7), 1240–1245.

Souder, E., Saykin, A.J., & Alair, A. (1995). Multi-model assessment in Alzheimer's disease: ADL in relation to PET, MRI and neuropsychology. *Journal of Gerontological Nursing, 21*(9), 7–13.

Tapp, J.T. (1989). Introduction. In R. Davis: *My journey into Alzheimer's disease.* Wheaton, IL: Tyndale House.

Welsh, K.A., Bulters, N., Mohs, R.C., Beehly, B.S., Edland, S., Fillenbaum, G., & Heyman, A. (1996). The Consortium to Establish a Registry for Alzheimer's Disease (CERAD). V: A normative study of the neuropsychological battery. *Neurology, 44*, 609–614.

Whitehouse, P.J., Lerner, A., & Hedera, P. (1993). Dementia. In K.M. Heilman & E. Valenstein (Eds.), *Clinical neuropsychology.* New York: Oxford University Press.

II

Providing Care in Alzheimer's Disease

Chapter 4

A Framework for Intervention

Be my friend, for I need one, but do not become my manager. And remember me, as my life and identity erode, as a person, not a case.

J. Ossofsky (1993)

The treatment of people with Alzheimer's disease and related dementias once was primarily a trial-and-error affair focused on controlling "problem" behaviors rather than on helping the individual. Often, it seemed as though concern was directed solely toward the family, with little regard for the distress felt by the individual with the disease. Restraints, drugs, and placement in a long-term care facility for the person with Alzheimer's disease were seemingly the only solutions offered to these distraught families, who did not know where to turn for help for themselves or for their family member with dementia.

Because the disease cannot be cured, any untoward response, physical or emotional, was blamed on the disease itself, not on the kind of treatment provided. Care was considered adequate if the person was kept clean and well fed and was protected from harm. It did not matter where the person was, what the person did, or whether anyone visited because he or she was not aware of what was happening. When care went beyond these limited attempts to help, it tended to be condescending, controlling, and overprotecting.

Most people did not know the difference between the benign memory declines of old age and the vicious degeneration of Alzheimer's disease. Even professionals called the person with Alzheimer's disease "senile" and believed that dementia was the inevitable consequence of growing older. That the care provided was spectacularly unsuccessful, even inhumane (although unintentionally so), should be no surprise.

Alzheimer's disease is now recognized as a disease associated with, but not an inevitable part of, aging. New drugs are rapidly being developed and tested. Nonpharmacological interventions are increasingly successful. The "problem" behaviors associated with the disease are recognized as understandable emotional responses to a frightening loss of mental abilities. Care that simply maintains life is no longer thought adequate; enhancing function and improving quality of life are the new goals. Cautious optimism has replaced profound pessimism.

USEFULNESS OF A FRAMEWORK FOR INTERVENTION

It would be interesting to ask caregivers why they are doing what they are doing for people with Alzheimer's disease. How many could give a reason for what they are doing?

In some instances the answers would be quite revealing about the limited understanding of the disease and its effects on people.

> At the CRS Alzheimer's Day Care Center, clients were not allowed to help each other. When asked why, the administrator hesitated a moment and then said, "Because they are paying us to do these things."

This administrator provided a business-oriented response rather than a therapeutically oriented one. The response was nontherapeutic because people with Alzheimer's disease have limited opportunities to "shine." Helping another person open a milk carton or move a chair is an opportunity not only to shine but to do something for another person, to be in the adult role of help provider for a change, rather than in the role of help receiver. It is more therapeutic to encourage the day center's clients to help each other than to ensure that they "get their money's worth" in personal service.

This kind of reasoning about what may be therapeutic or nontherapeutic is easier and more consistently successful if one uses a framework for intervention. A framework grounds the decision-making process in well-thought-out rationales and research results.

CENTRAL CONCEPTS OF INTERVENTION

The important concepts underlying intervention approaches are excess disability, enablement, and progressively lowered stress threshold.

Excess Disability

Probably the best-known framework for intervention with people with Alzheimer's disease and related dementias is the concept of *excess disability*. The concept of excess disability has been used since at least 1965, when Kahn and Goldfarb employed it to describe the sometimes striking difference between the amount of disability observed in the individual and the actual degree of underlying impairment (Brody, Kleban, Lawton, & Silverman, 1971). In other words, the person appears and acts far more disabled than is necessary given the extent of the damage done by the disease. For example, people being fed may be quite capable of feeding themselves given enough time and appetizing food in a form easy to handle and to swallow. Others may have been mute for months and yet can speak when provided treatment to reduce the excess communication disability.

Potential contributors to excess disability include a wide range of medical, interpersonal, and environmental factors. For example, overmedication may compromise mental function. Depression may contribute to a reduction in interest in participating in any activities, including the basic self-care activities of daily living (ADLs) (Peters, Reifler, & Larson, 1989). Constant correction of errors may cause a person to stop trying altogether, even to withdraw from social interaction.

A variety of behavioral and environmental interventions have been shown to reduce excess disability. Large-print signs and clear, concrete pictorials, for example, may help a nursing facility resident find the bathroom in time to prevent incontinence.

Although excess disability in relation to dementia was examined in professional journals as early as 1965, it was not widely recognized or tested until the late 1980s. Until that time, the prevailing societal attitudes toward Alzheimer's disease and other dementias simply could not encompass this important concept.

Enablement

A related concept is that of enablement. Dawson and colleagues introduced this term to emphasize a positive approach that focuses on remaining abilities rather than on losses (Dawson, Wells, & Kline, 1993). Unfortunately, and perhaps understandably, given the devastating changes that occur, the more common viewpoint has been the negative one, in which people with Alzheimer's disease and related dementias are assessed only in terms of what they cannot do. This type of assessment leads to an expectation of incompetence and often contributes to excess disability. It also tends to lead to *objectification* of the person, that is, treating the person as an object rather than as a human being. An example of objectification is to think of the person as the "demented patient in Room 409" rather than as "Emma, who was a dress designer and likes to comment on the colors people are wearing."

An enabling approach "emphasizes the person's capacity to engage as fully as possible in day-to-day living" (Dawson et al., 1993, p. 2); a nonenabling approach restricts the individual's range of activities unnecessarily and induces excess disability. Enablement is a holistic, humanistic, and optimistic framework for intervention. In contrast, a nonenabling framework is nihilistic, mechanistic, and pessimistic.

When using an enabling framework, efforts are made to *enhance* any ability that remains, even if it is unused. When ability is absent, *compensatory* interventions are appropriate (see Figure 4.1). Kitwood (1993) has been critical of the pessimism that has characterized care of the individual with Alzheimer's disease. Kitwood believes that many of the problems associated with the progression of the disease may be as much the result of inept, insensitive care as of neurological damage:

> "We"—professionals of all kinds, caregivers, family members, and the pattern of everyday life to which we are committed—are part of the problem too. Those who are dementing [*sic*] are a problem to "us"; they do not fit comfortably into .the structures to which we are accustomed. But conversely, "we" are a problem to "them," as a result of our fears, distractions, rigidities, insensitivities, and even the professional training that creates so deep a division between "us" and "them." (Kitwood, 1993, p. 543)

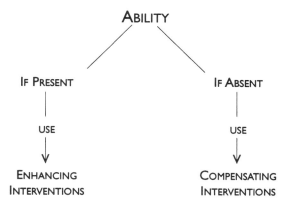

Figure 4.1. An enablement approach to treatment of people with Alzheimer's disease and related dementias. (Adapted from Dawson et al., 1993.)

Some of the ways in which this division is created include objectification, infantilization, and removal of the individual with dementia from everyday life. The idea that the progression of Alzheimer's disease represents a slow but steady death of the self, leaving only the physical body behind, is rejected by Kitwood. Instead, he believes that the personhood of the individual can be maintained, even replenished, through care that promotes the following (Kitwood & Bredin, 1992):

- Personal worth—a global feeling of self-value or self-esteem
- Agency—a sense of having some control over one's life
- Social confidence—feeling at ease in the company of other people
- Hope—a general feeling that the future will be good

Progressively Lowered Stress Threshold

Reducing or preventing the stress related to the frustrations and fears associated with Alzheimer's and related dementias is the emphasis of Hall and Buckwalter's (1987) concept of *progressively lowered stress threshold* (PLST). As the disease progresses, information becomes increasingly difficult to process and the effort becomes increasingly fatiguing. Reality orientation is an example of a potentially stress-inducing intervention; the continuous demands for correct information about the day, time, and place, and constant corrections when a mistake is made place a heavy cognitive burden on the individual who cannot answer these questions correctly. Stress builds rapidly as many demands are made all at once or a continuous stream of demands is made on the individual. Too many changes at once, too many demands, and too much resultant fatigue may precipitate a stress response.

Under conditions of minimal stress, the individual with Alzheimer's disease is calm and accessible; that is, he or she can be reached, spoken to, worked with. As stress increases, the person is likely to become anxious but is still accessible. If the stress levels become too high, however, the person may become very agitated, inaccessible, and dysfunctional. This reaction to high stress has been called a *catastrophic reaction*. The individual becomes tense and rigid, and may scream or hit him- or herself or others. The person's level of anxiety may be used as a barometer of the level of stress being experienced.

In place of the demanding types of therapy, such as reality orientation, more "reassuring" types of therapy are suggested (Hall & Buckwalter, 1987). These include validation therapy, music therapy, and relaxation exercises. In addition, consistent (rather than changing) routines, places, and people; frequent rests or "time-outs"; and a low-stimulus, low-demand environment reduce potential sources of stress. All of these techniques should be used within a psychological climate of unconditional positive regard. (More details on these various interventions can be found in Chapters 10 and 11.)

The PLST framework is sometimes interpreted to mean that a no-stimulus environment is best: low light, rest, quiet, time alone. However, most people with Alzheimer's disease and related dementias seem to enjoy undemanding, positive experiences: their favorite music, the company of other people, a walk at sunset. They do, however, seem to be stressed—sometimes very distressed—by too many demands or demands that are too difficult. Rather than argue low versus high stimulus, it seems that carefully selected stimuli adjusted to the person's level of tolerance may be the most therapeutic.

REHABILITATION PERSPECTIVE

Many important terms related to the treatment of Alzheimer's disease are used in different ways by different people. *Disability, impairment, dysfunction,* and *handicap* are a few examples of important terms with indistinct meanings. Nagi's (1991) model clearly distinguishes these terms and defines them as various dimensions of the effects of a disease such as Alzheimer's disease on an individual (see Table 4.1).

In Nagi's model the *pathology* dimension is the disease itself, which occurs at the cellular level (microlevel)—the neuron in the case of Alzheimer's disease. The disease process causes some type of trauma or degeneration of vital tissues. *Impairment* occurs at the organ or system level (macrolevel). For example, in Alzheimer's disease impairment is found in several specific areas of the brain, particularly in the temporal and parietal areas of the cortex, more specifically the hippocampus and nucleus basalis of Meynert. At the *functional* level Alzheimer's disease affects important functions of the brain, such as memory, abstraction, calculation, language, and judgment. The individual with this progressive pathology finds it increasingly difficult to perform these functions. Finally, the *disability* that results from the pathology is the effect that the disease ultimately has on the person's place in society. In the case of Alzheimer's disease the effect is a devastating loss of ability to work, drive a car, conduct one's affairs, and perform the everyday tasks of life, eventually even to care for oneself.

Some differences between Nagi's model and the definitions recommended in the World Health Organization's (WHO) International Classification of Impairments, Disabilities and Handicaps are noted (Lawrence & Jette, 1996). The WHO uses the term *disease* for the pathology level and *handicap* for any disadvantage the individual experiences as a result of the disease process. Because of the negative connotations associated with the word *handicap*, the term *disability* is used here, as it is in Nagi's model. More important, however, is the growing evidence that intervention focused on minimizing functional limitations may limit disability (Lawrence & Jette, 1996).

Rehabilitation Models

The approach to treatment that one chooses depends also on how the dysfunctions and disabilities are conceptualized. For example, the *deficit* model focuses on the losses or weaknesses that result from the disease. In contrast, a *competence* model focuses on the abilities demonstrated. The latter approach is not only more positive but also may be more useful in understanding how the individual copes with his or her disabilities and in planning a treatment program for that person (Tupper & Cicerone, 1991).

More specific direction for planning a treatment program comes from the interference, absence, and deficiency models for rehabilitation (Meier, Benton, & Diller, 1987). The *interference* model assumes that the disability is the result of some type of disturbance or breakdown that can be bypassed. For example, memory problems could be ameliorated by the use of mnemonic devices or verbal rehearsal, which circumvent the breakdowns in the storage and retrieval of information.

Table 4.1.   Nagi's model of disability using Alzheimer's disease as an example

Dimension	Level	Example
Pathology	Cellular	Neuronal damage
Impairment	Organ/system	Cortical areas of the brain, particularly temporal and parietal
Functional limitation	Person	Memory, abstraction, language, etc.
Disability	Society	Inability to perform tasks of everyday life

Adapted from Pope & Tarlov (1991).

The *absence* model assumes that the disability is the result of a deficit that cannot be repaired. Because the damage cannot be reversed, a substitute is provided. An example would be the use of a flashing light to alert a person who cannot hear the telephone. Reminder notes and maps of frequently used routes can be useful substitutes when memory and spatial orientation become a problem in the early stages of Alzheimer's disease. In later stages the lists are too often lost and the maps become too difficult to interpret to be useful.

A *deficiency* model assumes that the disability is the result, at least in part, of a lack of opportunity to practice. For example, muscles atrophy unless they are used. The treatment response is to provide guided practice. As the person's ability to perform the task improves, the amount of support is gradually reduced until independence is achieved.

Recognizing the assumptions behind a treatment as these models do is often helpful in evaluating its potential for success. As an example, if a person can no longer store complex new ideas, then no amount of practice will help retrieve these ideas. However, if storage and retrieval are compromised primarily by a short attention span and distractibility, then breaking down the idea into simpler components and reducing distractions may help the person learn it.

AN INTERVENTION FRAMEWORK

This section presents some additional fundamental ideas about the effects of the disease on the individual and a selection of strategies for treatment.

Fundamental Ideas

The person with Alzheimer's disease or a related dementia is still an adult and wishes to be treated as one.   Among many otherwise well-meaning caregivers there is a tendency to treat the individual with diminishing cognitive abilities as if he or she were retreating back into childhood. Infantilization is especially difficult to eliminate because of the increasing dependence of the person with Alzheimer's disease or related dementias and because of its apparent harmlessness. It may be difficult to recognize the pain inflicted on an adult by treating him or her like an infant or young child.

> In a recreationally oriented group for people with advanced Alzheimer's disease, the recreational therapist brought out some sponge balls to toss across the table. "Isn't this a kid's game? I'm not a child any more," said one of the group members. "Children do play this game," answered the therapist, "but adults do too. Don't grown men play baseball? And get paid for it?" The group member was satisfied with the answer and joined the game.

Although the person may eventually need help with eating and keeping clean as a young child does, this person has lived 50, 60, even 80 or 90 years and retains the memories and experience of those years. He or she is physically an adult and is emotionally more complex than an infant. Treating the person like an infant is inappropriate and demeaning.

It is said that the roles of parent and child are reversed when a parent develops dementia: The parent becomes the child and the child becomes the parent. The roles do change, but they do not reverse. The parent who once provided personal care to the child now is in need of that care from the adult child. However, emotionally and biologically the parent is still the parent and the child is still the child, although now an adult. Neither is a youngster and neither should be treated as one.

Some capacity to learn continues until the latest stages of the disease.
Completely obscured by the enormous losses experienced in Alzheimer's disease and the related dementias is the fact that some capacity to learn remains. The learning may be very limited and may require repeated practice, but it can and does occur.

> A locked Alzheimer's unit in a nursing facility had a very stable nursing staff. Most of the nurses and nursing assistants had worked there for 5 years or more. Occasionally, however, a staff member left and needed to be replaced. Invariably, the new person experienced a great deal of difficulty with the residents for the first few weeks. They rejected the new staff member's approach and refused to be cared for by him or her until they became acquainted. It was clear that they had learned who their caregivers were and that they recognized that the new person was a stranger to them and did not immediately trust this new person as they did the other staff members.

When the capacity to learn becomes limited and requires a great deal of effort to achieve, it becomes more important than ever that the information presented for learning be important, not trivial, to the individual.

People with Alzheimer's disease and related dementias continue to feel and respond to affection, joy, anger, sadness, and fear.
How long and to what extent the emotional life of a person with Alzheimer's disease and the related dementias continues is difficult to assess (Tappen & Williams-Burgess, 1997a). It is evident, however, that people with dementia do indeed experience emotions well into the later stages of the illness. In fact, their capacity for emotional response may be preserved longer than are other functions. This information is entirely contrary to earlier beliefs that they (mercifully) did not realize how bad their situation was and did not experience any distress over it, that only their families and friends felt the distress of seeing them in this condition. The following is an example of a change in emotional response of a group of people with severe dementia:

> When a new group of nursing facility residents with severe dementia was first formed, many sat in their wheelchairs with their heads down, rocking to some inner rhythm and responding little if at all to external stimuli. They did not say that they were unhappy and they did not shed tears, but they did appear sad, if not depressed. This therapeutically oriented group provided each resident who attended the opportunity to practice self-care skills such as feeding themselves, combing their hair and brushing their teeth in an environment designed to provide some success and avoid experiencing failure.
>
> As the weeks went by, fewer residents sat with their heads down during the group sessions and less rocking occurred. After 12 weeks, the residents entered the therapy room still in their wheelchairs but with heads up and smiles on their faces, even before they were greeted by the group leader. Apparently, the pleasurable anticipation of entering the group session was sufficient to improve their moods.

Awareness of the environment and of the people in it continues into the late stages.   Although eventually diminished and somewhat confused, some level of awareness of the environment and of the reactions of the people in it continues into the late stages of Alzheimer's disease. Sensitivity to people and surroundings may actually increase, according to the PLST theory. This increased sensitivity is particularly important when considering changes in routine, in living quarters, or in caregivers. What may seem a small change to the individual who is cognitively intact may overwhelm the capacity for adjustment of the person with Alzheimer's disease or a related dementia. A common example is the reaction to being moved from one residence to another or even from one unit to another within a nursing facility: function declines and anxiety increases. Recovery to previous levels of function may take several weeks.

A sense of self remains.   In a moving narrative about her own struggle with dementia Diana McGowin talks about feeling diminished by the disease, that there was "less of me every day than there was the day before" (1993, p. 33). Yet she still existed as Diana McGowin, still had a life worth living. As she wrote:

> If I am no longer a woman, why do I still feel I'm one? . . . If no longer sensitive, why do moving song lyrics strike a responsive chord in me? My every molecule seems to scream out that I do, indeed, exist, and that existence must be valued by someone! (p. 114)

Several events may occur in the later stages of Alzheimer's disease that lead family members and professional caregivers to believe that the sense of self is gone entirely. The first, and more common, event is the individual's inability to state his or her own name when asked. Certainly, this is evidence of failure to retrieve the requested word (the name), but it may well be an advanced degree of the anomia that appears early in the disease process. A second, less common event is a failure to recognize oneself in the mirror. People with Alzheimer's disease have been observed talking to the person seen in the mirror as if it were someone else, a stranger or a close relative of the same sex. This may be a perceptual problem of the same type that leads people to walk into closed sliding glass doors or to think that a mirrored room is larger than it is, or it may be a failure to recognize the way one looks.

Research and reflection on the maintenance of personal identity, or awareness of self, in Alzheimer's disease and related dementias indicates that it does continue, at least until the very late stages (Sabat & Harré, 1992; Tappen & Williams-Burgess, 1997b). In the absence of evidence that the sense of self is lost, treating the individual as if a sense of self remains is preferable to ignoring the very core of the person's being.

Maintaining Personhood Through Disease Progression   Most of these ideas are easy to accept when working with people in the earlier stages of the disease. People in the early stages of dementia are able to communicate freely and are capable of performing a wide range of everyday tasks. However, in the later stages it may require more effort to accept these ideas and to respect the person's right to be treated with dignity and to retain as much independence and control as it is possible to provide.

Strategies to Guide Treatment

Three basic strategies should be kept in mind in the treatment of people with Alzheimer's disease and related dementias. First, Alzheimer's disease and related dementias are fundamentally the result of organ failure. As for heart or liver failure, the goal of treatment is to slow, stop, or, if possible, reverse the physical degeneration that has occurred and prevent further degeneration. Little information exists to guide treatment decisions in this regard. However, new drugs are appearing rapidly and may provide the means to accomplish some or all of these goals. Until then, maintaining the physical health of the individual and avoiding any treatment that would further compromise brain function (such as overmedication) are recommended (see Chapters 8 and 12).

Second, the person with Alzheimer's disease or a related dementia was once a competent individual and wishes to be remembered for those competencies and accomplishments, as well as to be appreciated for his or her present self. To achieve this goal, some knowledge of the person's past is essential (see Chapter 5). Assessment of present capabilities also should be done so that these abilities can be enhanced and maintained for as long as possible (see Chapter 9).

Finally, the caregiver, whether a family member or paid staff member, is responsible for doing for the person with Alzheimer's disease whatever he or she can no longer do for him- or herself. This service requires considerable sensitivity to the pain that accompanies relinquishing control (over finances, driving a car, and later, one's own bathing and toileting). Keeping restrictions to a minimum and encouraging as much choice and independence as possible will contribute a great deal to maintaining some quality of life for the individual with Alzheimer's disease or a related dementia (see Chapter 9).

REFERENCES

Brody, E.M., Kleban, M.H., Lawton, M.P., & Silverman, H.A. (1971, Summer). Excess disabilities of mentally impaired aged: Impact of individualized treatment. *Gerontologist, 11*, 124–133.

Dawson, P., Wells, D.L., & Kline, K. (1993). *Enhancing the abilities of persons with Alzheimer's and related dementias.* New York: Springer Publishing.

Hall, G.R., & Buckwalter, K.C. (1987). Progressively lowered stress threshold: A conceptual model for care of adults with Alzheimer's disease. *Archives of Psychiatric Nursing, 1*, 399–406.

Kitwood, T. (1993). Persona and process in dementia. *International Journal of Geriatric Psychiatry, 8*, 541–545.

Kitwood, T., & Bredin, K. (1992). Towards a theory of dementia care: Personhood and well-being. *Ageing and Society, 12*, 269–287.

Lawrence, R.H., & Jette, A.M. (1996). Disentangling the disablement process. *Journal of Gerontology: Social Sciences, 51B*(4), S173–S182.

McGowin, D.F. (1993). *Living in the labyrinth: A personal journey through the maze of Alzheimer's.* San Francisco: Elder Books.

Meier, M., Benton, A., & Diller, L. (1987). *Neuropsychological rehabilitation.* New York: Guilford Press.

Nagi, S.Z. (1991). Disability concepts revisited: Implications for prevention. In A.M. Pope & A.R. Tarlov (Eds.), *Disability in America: Toward a national agenda for prevention.* Washington, DC: National Academy Press.

Ossofsky, J. (1993). Quoted in *Gerontologist, 33*, 3.

Peters, D.W., Reifler, B.V., & Larson, E. (1989). Excess disability in dementia. *Advances in Psychosomatic Medicine, 19*, 17–30.

Pope, A.M., & Tarlov, A.R. (Eds.). (1991). *Disability in America: Toward a national agenda for prevention.* Washington, DC: National Academy Press.

Sabat, S.R., & Harré, R. (1992). The construction and deconstruction of self in Alzheimer's disease. *Ageing and Society, 12*, 443–461.

Tappen, R.M., & Williams-Burgess, C. (1997a). *Expression of emotion in advanced Alzheimer's disease: Family and caregiver perspectives*. Manuscript submitted for publication.

Tappen, R.M., & Williams-Burgess, C. (1997b). *Not an empty shell: The lived experience of late Alzheimer's disease*. Paper presented at Dimensions of Caring and Spirituality in Health Care: Practice, Research and Theory Conference, Gainesville, Florida.

Tupper, D.E., & Cicerone, K.D. (1991). *The neuropsychology of everyday life: Issues in development and rehabilitation*. Boston: Kluwer Academic Press.

Chapter 5

Cognitive Retraining

Memory is the diary that we all carry with us.

Oscar Wilde

I can think of nothing but vanished memories, and therefore dare not think of the past any more. . . .
Memories can sometimes be temporarily inaccessible, like words, but surely they can never disappear completely during your lifetime?

J. Bernlef, quoted by Foley (1992)

The scene from the movie *On Golden Pond* is memorable: Henry Fonda portrays an older man leaving his lakeside cabin to pick berries. The berry patch is a familiar place, but suddenly, terrifyingly, he cannot find his way back. What was once a simple cognitive function (finding one's way home) had become an intellectual challenge that could no longer be met without some assistance. This is a common experience of people in the earlier stages of Alzheimer's disease.

Following an examination of information processing and a review of the cognitive dysfunctions that occur in Alzheimer's disease, several cognitive strategies that may be used to help the individual with Alzheimer's disease cope with these deficits are described in this chapter.

AN INFORMATION-PROCESSING MODEL OF COGNITION

The various types or *structures* of memory that have been theorized to exist (e.g., declarative memory, procedural memory, and their subtypes) were described in Chapter 4. Another way to think about memory is as a *process*. This process is often compared to the way a computer works: Information is put in (input), worked on in some way (processed), and the results (output) are then reported. The input, processing, and output also can be stored and retrieved for later use.

The information-processing model traces the flow of information through the system, but it does not consider the equipment (the millions of transistors on the computer chips) or the energy source (electricity) used in this processing. In the same way, the information-processing model of human cognition does not consider either the equipment (the neural networks of the brain) or the energy source (oxygen and glucose) that performs this processing. Only the processing of the information is considered. The disconnection between these various levels of thinking about cognition has presented a problem for some time, one that many scientists are working to remedy (Trehub, 1991).

The information that is processed by the human brain originates in the environment (see Table 5.1). This information can be described as a stimulus that is detected by one

Table 5.1.   An information-processing model

	In the . . .	Information is . . .
Stimulus to individual	Environment	Sent
	Sensory ports	Detected/received
	Immediate memory	Selected and attended to
	Short-term memory	Encoded
	Long-term memory	Stored and later retrieved
	Working (active) memory	Reactivated and used

Adapted from Anderson (1985).

of the senses: vision, hearing, smell, touch, or feel (Anderson, 1985). Our sensory ports (e.g., eyes, ears) continually receive huge amounts of information from the environment, far too much to process thoroughly. Because we cannot (and do not need to) pay attention to all of the information received through the senses, a selection process must occur (Trehub, 1991) through which much of the information received is filtered out and fades quickly from memory.

At this point in the processing of information, cues regarding what needs to be attended to can influence the selection process and prevent this fading.

> If a man and his young son walked past you on the street and your companion said, "Look at the boy's knees," you would probably remember later that the boy had badly skinned both knees. However, if your companion said to you after the two had walked past you, "Did you notice the little boy's knees?" and you had not noticed, you would not be able to attend to this detail and would not recall it later. Of course, you may remember that you missed this detail because your companion cued you (called your attention to it) too late.

Whether or not additional cues are provided, the person with normal (i.e., unimpaired) cognitive function then encodes the information that was selected and attended to. The immediate memory of the event will include many details, for example, how the boy was dressed or that he held his father's hand. However, these details are usually forgotten rapidly and a more general representation of what was observed remains. To cite another example, if a friend asked a question at a party, this is how a person's immediate and long-term memories of that question could differ:

> *Immediate memory of the event*: Dorothy said to me, "Mmmm . . . delicious. How do you make that wonderful chocolate walnut torte that you're so famous for?"
> *Long-term memory of the event*: Dorothy asked for my chocolate torte recipe.

The meaning of the event was retained but the specific details of what Dorothy actually said were not. Much of this process occurs automatically, without conscious effort on the part of the individual. However, a conscious effort can be made to observe and remember more than the usual number of details of a particular event.

This encoding and storage of information can be strengthened in several ways so that the information is easier to retrieve later. The more *meaningful* the information is, the more likely it is to be retained. For example, a telephone number is hard to remember unless it has some meaning. If the telephone number is the one you need to call to collect on a winning lottery ticket, you will certainly make a greater effort to remember it.

Rehearsing the number repeatedly helps to a certain extent. Reviewing it at *intervals* (every hour or so, all day long) is more effective than repeating it 20 times at once. If the numbers can be converted to a meaningful phrase, such as 1(800) WIN-$NOW, it will be much easier to remember because it has been *rephrased in a more meaningful form* (Anderson, 1985).

Imagining what you will do with the prize money and how exciting it will be to receive it also helps in retention. This is one form of what is called *elaborating* a memory, that is, connecting it to other memories so that there are several paths that can be used to retrieve it later. You might also link this information (the telephone number) to a *rhyme* (Holy cow! I'm going to WIN $NOW!) or to an *organizer* (relating it to other 1(800) numbers you know). Finally, thinking about the *context* in which you learned that you held a winning ticket and had to call this number to collect the prize improves retention: where you were at the time, who was with you, and how excited you were (Anderson, 1985). Many of these strategies for strengthening encoding and storage can be used to help people in the early stages of Alzheimer's disease remember important information such as their own telephone number or address.

Only information in an active state can be used by the individual, so information that is stored in long-term memory must be reactivated before it can be used. This is somewhat analogous to information stored in a computer that cannot be accessed unless the computer is turned on and the file in which the information is kept is located and opened. As with encoding, much of this reactivation is automatic, but it can also be done with conscious effort by the individual.

Ease of retrieval from storage seems to be affected by the number of paths or associations available that can lead to the particular piece of information needed and by the strength of these paths. For these reasons, recognition of an item is easier than recall because it provides a number of associations that can lead to the information. For example, it is usually easier to recognize the name of a high school friend from an alumni list than it is to recall it without any cues. A picture of that friend would also provide cues, especially if he or she was pictured with other people who could serve as cues to the person's identity. If the person was not a close friend, however, the association may be too weak and the search for the name could fail. *Interference* can also occur: If this person looks like a close friend or has a name similar to that of a close friend, the name of that close friend could interfere with the search for the other person's name (Anderson, 1985).

There is some evidence that "forgotten" memories may still exist, even if they are not easily retrieved. Anderson (1985) reports an experiment by Nelson that supports this idea. The research subjects were given a list of 20 number–noun pairs to learn. They practiced until they could recall every noun response to the number stimulus. Two weeks later, they recalled only 75% of the list. Some of the pairs they missed were then changed and the subjects were asked to relearn them. After studying the new list, they recalled 78% of the unchanged pairs but only 43% of the changed pairs. Anderson suggests that these results indicate that apparently forgotten memories are still there, at least in healthy individuals.

INFORMATION PROCESSING IN ALZHEIMER'S DISEASE

How does Alzheimer's disease affect the processing of information by the human brain? The evidence is incomplete and sometimes contradictory but it can still provide some direction for intervention.

Memory problems are usually the first indication of Alzheimer's disease. Finding the right word is an early and vexing problem. This problem could be caused by difficulty in gaining access to the information, to disrupted organization of the information in long-term memory, or to actual loss of this information. Evidence indicates that the stored information is not destroyed but that its retrieval becomes increasingly difficult. It also appears that, in the early stages of Alzheimer's disease, more information is available to the person than was previously thought possible. For example, although individuals with Alzheimer's disease consistently perform poorly in comparison to un-impaired controls when asked to name objects, they demonstrate greater preservation of access to information when asked to recognize an item by its functional use. McGlinchey-Berroth and Milberg (1993) note that if the information about the object was really lost, people with Alzheimer's disease should experience the same amount of difficulty with both tasks.

Another interesting aspect of cognition is *metamemory*, or the person's assessment of the strengths and weaknesses of his or her own memory. Confidence in the ability to provide a correct answer and ability to predict whether the correct answer would be recognized (*feeling-of-knowing*), both aspects of metamemory, were tested on a group of individuals in the middle stages of Alzheimer's disease (Pappas et al., 1992). Participants in the study were asked to indicate how confident they were of their answers to general information questions and an episodic memory (defined in Chapter 1) test and whether they would recognize the correct answer if it was shown to them. Although the individuals with Alzheimer's disease had much more difficulty answering the questions than did the controls, their confidence ratings were as accurate as those of the control. However, they were not as accurate in predicting their feeling-of-knowing (i.e., ability to recognize the correct answer).

Searching for information is a great deal slower in people with Alzheimer's disease than it is in other individuals, and successful retrieval of given words is quite impaired. The more complex a cognitive operation, the greater the slowing evidenced. Completion of simple tasks may not be affected at all in the earlier stages of the disease, although complex tasks become difficult (Parasuraman & Nestor, 1993).

Attention is also affected by Alzheimer's disease, again more during complex tasks than during simple ones. Selection processes appear to be adequate, at least early in the disease. The automatic processes are fairly well preserved but the effortful ones are im-paired. A single, simple task on which the person can focus undivided attention is not problematic until late in the disease. However, shifting focus from one task to another or trying to attend to two events at once is very difficult for the person with Alzheimer's disease (Parasuraman & Nestor, 1993).

> Margaret enjoyed walking through the gardens of a local park every Sunday with her daughter. They would often talk as they strolled. However, her daughter noticed that whenever she called her mother's attention to a particularly beau-tiful flower or interesting bird ahead of them, her mother would stop to look at it rather than continuing to walk toward it. It seemed as if she could not attend to an interesting object and proceed with the walk at the same time. Her daughter found that she had to cue her mother to begin walking again ("Let's keep walking").

Some experts in the neuropsychology of Alzheimer's disease believe that the central executive system that coordinates the use of the brain's resources for carrying out various mental tasks is affected by the disease (LaRue, 1992). This central executive system is thought to control the various processes of working (active) memory (Parasuraman & Nestor, 1993). If it is disrupted, shifting attention (i.e., the cognitive resources) from one event to another would be difficult, as would allocating cognitive resources to two tasks at a time. The disruption also could affect disengaging attention once it has been directed to some task or event.

The disruptions in information processing are not universal; there are still some processes the individual can do without difficulty. For example, the person with Alzheimer's disease can learn a simple task and can improve with practice, especially if the task is primarily automatic rather than effortful.

Declarative learning is far more impaired than is procedural learning (see Chapter 1 for definition). For example, practice in sanding furniture would lead to more improvement than would practice in repeating the items on a grocery list. Caregivers may also find that it is easier to engage the person's attention than to disengage it (Parasuraman & Nestor, 1993).

> Theresa found that it was fairly easy to get her husband Edward to comb his own hair. Usually, she just handed him the comb after he dressed and said, "Now, comb your hair." Often, though, if she did not tell him when to stop, he would just keep combing his hair.

Finally, using cues during learning and recall does seem to be of some help but does not overcome the deficits of the person with Alzheimer's disease in remembering and recalling information (LaRue, 1992). A number of other factors have been identified that may further impair or interfere with the memory process at any age. These factors include fatigue, anxiety, depression, illness, some medications, vision and hearing impairments, alcohol, and inadequate nutrition (Fogler & Stern, 1994). The impact on the individual with Alzheimer's disease may be greater than it is on the person who is cognitively intact.

In summary, single, simple, automatic tasks are easier than multiple, complex, effortful ones. Effortful operations in particular are performed more slowly and are more likely to be performed incorrectly. Shifting attention from one task to another is difficult. Learning is still possible, but procedural memory-based tasks are easier than declarative-based tasks. Much information can be retrieved, especially in the earlier stages of the disease, but with greater difficulty and much more effort and time than in individuals who are cognitively intact.

GENERAL PRINCIPLES IN APPLICATION OF COGNITIVE RETRAINING TECHNIQUES

The results of a number of research studies indicate that cognitive remediation targeted to remaining abilities may be helpful to the individual with Alzheimer's disease, at least over the short term. For example, the effectiveness of a 12-week comprehensive cognitive stimulation program given by family caregivers was evaluated (Quayhagen, Quayhagen, Corbeil, Roth, & Rodgers, 1995). The intervention involved memory techniques (both verbal and visual recall and recognition), problem-solving exercises (planning, conceptualization, and classification skills), and conversation exercises. Specific activities included math problems, card playing, reminiscence, and picture recognition. Quayhagen and colleagues found improvement in overall cognitive function (using the Mattis Dementia

Rating Scale), conversational fluency, and recall of nonverbal material (using the Visual Reproduction Test). Logs kept by the caregivers indicated that there was some transfer to daily life.

The following are some general principles, based primarily on the work of Arkin (1993) and Backman (1992), that may be used as guides to the selection and use of cognitive retraining strategies.

1. *Acknowledge the cognitive deficit*   Although raising the subject of a person's memory problems would not be acceptable in a social situation, many people with Alzheimer's disease respond with relief to an open discussion with a health care professional in a nonthreatening environment. Most appreciate the opportunity to obtain some assistance and will work diligently to maintain their level of independence. In fact, pretending that there is no problem when one exists may be a disservice to the individual who is frightened by these changes.
2. *Base intervention on relatively well-preserved skills*   The purpose of these interventions is to maintain as high a level of function as possible, not to return the person to normal function. Improvement in ability to maintain independence and in the person's quality of life are the primary goals. The choice of memory tasks to work on should be realistic. Highly complex, effortful tasks that require rapid responses may simply not be realistic choices for people with Alzheimer's disease.
3. *Enhance the encoding and retrieval processes of memory*   All of the cognitive strategies described later are based on attempts to either improve the encoding and retention of new information or aid retrieval of previously stored material.
4. *Select relevant tasks*   The object and content of the training should be both practical and personally relevant to the person with Alzheimer's disease. It is important not to burden the compromised brain and assault the reduced self-esteem of the individual by presenting difficult, meaningless tasks, such as practicing lists of words or memorizing strings of numbers. These tasks are as relevant and meaningful as reading the telephone book (Arkin, 1991). Some evidence from work with individuals with brain injury shows that targeted, process-specific remediation can improve attention (Sohlberg & Matier, 1987).
5. *Involve family caregivers in training when appropriate*   Many family caregivers are patient administrators of cognitive retraining after they have been taught how to do it. However, some people with Alzheimer's disease are less cooperative with a spouse or adult child than they are with an outsider. Moreover, some family caregivers have neither the energy nor the patience to provide regular training. Some judgment is thus needed in determining whether it is appropriate for a given family to provide retraining.

COGNITIVE RETRAINING STRATEGIES

The approaches to maximizing use of remaining cognitive capacities can be divided into two categories: use of external memory aids and enhancers of internal cognitive operations. Many of the external aids to memory are familiar. Lists, maps, reminders, and notes are used by everyone. Some of the internal operations enhancers are also familiar; mnemonics, rhymes, and imagery are examples. Other techniques, such as spaced retrieval and memory wallets, were designed especially for people with memory loss. In general, the internal approaches require a motivated individual, guidance of a well-prepared trainer, and considerable remaining cognitive capacity to succeed. None of these interventions can restore lost function. They can, however, help the individual better utilize remaining function.

External Memory Aids

The proverbial string around the little finger is a classic example of an external memory aid. It is not a very helpful one, however, because the string usually has no relationship to whatever it is the person is trying to remember. Such a device would probably be more frustrating than helpful for a person with Alzheimer's disease.

Reminders   More helpful reminders are those that have some relationship to what the person needs to remember. *Object cues*, for example, are directly related to what needs to be remembered. Placing boots by the front door is a reminder that because it is snowy outside some shoe protection is needed. Setting a kitchen timer when heating soup or boiling an egg reminds the person to turn off the stove before something is burned. Probably the most popular object cues used by older people are reminders to take medications. A small cup filled with the morning's medications placed on the breakfast table is helpful even for people without cognitive impairment.

Written reminders are also helpful memory supports. A note on the refrigerator door to "Have some orange juice" or "Eat some fruit" helps the person remember to eat a balanced diet. "Lock the door when you leave" or "Did you turn off the stove?" are helpful reminders that can be posted inside the front door.

Important telephone numbers can be taped next to the telephone so it is not necessary either to remember the number or to remember where the numbers are written down. Grocery lists circumvent the need to remember eight or nine separate items. It is also easier to follow written directions than it is to remember a verbal list of detailed instructions (Tappen, 1992).

Written reminders must be simply worded and prominently displayed. None of these reminders will work if the person does not notice them or cannot interpret them correctly.

Maps are a unique type of written reminder that may help the person in the early stages of Alzheimer's disease. A clear hand-drawn map of the route to the post office or a neighbor's house may help maintain independence. The map can also serve as a reminder of the person's destination if he or she becomes lost and needs to ask for help.

Telephone reminders may help the person with Alzheimer's disease remain independent longer or remain at home alone for several hours during the day. For example, a family member can call home and remind the person to eat lunch or to take a noontime medication. Reminders about appointments or other important tasks each day are also helpful. At the same time, the telephone calls provide a safety check for the person who is otherwise still capable of living independently.

Most of these reminders are useful primarily in the earlier stages of the disease. At some point, however, they will no longer be helpful.

> I sent my husband to the store with a list of what we needed. He took the condominium van so I didn't have to worry about him getting lost. He came back with five 10-pound bags of oranges and nothing else. He didn't even wait for his change.

Memory Wallets   Memory wallets were designed specifically for people with cognitive impairment. They may be more useful in later stages of the disease than the other types of reminders.

To prepare a memory wallet, family members assemble a list of facts about the person that are divided into several categories such as "My Life," "My Family," or "My Day" (Bourgeois, 1990). Biographical facts, such as the person's former occupation, number of children, or present address, are listed under each of the categories. To assist relearning, photographs of the person, family members, important events, and present living quarters are also collected and placed alongside the biographical statements. If possible, they are placed on small (3" × 4") pages that can be slipped into plastic covers or laminated and placed in a wallet.

The person for whom the wallet was designed can carry it and use it to self-prompt during conversations (Bourgeois, 1992). It can also be used to review current vital facts and reminisce. It is also used in training sessions (see "Memory Training" in the section "Methods to Enhance Internal Cognitive Operations").

In a small study of individuals with mild to moderate levels of dementia, Bourgeois (1992) found that use of memory wallets with and without daily training sessions helped these individuals to improve and maintain their conversational skills. Clearly, participants valued the wallets, and many used them to initiate conversations.

A larger scrapbook format also can be used to document important events in the person's life. The scrapbook may be used to stimulate conversation, and is particularly useful in long-term care settings, where staff do not know the person's history. The scrapbook, or *memory album*, emphasizes each resident's individuality in settings where it is often threatened by assembly-line approaches to providing care to large numbers of people with dementia, a situation that does not occur in the person's home. The visitor to a facility at which these memory albums are used may hear a staff member say, "Did you know Harold used to be a hat maker?" or "Harold, tell us about making hats. Was it hard work?" In this case the memory album serves as an external memory aid to staff, who can then provide cues to the resident.

Environmental Organizers   The environment or objects in the environment that specifically aid memory can be organized (the topic of environmental design is discussed fully in Chapter 11). Creating a *"memory place"* for things that are constantly being lost is one technique (West, 1985). The small table by the front door or a certain spot on the kitchen counter or the dresser in the bedroom may serve as the memory place for glasses, keys, watch, and other important items. Organizing the environment so that all essential papers are in one place, medications are easy to find, and glasses can be found (one person bought a dozen pairs of reading glasses and placed them in strategic spots all over the house, car, and office to cope with forgetting where they were) makes locating objects much easier. This works, however, only if the person remembers where the memory place is.

Maintaining routines is another way to organize the environment to support compromised cognitive function (Beck, Heacock, Rapp, & Mercer, 1993). The morning routine of rising, washing, dressing, and eating breakfast is a good example. Performing routines in the same order every day prevents the omission of important tasks, such as changing one's underclothes, well into the disease. Without routine, family caregivers are sometimes appalled to discover that the person with dementia has not brushed the teeth or washed the feet for weeks (occasionally months) before it was noticed.

Changes in routines may present challenges that the compromised brain cannot handle. A person who was capable of dressing him- or herself or getting the mail in familiar surroundings may suddenly appear incompetent to perform these tasks in a different setting.

We took a long drive to visit my sister in Milwaukee. It was late when we got there, so we just showed Mom her room, got her to bed, and went to bed ourselves. In the middle of the night, I heard her saying to herself, "How do I get out of here?" She was pacing the floor. She didn't know where she was.

Later, my sister woke me and said, "She's wrecking my room, pulling clothes out of the closet, knocking things over." Once she saw me, Mom was okay. She didn't remember any of this the next morning.

We were doing fine here in West Orange, but he [my husband] wanted to move out to Hillsdale. That was a mistake. All of a sudden, he couldn't find his way around. He would go knocking on every door, trying to find our apartment. He was frantic and the neighbors were upset. I couldn't let him go out alone anymore after we moved.

These changes in function occurred because the demand on limited cognitive resources increased in the unfamiliar setting. These people no longer knew where things were and their ability to reorient to the new surroundings was limited. Suddenly, tasks that had been automatic became effortful and the person could no longer do them.

Eliminating distracting stimuli is another way to reorganize the environment. Ensuring that only one jacket, one watch, and one pair of glasses is in view eliminates choices and makes it easier to prepare to go out. The number of decisions required of the person is reduced to a manageable level. Removing cleaning supplies from the bathroom cabinets eliminates the possibility of making a dangerous choice (e.g., choosing toilet bowl cleaner instead of shampoo, choosing cleanser instead of foot powder). Multiple stimuli compete for attention. Turning off the television during meals may help the person concentrate on eating, which is often a problem later in the disease process.

Undertaking only one task at a time (e.g., not trying to prepare a salad while grilling hamburgers) is a particularly important way to eliminate distractions. Another is giving instructions only one step at a time. For example, instead of saying, "George, get dressed and have breakfast quickly because we have to go to the doctor's this morning," the caregiver should remind George to get dressed, then remind him to eat breakfast, and then, when the meal is done, tell him it is time to go to the doctor's office.

Methods that Enhance Internal Cognitive Operations

Memory training is not new in the treatment of Alzheimer's disease. One of the earliest organized methods designed to improve memory in people with Alzheimer's disease was reality orientation (Department of Veterans Affairs, 1989; Folsom, 1985).

Reality Orientation   Designed by a nurse and a psychologist in the 1960s, reality orientation was intended to be a 24-hour approach to improving the person's memory for certain facts. It has been used primarily in institutional settings. The comprehensive approach includes individual, group, and environmental elements. In each of these elements emphasis is placed on remembering names, faces, places, time, day, date, and important events, such as holidays.

Group therapy sessions are the core activity of reality orientation. Participants are brought together every day for 20-minute sessions. During these sessions, they are asked to repeat one another's and staff members' names; recite the day, date, and time; and recall similar information, such as the name of the institution or the next holiday. They are praised for their success and corrected and asked to try again if they fail to produce the right answer.

Individual reinforcement of the facts learned during the group session is provided throughout the day. Although this reinforcement is intended to be helpful, the effect on the individual may not be what was intended.

> A visitor walking down the hall of Forest View Nursing Home was stopped by a resident who, on seeing the visitor go by, rushed to her door to ask a question. "Quick, mister, tell me what day it is."
> "It's Wednesday," answered the visitor.
> "Thanks. They'll be here asking me that any minute now."

Environmental reality orientation continues to be popular. Easily read signs, calendars, and clocks should be visible so that the person with dementia can self-prompt as to the day, date, and time, and can find his or her way around the facility. These sources of information are usually more available at home than they are in an institution.

An additional source of orienting information is the reality orientation board. A typical board may read, "Today is Wednesday. The weather is sunny." Additional information may include the day's menu, scheduled events, and the next holiday. It is important to maintain the currency and accuracy of the information. It is also important to avoid childish drawings (e.g., snowmen, pumpkins), phrases, or lettering that make the board look as though it belongs in a nursery school. The board can announce basic information in large letters and still appear to be an announcement board for adults.

Memory Training   As indicated earlier, there are limitations to the effectiveness of simply repeating the same information, particularly with people with Alzheimer's disease. A number of variations of the basic practice or *rehearsal* of information the person wishes to remember are available. Each of the variations described here attempts to improve on simple repetition, which is the basic approach of reality orientation groups.

Memory Enhancement General Training   Sandman's (1989) Memory Enhancement and General Awareness (MEGA) training program involves four 2-hour sessions a week for people with Alzheimer's disease and their significant others. The groups work on learning and remembering basic facts about other group members and the leader, recalling the details of a selected television program, planning an outing and carrying it out, and remembering segments of classic films. The approach involves drills in class, home study, and quizzes on the material assigned. Participants work hard. Some are able to recall almost as much as their cognitively intact partners but with great effort (Arkin, 1991). The tasks themselves are not especially relevant to everyday life, but participants may be encouraged to apply the same effort to information of greater importance to them.

Memory Wallet   Practice was also employed by Bourgeois (1992) to help people with Alzheimer's disease use their memory wallets. One of the 3 topics (e.g., "My Life") and 10 related statements are chosen by the person with Alzheimer's disease or the trainer. The person then reads each statement (e.g., "My husband, Raul, was born in Cuba") and elaborates on the statement by adding information (e.g., "His whole family came here from Cuba when he was a young man"). The trainer provides encouragement and praise for correct statements.

If the person cannot complete either of these tasks independently, the trainer provides a prompt such as, "Turn the page," "Read the next sentence," or "What else can you tell me?" If the person still cannot answer, the trainer provides some cues, either reading the first word or elaborating anew. The routine continues until all 10 statements have been read and elaborated upon by either the person or the trainer (Bourgeois, 1992).

This training should be conducted in a quiet, comfortable location. Short (15-minute) sessions help to keep frustration under control and prevent the person from becoming overly fatigued. (It is hard for people who are cognitively intact to imagine how fatiguing this work can be for someone with Alzheimer's disease.) The trainer also needs to be sensitive to the person's level of frustration to avoid over-stressing the person.

"Q and A" with Memory Tapes   After observing Sandman's approach, Arkin (1991) suggested some modifications. She noted that some people with Alzheimer's disease for whom the MEGA approach had not been helpful were more successful with a question-and-answer ("Q and A") format based on memory tapes.

Either audiotapes or videotapes can be used. These tapes are prepared for each individual; they contain brief narratives on personally relevant subjects, such as biographical information, important people, and major events (e.g., births, weddings). Questions follow the narratives on the tapes, with a pause for the person to supply the answer, followed by the correct answer on the tape (Arkin, 1991). This format is similar to that used on language-learning tapes created for people who plan to travel or live overseas. Providing the answers on the tape helps to keep frustration at a tolerable level. The emphasis is on information of personal significance to the individual with Alzheimer's disease, so that viewing or listening to the tapes is a pleasant and meaningful experience and the subject matter has a high level of emotional significance for the individual according to Arkin.

Most people with Alzheimer's disease need some encouragement to continue working with these tapes. This coaching can be done by family or friends after they have become familiar with the techniques. The sessions should be short, to limit fatigue and frustration, and frequent, to minimize forgetting.

Spaced Retrieval   Camp (1989) adapted the spaced retrieval method used with patients with brain injury for use with individuals with Alzheimer's disease. The information to be learned is presented and retrieved through questioning, as with the previous strategies. However, the interval between presentation and questioning is increased (from 5 seconds to 10, 20, 40, and 60 seconds and then by 30-second intervals) as the person becomes more successful in retaining the information (McKitrick, Camp, & Black, 1992). If the person cannot retrieve the information after an increase in the interval, the interval is reduced back to the level at which the person had been successful.

Enhancing the Encoding Process   A few additional strategies place less emphasis on rehearsal and more emphasis on enhancing the encoding process. Most of these strategies require conscious effort to use and are therefore of use only in the earliest stages of the disease.

Visual Imagery   Visual imagery uses interesting, humorous, and even absurd mental pictures to make something easier to remember. For example, the person with early-stage Alzheimer's disease could remember his or her dentist's name, Dr. Hertz, by imagining the dentist with an enormous pair of pliers aimed at someone's open mouth. The humor in imagining a dentist with a name that sounds like "hurts" makes it easier to remember.

Verbal Elaborations   Verbal elaborations are the word-based equivalents of visual imagery. Rhymes; mnemonics; stories; associations with familiar people, places, or events; and a high emotional content all lead to more effective encoding and subsequent retrieval. The following are examples of each of these:

> *Rhymes*—If the person needs to remember to take the Number 10 bus back home, a rhyme such as "Ten, ten, the big fat hen," can be repeated several times before leaving home and at intervals before going to the bus stop.
>
> *Mnemonics*—Mnemonics can be used to organize a more complex set of information into a retrievable "chunk." Grandchildren's names, for example, can be organized into mnemonics (e.g., GROWL for Geri, Rita, Ollie, Will, and Luke; KIDS for Katie, Iris, Dean, and Sue). Caregivers can suggest rhymes and mnemonics if the person can no longer create them. Studies of the use of various mnemonics techniques by cognitively intact older adults have generally produced positive effects, at least over the short term (up to 6 months) (Neely & Backman, 1993).
>
> *Stories*—Stories should not be too long or too complex. For example, to remember a new neighbor's name, the caregiver can say, "Your new neighbor's name is Kate. Remember, she's the one who thought she lost her cat but found it hiding in the closet."
>
> *Familiar places, people, or events*—Familiar information can be used in the same way as simple stories. For example, the new neighbor can be remembered in a different way: "You remember that Kate comes from Chicago, like you do."
>
> *Information with high emotional content*—Like personally relevant information, information with a high emotional content is easier to remember and on which to elaborate. For example, the loss of a beloved pet is an event more easily recalled than an ordinary trip to the bank. The excitement of a Super Bowl game is also more memorable than an ordinary television quiz show.

Caregivers can use each of these elaborations as cues to help the person with Alzheimer's disease remember and later retrieve needed information.

Peg Systems   Peg systems are even more complex and should be reserved for vital information for people in the very earliest stages of the disease. The numbers 1–10 can be used as a set of mental "pegs" on which to hang important words or images related to those words. Often, rhyming words are used. For example, if a person with Alzheimer's disease needs to remember a routine for entering the condominium pool every afternoon, the following could be used:

> ONE . . . SUN—Put on sunscreen.
> TWO . . . SHOE—Take off shoes and shirt.
> THREE . . . SEE—Is the lifeguard there?
> FOUR . . . MORE—Are people in the way?
> FIVE . . . DIVE—OK to dive in.

The advantage of peg systems is that they provide a way to organize fairly complex information. The disadvantage is that they require learning a considerable amount of information; thus they are useful only in the earliest stages of the disease even if the caregiver creates the mental "pegs" for the person.

REFERENCES

Anderson, J.R. (1985). *Cognitive psychology and its implications.* New York: W.H. Freeman.

Arkin, S.M. (1991). Memory training in early Alzheimer's disease: An optimistic look at the field. *American Journal of Alzheimer's Care and Related Disorders and Research, 6*(4), 17–25.

Arkin, S.M. (1993). *Memory training in early Alzheimer's.* Poster presented at the American Psychological Association Conference, Washington, DC.

Backman, L. (1992). Memory training and memory improvement in Alzheimer's disease: Rules and exceptions. *Acta Neurologica Scandinavica Supplementum, 139,* 84–89.

Beck, C., Heacock, P., Rapp, C.G., & Mercer, S.O. (1993). Assisting cognitively impaired elders with activities of daily living. *American Journal of Alzheimer's Care and Related Disorders and Research, 8*(6), 11–20.

Bourgeois, M.S. (1990). Enhancing conversation skills in patients with Alzheimer's disease using a prosthetic memory aid. *Journal of Applied Behavior Analysis, 23*(1), 29–42.

Bourgeois, M.S. (1992). Evaluating memory wallets in conversations with persons with dementia. *Journal of Speech and Hearing Research, 35*(12), 1344–1357.

Camp, C. (1989). Facilitation of new learning in Alzheimer's disease. In G.C. Gilmore, P.J. Whitehouse, & M.L. Wykle (Eds.), *Memory, aging and dementia: Theory, assessment and treatment* (pp. 212–225). New York: Springer Publishing.

Department of Veterans Affairs. (1989). *Dementia: Guidelines for diagnosis and treatment.* Washington, DC: Veterans Health Services Research Administration.

Fogler, J., & Stern, L. (1994). *Improving your memory: How to remember what you're starting to forget.* Baltimore: The Johns Hopkins University Press.

Foley, J.M. (1992). The experience of being demented. In R.H. Binstock, S.G. Post, & P.J. Whitehouse (Eds.), *Dementia and aging: Ethics, values and policy choices.* Baltimore: The Johns Hopkins University Press.

Folsom, G.S. (1985). Reality orientation: Full circle. *Bulletin of the New York Academy of Medicine, 61,* 343–350.

LaRue, A. (1992). *Aging and neuropsychological assessment.* New York: Plenum.

McGlinchey-Berroth, R., & Milberg, W.P. (1993). Preserved semantic memory structure in Alzheimer's disease. In J. Cerella, J. Rybash, W. Hoyer, & M.L. Commons (Eds.), *Adult information processing: Limits on loss.* San Diego: Academic Press.

McKitrick, L.A., Camp, C.J., & Black, F.W. (1992). Prospective memory intervention in Alzheimer's disease. *Journal of Gerontology: Psychological Sciences, 47*(5), 337–343.

Neely, A.S., & Backman, L. (1993). Long-term maintenance of gains from memory training in older adults: Two $3\frac{1}{2}$ year follow-up studies. *Journal of Gerontology: Psychological Sciences, 48*(5), 233–237.

Pappas, B.A., Sunderland, T., Weingartner, A.M., Vitiello, B., Martinson, H., & Putnam, K. (1992). Alzheimer's disease and feeling-of-knowing for knowledge and episodic memory. *Journal of Gerontology: Psychological Sciences, 47*(3), 159–164.

Parasuraman, R., & Nestor, P.G. (1993). Preserved cognitive operations in early Alzheimer's disease. In J. Cerella, J. Rybash, W. Hoyer, & M.L. Commons (Eds.), *Adult information processing: Limits on loss* (pp. 77–111). San Diego: Academic Press.

Quayhagen, M.P., Quayhagen, M., Corbeil, R.R., Roth, P.A., & Rodgers, J.A. (1995). A dyadic remediation program for care recipients with dementia. *Nursing Research, 44*(3), 153–159.

Sandman, C.A. (1989). *Memory training in Alzheimer's patients: Evidence for behavioral plasticity.* Paper presented at a meeting of the American Society on Aging, San Diego.

Sohlberg, M.M., & Matier, C.A. (1987). Effectiveness of an attention-training program. *Journal of Clinical and Experimental Neuropsychology, 9*(2), 117–130.

Tappen, R.M. (1992). An introduction to non-pharmacologic treatment strategies for Alzheimer's disease. *Aging and Neuroscience, 1*(1), 9–17.

Trehub, A. (1991). *The cognitive brain.* Cambridge, MA: MIT Press.

West, R. (1985). *Memory fitness over 40.* Gainesville, FL: Triad Publishing Co.

Wilde, O. (1996, August 12). Quoted in "Thoughts on the business of life." *Forbes.*

Chapter 6

Psychodynamics of Alzheimer's Disease

What gives her world inner cohesion is emotion.

D.D. Gray (1993)

I shatter psychologically in any pressure situation.

R. Davis (1989)

Although the cognitive effects of Alzheimer's disease have drawn the most attention, the emotional effects are at least their equal in causing distress for both people with Alzheimer's disease and their caregivers. Not only do emotional disturbances increase the sense of burden for caregivers but they are a principal reason for placement in a long-term care facility (Bolger, Carpenter, & Strauss, 1994).

This chapter examines the subjective experience of Alzheimer's disease, from the earliest stages, when people may be quite articulate in communicating their feelings, to the latest stages, when most people with Alzheimer's disease have limited means of communication left to them. The most common psychiatric problems associated with Alzheimer's disease—depression, anxiety, delusions, and hallucinations—and activity disturbances are then considered. Psychotherapeutic strategies, from effective communication to validation therapy, are examined in Chapter 7.

SUBJECTIVE EXPERIENCE OF ALZHEIMER'S DISEASE

How does it *feel* to have Alzheimer's disease? What is it like to have trouble remembering things, knowing one's memory will get worse, and that eventually one will not even be able to take care of oneself? The answers to these questions are important to both formal and informal caregivers of people with Alzheimer's disease. The better we understand the subjective experience of Alzheimer's disease, the more effective we can be in helping people cope with it (Cohen, 1991).

Initial Reaction

The emotional response to developing Alzheimer's disease has been compared to the grieving process. As individuals first realize that they have Alzheimer's disease and then begin to grieve their losses, they may move through the following stages (Cohen, 1991):

- Recognition and concern—"What is wrong with me?"
- Denial—"No, not me. It can't be Alzheimer's disease."
- Anger, guilt, sadness—"Why did it happen to me?"

- Adaptation—"I'll live each day until I die."
- Separation from self

(Disagreement has arisen about when separation from self occurs. Some researchers believe that it occurs gradually, as cognitive abilities decline; others believe that it occurs at the end of life.)

Finding out that one has Alzheimer's disease is a very stressful event. In their book *The Loss of Self*, Cohen and Eisdorfer (1986) relate how people react to the diagnosis of Alzheimer's disease: shock, anger, disbelief, fear, despair, hopelessness, desperation. Some angrily deny that they have developed the disease. Others are so frightened by the prospect that they are unable to talk about it or ask questions for a while. Still others may experience some relief to know that they are not "crazy."

Whatever the response, newly diagnosed patients need opportunities to learn more about the disease, to talk about their feelings, and to plan for the future before their ability to do so is too limited. All of this should be done at their own pace. People should not be rushed or pressured to "face reality" before they are ready. It is important that they know someone is available and willing to talk with them when they are ready to do so.

False reassurance that everything will be all right is usually seen as just that. Genuine reassurance that others will continue to love and care for the person is probably the most helpful and deeply desired response.

Some health care professionals have developed the habit of speaking primarily to the family rather than to the older person, even when the older person does not have dementia. Some families encourage this habit to protect the older person or avoid upsetting him or her. Although the intent is well meant, the outcome is harmful. Excluding older people from discussions concerning their well-being is not only a violation of their right to be involved in their own medical care but it also denies them the opportunity to share their fears and to make financial, legal, and other arrangements while they can still articulate their wishes and make known their preferences for future care.

Although each older person will react to the diagnosis of Alzheimer's disease in terms of his or her own personal experience, hopes, and fears, some concerns are commonly expressed. Many people fear the loss of independence that comes when they are no longer able to drive a car, earn a living, or maintain their own checkbook. Others fear the loss of dignity and self-respect that comes when they can no longer feed or clothe themselves. For some, it is the loss of control over their lives that is frightening: Eventually unable to make decisions, they will have to depend on others to make decisions for them. Many fear that they will be abandoned by their families when the disease renders them unattractive, incoherent, and incapable of giving anything back to those who care for them.

Early Stages

The early stages of Alzheimer's disease are a time of terrible awareness. The individual notices the changes taking place, although he or she may try to hide them or deny them publicly (Cotrell & Lein, 1993). Many try to continue their usual activities. Often, they succeed for a while, even continuing to work, sometimes with help from co-workers or family. Eventually, however, they will have to relinquish work and other responsibilities or have them taken away.

Although people in the early stages may experience diminished energy, irritability, and a tendency to withdraw, judgment and social skills are maintained (Miller, Chang, Oropilla, & Mena, 1994). Some people with the disease avoid the use of the term *Alz-*

heimer's disease, preferring to call it their "memory problem" or their "forgetfulness" (Bahro, Silber, & Sunderland, 1995). The challenge in these stages is to reorganize and adapt to the life changes that come with the progression of the disease (Cotrell & Schultz, 1993).

Diana McGowin (1993) wrote a personal account of her entry into the world of Alzheimer's disease, in which she vividly describes the emotional ups and downs of the early stages. Using a term reminiscent of Cohen and Eisdorfer's "loss of self," she writes that there was "less of me every day than there was the day before" (p. 33), as she struggled to learn how to live with this disease. At times, she became so depressed and fearful of losing her mind that she retreated to her bedroom, pulling the drapes and locking the door. At other times, she valiantly struggled to go on with her life, bluffing her way through memory lapses, reading literature on Alzheimer's disease that she originally found repugnant, and relearning the meaning of such ordinary objects as traffic signs and signals. Small victories brought her some satisfaction during this stressful time.

Some of McGowin's efforts had drawbacks, however. Covering up her memory lapses to avoid embarrassment prevented her from confiding in friends or family members, creating a sense of isolation and loneliness and reducing opportunities to draw on their strength. She needed to know that these people would stand by her later, that she would not be deserted in her time of greatest need, which was still to come. She also wrote of her fear that she would lose her "last shred of dignity and control over myself" (p. 82), realizing that the rights and responsibilities she had as a responsible adult in society, such as a driver's license or the privilege of managing her own money, were becoming "tenuous and delicate" (p. 83). McGowin knew they would continue only if nothing untoward happened, and she knew also that eventually it would.

Middle Stages

At some point, the coverups and tenacious protection of adult rights and responsibilities no longer succeed. Abilities diminish to the point at which insistence on independence becomes dangerous: Perhaps an auto accident, burns from cooking, or financial disaster occurs. Eventually, every person with Alzheimer's disease must work out new ways to handle life's challenges and find new meaning in their lives, even a reason to live. Faced with these challenges, some withdraw and others lash out at whomever is nearby. Although either response is understandable, neither is healthy and intervention may be needed to help people find more satisfying ways to cope with their problems (see Chapter 7).

Feelings of insecurity are often evident even in people who do not withdraw or lash out. The following is a sample of a conversation between a newcomer to an Alzheimer's day center and a regular attendee, both in the transition from early to middle stage:

NEWCOMER: (A little worried) Do you know what time we leave?

REGULAR: I leave when my daughter picks me up.

NEWCOMER: My son is supposed to come back for me.

REGULAR: Then you'll leave when he comes.

NEWCOMER: How will he know when it's over? What if he doesn't come?

REGULAR: Maybe he won't.

NEWCOMER: What will I do?

REGULAR: You'll have to stay here.

NEWCOMER: (Now very worried) I can't do that. I hope my son knows where I am.

The newcomer's worry is palpable. Visions of being locked in a strange building overnight were clearly developing in the newcomer's mind until a staff member intervened. The newcomer had sufficient cognitive ability to recognize being in a new and unknown place but not enough to figure out how to arrange to be taken home. Without some reassurance, the newcomer might have become very worried and upset. It is also interesting that the regular attendee was able to provide some concrete information but was not able to relate to the newcomer's worries or to help solve the problem.

Many people in the middle stage of Alzheimer's disease begin to experience difficulty expressing themselves clearly and fully. Their narrations become shorter, less descriptive, even emptier, but nevertheless eloquent sometimes in communicating their feelings. A number of individuals with Alzheimer's disease use the words "crazy" or "losing my mind" to describe what they are experiencing. "What is happening to me? I must be losing my mind," or "Why am I here with all these crazy people? Am I crazy, too?" are common questions asked of caregivers.

This phase can be very difficult for both the person with Alzheimer's disease and the caregiver. Sudden shifts in mood are common. People at this stage still recognize what is happening and are likely to become upset when they are unable to handle a situation. As the disease progresses, some people begin to overreact, becoming agitated over what seems to caregivers to be a minor frustration. These overreactions are sometimes called *catastrophic reactions*.

Misperceptions are also more likely to occur in this stage than in the early stages, sometimes leading to serious problems. For example, the individual may misplace a treasured watch and then accuse a friend of having stolen it. Some have ordered spouses out of the bedroom, claiming they are strangers and threatening to call the police. Others have approached strangers and claimed that they are being held against their will, causing considerable consternation on the part of their family members.

Not everyone experiences this high degree of distress. Some seem to accept the changes with astonishing equanimity. They relinquish responsibilities easily and find renewed pleasure in closeness to loved ones. They trust fully in their caregivers and show little fear or insecurity. Some caregivers describe them as "pleasantly demented," an ironic but accurate description of their demeanor. Much probably can be learned from these apparently well-adapted individuals, who seem to have learned how to live with their lower level of cognitive ability and to be able to derive some satisfaction from what many would consider a diminished life.

A minister describing his own experience with Alzheimer's disease wrote eloquently of the limited alternatives a person faces at this juncture: "I can either struggle angrily and uselessly against the inevitable, or else I can admit my inadequacy and humbly ask for help" (Davis, 1989, pp. 56–57). The choice, he wrote, was up to him. He could either submit peacefully or continue to be frightened and frustrated by his diminished capabilities. The importance of choosing to trust in other people emerges forcefully from his writing: Either he limited himself to familiar places or he could venture beyond them in "blind trust with someone who will take care of me" (p. 5).

Late Stages

Both formal and informal caregivers indicate that many individuals with Alzheimer's disease seem less distressed in the late stages than they had been in the middle stage (Tappen & Williams-Burgess, 1997). Whether this perception exists because they have adapted to their situation, become resigned to it, or are simply less aware of their losses is not clear.

Verbal expressions of emotion in the later stages tend to be brief and often direct:

"I love you."

"I'm going to kill you."

"I wish I were dead."

Certain types of incidents seem to precipitate emotional outbursts: invasions of personal space, loss of privacy and modesty, and frustration over the inability to do or say something. Shifts in emotion continue to occur with some individuals. "Sometimes they're angry, sometimes happy or sad," residential facility staff say when asked. "It takes only a second to go from one to the other."

As the ability to communicate verbally diminishes, the reliance on nonverbal communication of emotion increases. Smiles, laughs, frowns, screaming, and calling out occur. Clenched teeth, clenched fists, and shaking hands indicate anger and frustration. Hanging their heads, keeping their eyes closed, giving up favorite activities, staying in their rooms, and sleeping all day frequently signal sadness or depression. Rubbing a forehead or other body part or moaning may indicate pain. Smiling, laughing, and reaching out to people are usually signs of pleasure and happiness; "big eyes," tension, and a frightened expression are indicators of worry or fear.

Family and facility staff use hugs, gentle words of affection and reassurance, and questions about what is wrong to respond to these nonverbal communications. They also use redirection when something upsets the person; changing the subject, giving the person a snack, taking the person for a short walk, providing a distracting task, or leaving the person until he or she is calmer are often helpful responses.

By the very late stages of the disease, people with Alzheimer's disease are rarely able to express directly what they are experiencing. Reliance on nonverbal communication increases to the point at which one must depend on the caregivers who know the people with the disease well for an interpretation of how they feel or what they want. The results of research by Lawton, Van Haitsma, and Klappa (1996) on affect in people with moderately severe Alzheimer's disease support the idea that this evidence of mood is "legible" (i.e., readable by other people).

Although it is often said that a person's personality changes with Alzheimer's disease (Bahro et al., 1995), continuity of premorbid (preillness) personality and coping styles is also observed by caregivers (Cotrell & Lein, 1993). This observation is of particular interest in the late stages: Is this individual recognizable, still the same person he or she once was, or is he or she an entirely different person now? Gray (1993) says of his mother that there were "blurred but distinguishable continuations" of who she once was (p. 8). He wondered if it was like looking in a broken mirror. Perhaps it was more like trying to find data in a computer whose files are damaged so that some of the information could no longer be accessed. One of the differences from computers is that humans also have emotions, and this, according to Gray, is the core of the person's continued humanity. Emotion mattered more to his mother than words or ideas in her final days. He believed that as his mother lost her ability to think, she turned increasingly to operating on the underlying stream of emotions that is a part of all of us.

In order to communicate with someone in the very late stage of Alzheimer's disease, Gray recommends listening to the emotion expressed. This type of communication is different from our usual mode of communication, either professional or social. People must sift through the garble, he says, to reach the core of the communication hidden within a confused flow of thought fragments. Trying to understand exactly what has been said or attempting to clarify what the person means may be very difficult. Gray likens this kind of communication with a person in the latest stages of the disease to trying to see at night: A shape can be discerned but the details are lost.

EMOTIONAL PROBLEMS ASSOCIATED WITH ALZHEIMER'S DISEASE

In this section selected mood disturbances (e.g., depression, anxiety, delusions, hallucinations) are examined first, followed by activity disturbances (e.g., sleep disturbances, pacing, aggression, changes in sexual behavior) that may occur.

Mood Disturbances

Mood disturbances are common in people with Alzheimer's disease. Where do these emotional disturbances come from? Are they a *result* of the disease or a *response* to the disease? These questions have no answers yet, but answers are on the horizon as research in this area continues.

Cohen (1991) suggests that, with the exception of psychosis, much of the negative emotional response is caused by our inability to understand and help people with Alzheimer's disease cope with losses and their reactions to these losses. Others (e.g., Flint, 1991), however, emphasize the biological mechanisms that may underlie much of the emotional disturbance observed, implying that they are a part of the disease itself rather than merely a response to the disease.

Clearly, the relationship of cognition, mood, behavior, and neuropathology is not well understood. As with many other health concerns, there are probably multiple factors involved. These factors may include genetics, premorbid personality, neuropathology of the disease, reaction to the effects of the disease, and changes in the individual's living situation (Bolger et al., 1994):

- *Genetics:* A positive family history of depression has been related to increased risk of depression.
- *Premorbid personality:* Recurrence of depression in the same individual is quite common.
- *Neuropathology of Alzheimer's disease:* Impaired function of neurotransmitter systems has been linked to emotional disturbances. Injury to various brain structures has also been linked to behavior disturbances.
- *Reaction to the effects of the disease:* The progression of losses, compared by some to a "living death," may be sufficient cause for emotional disturbances.
- *Changes in living situation:* The death or even the emotional withdrawal of the person on whom the individual depends for support or a move to a nonsupportive environment may precipitate or exacerbate emotional disturbance.

More research is needed to disentangle the interaction of these factors and evaluate their effect on the mood and behavior of people with Alzheimer's disease.

An interesting research study examined the mood and behavior changes reported by caregivers of 50 people in the mild, moderate, and severe stages of Alzheimer's disease (Mega, Cummings, Fiorello, & Gornbein, 1996). All of the participants were undergoing evaluation at a dementia clinic. Five in the mild stage and one in the moderate stage reported no psychological problems at all, but 88% of the group did. The most commonly reported problem was apathy, which was observed by the caregivers in 72% of the group. This was followed by agitation (60%), anxiety (48%), irritability (42%), dysphoria (38%), and delusions (22%). Hallucinations were observed in only 10% and euphoria in only 8% of the participants in the month preceding the interview. The problems were not related to age but there was some difference by gender: The men were more likely to be agitated than the women. Some differences by stage of the disease were also found. Agitation (e.g., crying, kicking, resistance), dysphoria, apathy, and aberrant motor behavior (e.g., rocking, picking at one's clothes) were reported more often in people in the later stages. Dysphoria increased from 10% in the mild stage to 60% in the severe stage, but major depression was infrequent. Delusions were more common in the later stages but hallucinations were more common in the earlier stages. These researchers concluded that psychological problems are not determined by the degree of cognitive impairment, that some problems are transient, and that they vary considerably from one person to another.

Depression   Although estimates of the prevalence of depression among people with Alzheimer's disease vary wildly (from 0% to 87%), there is general agreement that depression is both a common and a serious problem for people with Alzheimer's disease (Liebson & Albert, 1994; Teri & Truax, 1994). One of the reasons for the discrepancies in the estimates is the failure to distinguish between major and minor depression and depressed mood. Another reason is the difficulty of diagnosing depression in a group of people experiencing increasing communication impairment. It has also been suggested that depression may be phenomenologically different in people with Alzheimer's disease (Patterson et al., 1990). Even in groups of older adults with a wide range of cognitive abilities, there seems to be a relationship between diminished cognitive ability and depression (Lichtenberg, Ross, Millis, & Manning, 1995). Some researchers believe that depression usually appears after the disease is established (Wands et al., 1990), but the precise relationship between depression and cognitive impairment is still a matter of some debate.

    To further complicate matters, cognitive impairment resulting from depression may resemble Alzheimer's disease, and some of the behavioral manifestations commonly associated with depression—weight loss, slowing, insomnia, agitation—may occur in Alzheimer's disease in the absence of depression (McGuire & Rabins, 1994). Both depressed individuals and individuals with Alzheimer's disease evince reduced ability to concentrate, reduced attention span, and generalized loss of interest (Bolger et al., 1994).

    Depression is characterized by depressed mood, loss of pleasure and interest in one's surroundings, weight loss or gain, insomnia or hypersomnia, psychomotor agitation or retardation, fatigue, low energy, feelings of worthlessness and guilt, impaired ability to think, impaired ability to concentrate, and recurrent thoughts about death (American Medical Association, 1993). The American Psychiatric Association (1994) guidelines for depressive disorder state that the individual must exhibit depressed mood or loss of interest or pleasure in all activities as well as four other depressive symptoms, such as significant weight loss or insomnia, for at least 2 weeks. A milder form of depression called dysthymia involves persistent sadness for at least 2 years. Other forms include minor depression, brief depressive disorder, and mixed anxiety and depression.

    The depressed individual may express more feelings of worry, sadness, hopelessness, and displeasure than the nondepressed person with Alzheimer's disease. Most of the time, the nondepressed person with advancing Alzheimer's disease will at least attempt to answer a question, sometimes offering rambling answers, whereas the depressed person is unlikely to attempt any answer at all (Bolger et al., 1994).

> Jacob sat near the elevator every afternoon, greeting everyone who entered
> the Alzheimer's unit. He really did not have much to say, but he always asked
> people how they were or what the weather was like. If a visitor resembled his

son, he would invariably ask him, "When are you going to take me home?" If the visitor resembled his granddaughter, he would ask her, "Did you bring me some cookies?"

In contrast, Frank rarely looked up at anyone, even when he was moved out into the hallway of the same unit. If someone greeted him, he would nod his head without looking up. If the visitor persisted, he would shake his head and wave a hand as if to say, "Leave me alone. Go away." When he was engaged in conversation, he often said, "Why don't you just shoot me" or "Let me die."

Factors Related to Depression   Both physiological and psychological factors related to depression in Alzheimer's disease have been identified. On the physiological side, there is some evidence that depression in Alzheimer's disease is associated with the loss of noradrenergic and serotonergic neurons (Flint, 1991). The resulting transmitter deficit may precipitate depression (neurotransmitters are described in Chapter 2). A genetic predisposition unrelated to Alzheimer's disease may also be present (McGuire & Rabins, 1994).

On the psychosocial side, depression may be related to the experience of continuing failure, perceived stigma, reduced self-esteem, loss, and social isolation resulting from the disease (Cotrell & Schultz, 1993). A number of factors within the individual may also shape his or her response to Alzheimer's disease and the consequent risk for developing depression: the individual's past and present ability to manage change and loss, his or her own personal appraisal of the meaning of the illness, and the response of significant people around him or her.

The experience of continuing, even escalating, failures may be reason enough to stop trying to function, resulting in excess disability and, sometimes, in depression. Stigma comes primarily from the loss of intellect that leads to a sense of inferiority and social unacceptability. Cotrell and Schultz (1993) suggest that some behavior labeled as "problematic" may actually be unsuccessful attempts to avoid being stigmatized. Compounded with an increasingly restricted lifestyle, the isolation that can occur when friends and family withdraw, inability to reciprocate in the give-and-take of personal relationships, and discrediting by self and others results in a substantial list of psychosocial factors that may contribute to the development of depression.

Treatment   Supportive psychosocial therapies, medication, and electroconvulsive therapy have been used to treat depression in people with Alzheimer's disease (Flint, 1991). Psychosocial interventions should be initiated as soon as possible in order to make the most of the insight and communication skills that remain. *Cognitive* approaches to treating depression emphasize redirection of negative thoughts. *Behavioral* approaches emphasize increasing the level of positive experiences (Bolger et al., 1994). Strongly confrontational approaches (e.g., forcefully countering denial) are not recommended unless the individual's behavior presents a danger to him- or herself or others (Bahro et al., 1995).

Antidepressant medication has generally been found effective in treating depression in people with Alzheimer's disease. Several precautions are necessary in prescribing antidepressants: avoiding medication with any anticholinergic effect, which would exacerbate the cognitive deficits; selecting a drug with the appropriate degree of sedating effect; and keeping the dosage as low as possible because of the frailty and advanced age of the majority of these individuals (Ashford & Zec, 1993).

Electroconvulsive therapy is usually reserved for people who are severely depressed or suicidal.

Unfortunately, the amount of research on the effectiveness of these interventions remains limited. The general impression, however, is that depression is treatable and should not be ignored in even the most cognitively impaired individual.

Anxiety   Far less attention has been paid to either the prevalence or the treatment of anxiety in people with Alzheimer's disease. This fact is particularly surprising given the frequency of agitation and acting-out behaviors, which greatly distress caregivers. Attribution of these behaviors to the disease rather than to an emotional response to the disease may be one reason for the failure to study the problem. Another reason may be the problem of distinguishing minor phobias, found in as many as 15% of older adults, from major phobias and panic disorders, found in only 0.1% of older adults. One study found more anxiety than depression in the earliest stages of dementia (Wands et al., 1990), leading the researchers to speculate that the initial emotional response to a decrease in cognitive function was primarily anxiety. Anxiety also can have a negative effect on attention span, exacerbating the cognitive impairment (Burger, Kee, & Alden, 1993).

Factors Related to Anxiety   Anxiety may be habitual, situational, or related to disability in people with Alzheimer's disease. It may be related to the fears engendered by the disease that were described earlier in the chapter: being abandoned, losing one's independence, losing one's mind, becoming a burden. Increasing difficulty in coping with the demands of everyday living, such as finding one's way home, may lead to panic attacks in some individuals. The "catastrophic reactions" to what appear to be minor frustrations in the later stages may be a manifestation of extreme anxiety (Bolger et al., 1994).

Treatment   Counseling may be effective in treating anxiety in the early stages, particularly if the anxiety is related to the fears noted previously. Supportive psychosocial therapies may help the individual regain some sense of order and control over his or her environment. In the later stages limiting the demands placed on the person, maintaining consistency in routines, and providing reassurance that the person will not be forced to cope alone may reduce the occurrence of catastrophic reactions (Bolger et al., 1994). If these interventions are not sufficient, medication with antianxiety drugs (examined in more detail in Chapter 8) may be necessary, but oversedation should be avoided.

Delusions and Hallucinations   Both delusions and hallucinations appear to be fairly common in people with Alzheimer's disease (at least in comparison with people who are cognitively intact), occurring in 10%–73% at some point in the progression of the disease (Liebson & Albert, 1994). The delusions and hallucinations experienced by people with Alzheimer's disease may differ in some respects from those observed in other people experiencing psychiatric problems.

Delusions are false cognitions (i.e., incorrect or inaccurate beliefs firmly held by the individual). The delusions associated with Alzheimer's disease are generally simple, straightforward, and related to the person's family or environment rather than the more bizarre, complicated, integrated systems of delusions found in people with schizophrenia (Flint, 1991). Common examples in people with Alzheimer's disease are beliefs that their spouse has been unfaithful, their caregiver is an imposter, or someone has stolen a prized possession or taken money from their bank account (Bolger et al., 1994).

Felicia was convinced that her husband was a stranger in her house. When they went shopping together, she often asked a clerk or customer to help her escape from her kidnapper, much to her husband's chagrin. At night, she would scream, "Help! Rape!" if he came into their bedroom. One night, she ran to the kitchen for a butcher knife when he yelled back, "That's enough of this! I'm going to sleep in our room tonight whether you like it or not!" For months after that, her hurt and angry husband slept in the spare room to keep her calm.

Hallucinations are false sensory experiences. They appear real to the patient but have no basis in fact. Visual hallucinations are more common than auditory ones in people with Alzheimer's disease.

Murray leaned over the side of his chair and began to call "Here boy! Come here. That's a good boy." When his wife asked him what he was doing, Murray answered, "I'm just talking to the dog." "There's no dog there!" his wife exclaimed. "Yes, there is," Murray responded. "Here boy, come on now. That's a good dog."

Factors Related to Delusions and Hallucinations   Some of the delusions and hallucinations observed in people with Alzheimer's disease actually may be illusions or misidentifications. *Misidentifications* may be either cognitive or sensory. The individual may not recognize his or her own home, relatives, personal possessions, pet, or even his or her own reflection in the mirror.

Lillian often spoke to her reflection in the mirror in the washroom at the day center. "Who are you talking to?" the aide asked her one day. "My sister, Ethel," Lillian replied.

The aide mentioned this incident to Lillian's daughter when she came to pick Lillian up from the center. Her daughter told the aide, "Aunt Ethel was older than my mother. They were both the same size and both had the same gray eyes. Now that you mention it, my mother does look like Aunt Ethel."

Illusions also occur: marks on the wall may look like insects, colorful wallpaper designs may look like birds or snakes. People with Alzheimer's disease are often seen leaning over to pick up something off a patterned floor when nothing is there or stepping over a dark spot as if there were a hole in the flooring.

Visual problems may be responsible for some of these symptoms. Sensory deficits are common in older adults, and visuospatial deficits occur frequently in Alzheimer's disease. In combination, they may make it difficult for the older person with dementia to understand what it is he or she is seeing. It is possible that the individual's attempts to make sense out of confusing visual or auditory inputs may lead to the development of delusions or hallucinations (Bolger et al., 1994).

Language problems may also contribute to situations in which it appears that the individual is delusional or hallucinating. For example, the individual may actually recognize a family member or friend but be unable to retrieve the name from memory.

Flint (1991) suggests that most delusions and hallucinations are a result of the disease itself, not of new or preexisting psychiatric illness, sensory deficits, or cognitive impairment. Disease-related damage to the basal ganglia, thalamus, and limbic structures may be responsible, as well as impaired dopamine function, which has been related to delusions and hallucinations in people with Parkinson's disease.

The difficulty experienced in attempting to distinguish the effect of organic damage from psychological defenses reemphasizes the need to develop a psychobiological model to explain the psychiatric problems associated with Alzheimer's disease (Bahro et al., 1995).

Treatment   Both behavioral and pharmacological interventions may be used to treat delusions and hallucinations. Behavioral interventions may include reinforcement (i.e., providing rewards for desired behavior), differential attention (i.e., attending only to desirable, not undesirable, behavior), and modeling (i.e., acting as an example of the desired behavior) (Bolger et al., 1994). Antipsychotic drugs seem to be more effective in the treatment of delusions than in the treatment of hallucinations (Flint, 1991), perhaps providing some additional clues to their origin. Haloperidol is frequently prescribed for these problems. The antianxiety drugs are also used in some cases (American Medical Association, 1993), as examined in more detail in Chapter 8.

Activity Disturbances

Often lumped together with other symptoms in the category of "problem behaviors," most of the activity disturbances associated with Alzheimer's disease are poorly understood. This section considers four of the most common: sleep disturbances, pacing, aggression, and inappropriate sexual behavior.

Sleep Disturbances   Sleep disturbances appear to be closely related to the severity of the cognitive deficits of Alzheimer's disease. People in the advanced stages of Alzheimer's disease spend time in bed wide awake, take a longer time to reach REM (rapid eye movement) sleep, and have less slow-wave sleep than cognitively intact individuals (Miller et al., 1994). Some describe this problem in terms of turning night into day: People sleep most of the day but become awake and alert at night when caregivers want to sleep.

Hopkins and Rindlisbacher (1995) prefer to characterize the problem as a disruption and fragmentation of the normal pattern of rest and activity. Some evidence exists that normal circadian (sleep–wake) cycles are disturbed in Alzheimer's disease. This disturbance may be caused by damage to the optic tract, limbic structures, and brain stem (Bolger et al., 1994) or, more specifically, to a loss of cells in the suprachiasmatic nucleus of the hypothalamus that governs sleep–wake cycles (Hopkins & Rindlisbacher, 1995). The disturbance also has been ascribed to daytime napping, but there is increasing doubt that napping causes serious disturbances of the sleep–wake cycle.

> A retired night nurse in the middle stages of Alzheimer's disease was admitted to a long-term care facility. The staff quickly learned that their daytime routine of breakfast in the dining room, followed by bath and shower time and group activities at 10:00 A.M., would not appeal to this woman. After a few mornings of clenched fists and kicks when the staff tried to get her out of bed, staff members reconsidered the routine. The night staff reported that she enjoyed sharing their midnight lunch with them and spent most of the night quietly "making rounds" on all of the residents, carefully covering them and straightening the nightstands. Usually around 7:00 A.M. she was ready for a shower and bed, as was her lifelong pattern.
>
> On occasion the staff had problems explaining to administrators and federal inspectors why she was in bed all day, but her assessment and care plan always convinced them that their care was not negligent. The retired nurse was able to continue her lifestyle despite her disease and relocation to a long-term care

facility. She was not medicated for her aggressive behavior, the day staff avoided confrontation, and, most important, both she and the night staff thoroughly enjoyed the late night suppers and companionship.

If the neurophysiological hypothesis for the sleep disturbance is correct, the current behavioral and pharmacological treatments may be misguided. For example, instead of restraining the person at night, he or she would be better off if allowed to engage in safe, nondisruptive activities in a secure environment (Hopkins & Rindlisbacher, 1995). The traditional routines (especially the rigid mealtimes and rules about wake-up times and bedtimes) of a typical day center or long-term care facility would be entirely inappropriate for the individual with disturbed circadian rhythms. Exercise, eating, bathing, and bedtime routines in particular should be modified to accommodate the person's fragmented rest and activity patterns. This accommodation means that traditional staffing patterns, in which the greatest number of staff members are present in the daytime hours, should also be modified if patients are awake and active at night (Hopkins & Rindlisbacher, 1995).

Sundowning is another rest/activity disturbance that has drawn a considerable amount of attention. Restlessness and agitation have been noted to increase in some people with Alzheimer's disease as the sun sets. Soft music and dimmed lights have been used to counter the effects of sundowning with some apparent success.

Pacing   Pacing and wandering are common activity disturbances found in people with Alzheimer's disease and are associated with increasing impairment (Spector & Jackson, 1994). Some wandering appears to be purposeful: The goal is to find the exit, often interpreted as a desire to "go home" or to return to a time when they felt more comfortable and secure. Other pacing may simply be movement, a need for exercise, stimulation, or activity in general (Bolger et al., 1994). Unless individuals become exhausted as a result of excessive pacing, most caregivers believe that pacing should be allowed to continue within a secure environment.

Aggression   Physically aggressive (e.g., hitting, kicking) and verbally aggressive (e.g., screaming, cursing) behaviors are not only evidence of a distressed patient but also disturbing to caregivers. These problems are particularly common in the advanced stages of the disease (Cohen-Mansfield, Marx, & Werner, 1992).

As with most of the other problems examined in this chapter, aggressive behavior is probably the result of multiple psychosocial and physiological factors. These factors include neurophysiological changes, individual experience and predisposition, the quality of the person's social supports, and environmental triggers (Kolanowski, 1995). Decreased metabolism of serotonin has been associated with a number of impulsive behaviors, such as reckless driving and acting out. Past history may predispose some individuals to aggressive behavior. Conflicted, nonsupportive family relationships and limited social networks may also predispose some individuals to these behaviors. Consider the relevance of the following comments on this subject from a family caregiver:

> My wife never went through the problems that most of the people in the support group talk about. Before she got sick, she was a gentle, softspoken woman. We never raised our voices at each other, never raised a hand to our children. Now, if I get aggravated, I try to take a deep breath or to walk away for a few minutes until I calm down. Maybe that's why we haven't had more problems.

Many, although not all, aggressive and acting-out behaviors occur during completion of activities of daily living (ADLs): bathing, toileting, dressing. Often, frustration is the trigger in these situations, although the embarrassment of needing help with these intimate tasks also may trigger a reaction. Caregivers who protect a person's privacy and watch carefully to prevent the level of frustration from rising too high often can prevent these outbursts. Allowing a time-out for everyone to calm down before proceeding is often effective as well.

Changes in Sexual Behavior   Most of the information about the changes in sexual behavior associated with Alzheimer's disease comes from clinical observation and anecdotal (i.e., caregiver) reports. The most common problems reported are heightened sexual interest and activity, loss of sexual interest, and inappropriate behaviors. Some inappropriate behaviors appear to be related to the misperceptions described earlier: inability to distinguish friends from strangers, failure to recognize a spouse as a sex partner, and inability to distinguish public and private places and the behaviors that are congruent with each. Cohen and Eisdorfer (1986) related the experience of one caregiver whose wife apparently failed to distinguish correctly between private and public places: "I was shocked. My wife sat out in the lawn chair by the pool—stark naked reading a book!" (p. 169). The sexual urges are normal, say Cohen and Eisdorfer, but the manner in which they are pursued may be anything but usual or socially acceptable.

Caregivers' own experiences and feelings about intimacy are also an important factor. Some are alienated and repelled by their impaired spouses' forgetfulness, need for assistance in ADLs, and diminished ability to relate to the feelings and needs of other people. The quality of the sexual relationship before the effects of the disease were evident is another important factor.

Kuhn (1994) identified four common patterns of change in sexual behavior in the individual with Alzheimer's disease:

- *Sexual interest and ability continue as before.* In some cases couples continue to be satisfied with their sexual relationship. In others, loss of ability to relate to another individual diminishes the satisfaction of one or both partners. Some partners are able to assume the helper role for the person with Alzheimer's disease as they do in other aspects of everyday life and maintain a satisfying relationship; others find this difficult.
- *Difficulty in performance develops.* Some of these problems may be the result of other age-related changes or poor health. Other performance problems may result primarily from limited attention span, reduced physical coordination, or other physical changes related to Alzheimer's disease. The aids to sexual performance commonly suggested for older people (e.g., hormone creams, vaginal lubricants, penile implants) may be sufficient in this instance. Alternate sources of gratification (e.g., mutual masturbation, repositioning, oral sex) may prove helpful and satisfying to both partners. Evaluation of the effect of any medications the person may be taking is also important because they may have a powerful effect on sexual interest and performance.
- *Increased interest in sex, even hypersexuality, may develop.* For some people with Alzheimer's disease, sexual relations may be one of the few remaining activities they can perform well. The result can be an overemphasis on this aspect of the relationship to fill an increasingly empty life.
- *Diminished or no interest in sexual relations.* This loss of interest may be part of a general reduction in energy and loss of interest. Depression also may be involved.

Professional help for sexual problems begins with the ability to approach the subject with sensitivity to the needs and feelings of both partners. It is particularly important to provide an atmosphere in which the individuals involved can discuss their concerns comfortably and receive nonjudgmental guidance leading to a satisfying resolution of their problem. The goal is to help them understand the effects of the disease (to the extent that professionals understand them) and one another's responses to the problem and to resolve the problem in a manner satisfying to both.

REFERENCES

American Medical Association. (1993). *Medication.* Chicago: Author.

American Psychiatric Association. (1994). *Diagnostic and statistical manual of mental disorders (DSM-IV)* (4th ed.). Washington, DC: American Psychiatric Press.

Ashford, J.W., & Zec, R.F. (1993). Pharmacological treatment in Alzheimer's disease. In R.W. Parks, R.F. Zec, & R.S. Wilson (Eds.), *Neuropsychology of Alzheimer's disease and other dementias.* New York: Oxford University Press.

Bahro, M., Silber, E., & Sunderland, T. (1995). How do patients with Alzheimer's disease cope with their disease? A clinical experience report. *Journal of the American Geriatrics Society, 43,* 41–46.

Bolger, J.P., Carpenter, B.D., & Strauss, M.E. (1994). Behavior and affect in Alzheimer's disease. *Clinics in Geriatric Medicine, 10*(2), 315–337.

Burger, M.C., Kee, B.S., & Alden, J.D. (1993). *Affective symptoms and memory performance of early Alzheimer's disease.* Paper presented at the 46th Annual Scientific Meeting of the Gerontological Society of America, New Orleans.

Cohen, D. (1991). The subjective experience of Alzheimer's disease: The anatomy of an illness as perceived by patients and families. *American Journal of Alzheimer's Care and Related Diseases and Research, 6*(3), 6–11.

Cohen, D., & Eisdorfer, C. (1986). *The loss of self.* New York: Norton.

Cohen-Mansfield, J., Marx, M.S., & Werner, P. (1992). Agitation in elderly persons: An integrative report of findings in a nursing home. *International Psychogeriatrics, 4*(2), 221–240.

Cotrell, V., & Lein, L. (1993). Awareness and denial in the Alzheimer's disease victim. *Journal of Gerontological Social Work, 19*(3/4), 115–132.

Cotrell, V., & Schultz, R. (1993). The perspective of the patient with Alzheimer's disease: A neglected dimension of dementia research. *Gerontologist, 33*(2), 205–211.

Davis, R. (1989). *My journey into Alzheimer's disease.* Wheaton, IL: Tyndale House.

Flint, A.J. (1991). Delusions, hallucinations and depression in Alzheimer's disease. *American Journal of Alzheimer's Care and Related Diseases and Research, 6*(3), 21–29.

Gray, D.D. (1993). *I want to remember: A son's reflection on his mother's Alzheimer's journey.* Wellesley, MA: Roundtable Press.

Hopkins, R.W., & Rindlisbacher, P. (1995). Some clinical consequences of the rest and activity disturbance in Alzheimer's disease. *American Journal of Alzheimer's Care and Related Diseases and Research, 10*(1), 16–25.

Kolanowski, A. (1995). Aggressive behavior in institutionalized elders: A theoretical framework. *American Journal of Alzheimer's Care and Related Diseases and Research, 10*(2), 23–29.

Kuhn, D.R. (1994). The changing face of sexual intimacy in Alzheimer's disease. *American Journal of Alzheimer's Care and Related Diseases and Research, 9*(5), 7–14.

Lawton, M.P., VanHaitsma, K., & Klappa, J. (1996). Observed affect in nursing home residents with Alzheimer's disease. *Journal of Gerontology: Psychological Sciences, 51B*(1), 3–14.

Lichtenberg, P.A., Ross, T., Millis, S.R., & Manning, C.A. (1995). The relationship between depression and cognition in older adults: A cross-validation study. *Journal of Gerontology: Psychological Sciences, 50B*(1), 25–32.

Liebson, E., & Albert, M.L. (1994). Cognitive changes in dementia of the Alzheimer's type. In D.B. Calne (Ed.), *Neurodegenerative diseases* (pp. 615–629). Philadelphia: W.B. Saunders.

McGowin, D.F. (1993). *Living in the labyrinth: A personal journey through the maze of Alzheimer's.* San Francisco: Elder Books.

McGuire, M.H., & Rabins, P.V. (1994). Mood disorders. In C.E. Coffey & J.L. Cummings (Eds.), *Textbook of geriatric neuropsychology* (pp. 243–260). Washington, DC: American Psychiatric Press.

Mega, M.S., Cummings, J.L., Fiorello, T., & Gornbein, J. (1996). The spectrum of behavioral changes in Alzheimer's disease. *Neurology, 46,* 130–135.

Miller, B.L., Chang, L., Oropilla, G., & Mena, I. (1994). Alzheimer's disease and frontal lobe dementias. In C.E. Coffey & J.L. Cummings (Eds.), *Textbook of geriatric neuropsychology* (pp. 389–404). Washington, DC: American Psychiatric Press.

Patterson, M.B., Schnell, A.H., Martin, R.J., Mendez, M.F., Smyth, K.A., & Whitehouse, P.J. (1990, January–March). Assessment of behavioral and affective symptoms in Alzheimer's disease. *Journal of Geriatric Psychiatry and Neurology, 3,* 21–30.

Spector, W.D., & Jackson, M.E. (1994). Correlates of disruptive behavior in nursing homes: A reanalysis. *Journal of Aging and Health, 6*(2), 173–184.

Tappen, R.M., & Williams-Burgess, C. (1997). Expression of emotion in advanced Alzheimer's disease: Family and caregiver perspectives. Submitted for publication.

Teri, L., & Truax, P. (1994). Assessment of depression in dementia patients: Association of caregiver mood with depression ratings. *Gerontologist, 34*(2), 231–234.

Wands, K., Merskey, H., Hachinski, V., Fisman, M., Fox, H., & Boniferro, M. (1990). A questionnaire investigation of anxiety and depression in early dementia. *Journal of the American Geriatrics Society, 38*(5), 535–538.

Chapter 7

Psychotherapeutic Strategies

. . . surprise caught
in his voice
as if he's discovered words
are stitched to his skin
in a pouch just out of reach . . .

J. Hall (1994)

Are we playing tricks on ourselves and on the Alzheimer's patients . . . when we
attend support groups for ourselves . . . but fail to provide social peer support for
our confused, isolated and frightened care recipients with Alzheimer's?

S. Arkin (1995)

Following the discussion in Chapter 6 of the emotional consequences of Alzheimer's disease, this chapter considers a variety of nonpharmacological psychotherapeutic interventions that have been developed or modified for people with Alzheimer's disease. The diversity in approach reflects the various traditions from which the treatments have sprung: psychiatry, gerontology, speech-language pathology, recreation, and others. The common denominator is a concern with the emotional responses to the vagaries of Alzheimer's disease. The goals of the various approaches, however, differ substantively. Some focus on control, others on easing the psychological pain, still others on keeping the person constructively occupied. Does this matter? It could matter a great deal. For example, when the goal is control of behaviors that distress others, consideration of the long-term effect on the person with Alzheimer's disease may be lacking. Rather than addressing the discomfort that led to the behavior, the intervention is focused on suppressing or prohibiting it.

A number of strategies are available for treating the emotional problems associated with Alzheimer's disease, including behavior change, support groups, activity groups, reminiscence, remotivation, and validation. Some of these techniques are employed primarily in groups and others are more individually oriented. Some are more appropriate in the early stages of the disease; others are designed for people in the advanced stages. Consideration of techniques to facilitate communication between caregiver and care receiver precedes this discussion because communication is the fundamental process through which these interventions are accomplished.

COMMUNICATION

Being able to share one's thoughts, feelings, and opinions with other people is critical to emotional well-being. This ability slowly but relentlessly declines as Alzheimer's disease progresses.

Communication involves both cognitive and motor processes. The motor processes, such as movements of tongue and jaw or of air in and out of the lungs, do not seem to be much affected by Alzheimer's disease. The cognitive processes, in contrast, are profoundly affected by the disease. Supporting and enhancing use of the individual's remaining cognitive capacity and reducing the frustrations engendered by communication failures are the primary goals of the techniques described here.

Communication in the Early Stages of the Disease

Communicative difficulties appear early in the course of Alzheimer's disease, usually after memory deficits have become evident. From reports of family caregivers, the communication problems are first noted in difficulty writing a letter, finding the right word, and naming objects (Bayles & Tomoeda, 1991). Speech errors (e.g., saying "bagoon" instead of "balloon") may worsen the naming problem (Biassou et al., 1995). Production of apparently meaningless sentences (e.g., "So that makes it a make it?") or incomplete sentences, failure to understand what is read, and inability to recognize humor appear in the later stages of the disease.

The decline in ability to communicate is vividly portrayed in the results of a longitudinal (5-year) study of the changes in oral communication that occur over time (Tomoeda & Bayles, 1993). Asked to describe a Norman Rockwell picture (mother and children going off in Easter bonnets while father reads the paper, still in his bathrobe), subjects in the early stages provided lengthy, even wordy, descriptions of the picture. In fact, the subjects in the early stages of Alzheimer's disease used more words in their descriptions than did the controls (no cognitive impairment). The conciseness of their responses, however, was a different story. Participants with Alzheimer's disease were less concise, were more repetitive, made more incomplete statements, and conveyed fewer ideas altogether than did the controls.

As the disease progressed, verbal output diminished dramatically in the participants with Alzheimer's disease. People in the middle stages produced more incomplete statements than did those in the early or late stages. In the advanced stages there were few ideas to repeat (Tomoeda & Bayles, 1993). By the fifth year, one of the participants said only "Yeah" and "I like it" when asked to describe the picture (p. 16). In fact, the researchers believed that the participants were approaching muteness by the end of the study.

In the early stages of Alzheimer's disease the primary *expressive* communication problems are finding the right word and using too many pronouns with vague antecedents. The primary *receptive* (i.e., comprehension) problems are difficulty understanding long or very complex discussions and difficulty remaining focused on the main points rather than on secondary points. The individual with Alzheimer's disease can do much to facilitate communication. Clark and Witte (1991) suggest the person use the following types of statements to prevent communication failures:

- "Would you say that again more slowly?"
- "Wait a moment, I'm trying to think of the right word."
- "What were we talking about? I've forgotten."

People with these relatively minor communication impairments can (and often do) use their remaining abilities to make up for their deficiencies. The following are some examples adapted from Clark and Witte (1991):

- *Circumlocutions:* talking around the word the person cannot think of is often sufficient to convey meaning to a perceptive listener. For example, instead of saying, "Would you turn off the television for me?," the person who has forgotten the word TELEVISION can say, "Would you please turn off that noisy thing over there for me?"
- *Phonemic cueing:* Using another word that sounds like the word needed may also suffice in some instances. For example, if the person wants to ask for a cup but cannot retrieve the word, he or she may say, "May I have that, oh, it sounds like pup, sup . . . I've got it—cup." Rhyming may help the person find the word before the caregiver has figured it out.
- *Life experience strategy:* A concrete example from one's life experience may be used to illustrate an abstract idea that the person is having difficulty explaining. For example, in order to explain despair, the person may refer back to the time the family thought their dog had been lost, describing how they missed the dog and thought they would never see it again.

These strategies can be shared with the person with Alzheimer's disease and they can be practiced.

Caregivers can also support the person's attempts to communicate clearly. In the early stages, this is accomplished by attitude almost as much as it is by techniques. Attitude includes the following key points (several of these are adapted from Yale's [1994] work with people in early-stage Alzheimer's disease):

- Be patient. Allow the person a little extra time to finish a thought or respond to your questions.
- Ask permission to assist when the person cannot find the right word or is having trouble following someone else's story.
- Simplify your own explanations without being condescending. In other words, continue to treat the person as a rational adult, simply one who is having difficulty organizing his or her thoughts.
- Pay more attention to the nonverbal message that may explain the verbal message.
- Use more nonverbal channels when talking with the person, such as pointing to an object as well as saying its name.
- Adjust your expectations to the person's level of ability. As cognitive impairment increases, reduce the complexity and level of abstraction of your conversation.

Following these suggestions should not mean that certain topics can no longer be discussed. In fact, arbitrarily withholding any information from the individual in the early stages of the disease would be inappropriate. The manner in which information is conveyed should be adjusted to accommodate the impairment. Clearer, more carefully thought-out explanations and discussion are required.

Communication in the Middle Stages of the Disease

Far more effort is required to communicate effectively with the person in the middle stages of Alzheimer's disease than in the early stages. The responsibility for maintaining a conversation, clarifying misunderstandings, and filling in lost words or memories falls increasingly on the caregiver as the disease progresses. Efforts are focused on three primary goals: encouraging communication efforts, accurately interpreting what has been expressed, and facilitating comprehension. Key points are listed in the following description of each of these goals.

Encouraging Efforts to Communicate   This goal is based primarily on a *practice strategy*, that is, on the assumption that it is essential the person continue to use communicative skills in order to maintain them at the highest possible level. Some strategies to encourage communicative efforts include:

- Listening to whatever the person is saying and responding as appropriately as possible. Never ignore attempts to communicate.
- Speaking directly to the person with Alzheimer's disease, not to the spouse, friend, or caregiver.
- Allowing time for the person to respond to you. Remember that the work of comprehending what you have said and formulating a response is far more effortful for the person with Alzheimer's disease.
- Avoiding correcting the person unless absolutely necessary. It can be very discouraging to be reminded constantly of one's errors.

Facilitating Interpretation   A fundamental principle of communication is that there is meaning in every attempt to communicate, no matter how difficult it is to discern that meaning. This is easier to attempt than to accomplish when a message is garbled. If caregivers approach the task of interpretation with this principle in mind, they will be far more successful in accurately interpreting the person's meaning. The following suggestions may be helpful:

- Use your knowledge of the person to help you understand what he or she wants but do not allow this knowledge to lead you to erroneous assumptions. Remember that people's needs are not necessarily constant or consistent.
- Listen carefully and think about what the person is trying to say, keeping in mind that word substitutions may make a simple statement sound absurd at first. Bohling (1991) offers an example: a person with Alzheimer's disease said, "Right yes, on a button, very pretty," but meant to say "Right yes, on a shirt, very pretty" (pp. 252–253). The person may also switch from one frame of reference to another without warning, leaving the listener thoroughly baffled unless this switch is noted (Bohling, 1991). For example, the caregiver may ask the person if the movie shown at the day center was interesting and be confused by the response, "Yeah, but the kids wouldn't sit still," unless the caregiver realizes that the person has switched the frame of reference to a movie seen long ago.
- Use the nonverbal portion of the communication and the emotion expressed as clues to correct interpretation.

Facilitating Comprehension   Adapting one's own communication style to the level and type of impairment that occurs with Alzheimer's disease is also helpful. For example,

- Speak more slowly than usual.
- Do not speak louder unless compensating for uncorrected hearing impairment, when you may have to place your mouth quite close to the person's ear.
- Use simpler or more familiar words and expressions: "walk" instead of "ambulate," "memory" instead of "cognition."
- Repeat what you have said if the person does not understand it. Use the same words unless you realize that what you said was too complex or too abstract for the person.
- Keep the entire message relatively simple. For example, if you are going on vacation, say, "I'm going to Jamaica," instead of "I'm leaving next Tuesday for a week-long

vacation in Jamaica." You can add the elaborations after the person has processed the first bit of information.

- Ask for opinions rather than facts when possible. No opinion is wrong.
- Use concrete rather than abstract expressions. For example, you might say, "James lost his job and is worried about money now," instead of "James is having some serious financial problems because of unemployment."
- Use congruent nonverbal communication to enhance the verbal communication. For example, you might pick up the toothbrush while talking about getting teeth clean, or you might talk about dinner while in the kitchen rather than in the living room.
- Watch the person's level of frustration. Try to keep conversational demands within his or her level of tolerance.

Some evidence from research shows that these adaptations (e.g., shorter, less complex sentences) facilitate communication with individuals with Alzheimer's disease (Kemper, Anagnopoulos, Lyons, & Heberlein, 1994).

Communication in the Later Stages of the Disease

It *is possible* to communicate with the person with Alzheimer's disease in the later stages, but it requires great effort on the part of the caregiver and more reliance on nonverbal communication. Although it is difficult to say just how much the person can understand or express, clinical observation suggests that it is more than is generally assumed. The goals at this stage are to stimulate communication and to facilitate comprehension. Some strategies include:

- Use touch (as tolerated by the individual) to gain and hold the person's attention as well as to calm and reassure if necessary.
- Assume that the tone of your voice and your body language may convey as much of the message as your words, and act accordingly. Rough handling or a tense, tight-lipped reply may well convey anger even though your words are kind.
- Talk about things that are significant to the person: a treasured grandchild, beloved pet, passionate hobby, or favorite form of entertainment.
- Use props to enhance comprehension. If you are talking about a grandchild, show the person a photograph of the child. If talking about the garden or the weather, step outside or to the window and point to the object.
- Try singing and rhyming or saying familiar prayers if these please the individual. Often, these activities are easier to engage in than is verbal discourse.
- Do not give up communicating with the person. Allow an extended amount of time for a response, far longer than you would with a cognitively intact person, and accept positive nonverbal responses as encouragement to continue the conversation.

Family and friends who visit or care for people in the latest stages of the disease often need guidance and support to continue their attempts to communicate with the individual when the amount of comprehensible response diminishes.

INDIVIDUAL-ORIENTED INTERVENTION

Behavior Change

Although disruptive behavior (e.g., screaming, wandering, kicking, hitting) is not limited to people with Alzheimer's disease, its occurrence in older people has been found to be related to physical and cognitive impairment. The term *disruptive behavior* is considered to be preferable to "agitated behavior" or "problem behavior" (Jackson et al., 1989), although it still focuses on the needs of the caregiver rather than the care receiver. It also may be defined as "acting out behavior" (Spector & Jackson, 1994), a term that shifts the focus to the patient.

Much of the emphasis in the early literature on disruptive behaviors and Alzheimer's disease was on the burden it places on both family and formal caregivers. Little recognition was given to the distress that may be the cause of these behaviors. The result was that solutions were directed toward eliminating the behavior rather than toward correcting the cause of the behavior.

Factors Contributing to Disruptive Behavior

Newer thinking about disruptive behavior is directed toward analysis of the antecedents of that behavior and design of interventions based upon this analysis. Physiological changes, inappropriate environments, and inadequate treatment may be responsible for much disruptive behavior exhibited by people with Alzheimer's disease (Kolanowski, 1995). Jackson and colleagues (1989) suggest that disruptive behavior may have physical, psychological, and social or environmental antecedents. For example, in their survey of Rhode Island nursing facilities they found a tendency to engage in disruptive behavior among cognitively intact residents who were incontinent, an indication that humiliation and frustration may be responsible for some of this behavior. They also noted that women were more likely to scream or moan while men were more likely to become abusive, an indication that gender-based expectations of behavior influence the manifestations of disruptive behavior.

The physical damage exacted on certain areas of the brain by Alzheimer's disease also may contribute to the occurrence of these behaviors (Kolanowski, 1995), but the mechanisms by which this happens have not been thoroughly explored. Physical and chemical restraints applied to eliminate the disruptive behavior may, paradoxically, increase it.

An overstimulating or overdemanding environment, whether in the home or in a long-term care facility, also may trigger these behaviors and then sustain them if the environment is not modified (Mintzer et al., 1993). Invasion of personal space; overcrowding; competition over a desired object, person, or place; and gestures interpreted as threatening may all trigger disruptive behavior. It is also interesting to note that much of this behavior erupts during bathing and other personal care activities, especially but not only when provided by inexperienced staff (Kolanowski, 1995).

All of these factors must be considered when analyzing the reasons for disruptive behavior. Both immediate and long-term strategies to reduce disruptive behavior for the benefit of both the caregiver and the care recipient may be used.

Whatever the reason, the individual who displays disruptive behavior may be signaling a need or calling for help. On the basis of an analysis of factors associated with various disruptive behaviors, Cohen-Mansfield, Marx, and Werner (1992) believe that behaviors such as pacing may fill a need for exercise or stimulation. Screaming, complaining, and other verbal behaviors may indicate physical or emotional distress or both and should receive prompt attention. They should not be ignored.

Immediate Responses to Disruptive Behavior

Although it would be preferable if disruptive behaviors were prevented and never occurred at all, acting-out behaviors are a relatively common occurrence in the middle and late stages of Alzheimer's disease. Immediate responses to disruptive behavior are targeted to calm the individual and prevent injury. Longer term strategies should also be devised and implemented.

A number of techniques are generally recognized as useful during this immediate intervention phase. Distraction is probably the most widely recommended technique.

> Mae Jessup had been a client at the day center for several years. Her Alzheimer's disease had progressed to the point at which she needed some assistance with dressing and toileting, but she often resisted being helped. Based on their own observations and discussion with Mae's family, day center staff believed that her resistance stemmed primarily from embarrassment.
>
> When a new staff member tried to help her pull up her trousers after toileting, Mae became very upset. She began screaming wordlessly and shook her clenched fists at the staff member, who retreated in fear. A more experienced staff member familiar to Mae gently led her out of the restroom, but Mae continued to scream. Her whole body tensed, as if for a fight. The staff member took Mae to an empty room adjoining the main dining room, softly humming the "Tennessee Waltz." "Let's dance, Mae. This is your favorite song, isn't it?" Slowly, gently, she touched Mae's shoulder and began to lead her in a slow waltz around the room. As they moved together, the screaming subsided and the tension decreased. Eventually (it took almost 15 minutes), Mae began humming along with her.
>
> Day center staff met later that day to analyze the event and plan an approach to prevent triggering another outburst from Mae.

This example illustrates many of the techniques used to deal with outbursts of this type. These techniques and others, some of which are adapted from Teri and Logsdon (1990), include the following:

- Approach the person slowly and quietly. Stay calm yourself to avoid escalating the tension.
- Speak calmly and quietly, but not condescendingly, to the person. Avoid words or gestures that could be interpreted as threatening in any way.
- Use a light touch on the arm or back, which may be calming.
- Use quiet music and soft lighting, which may also be calming.
- Distract the person's attention from the unpleasant situation to a pleasant, attractive one. An offer of a tempting snack or desirable activity (e.g., going outside, feeding the cat, looking at photographs) may be sufficient distraction.
- Move the person away from the place, people, and/or objects that triggered the outburst.
- Avoid arguing, reasoning, or confronting; this type of response usually exacerbates the problem.
- Avoid physically restraining the person; restraints may exacerbate the problem.
- Ask for help if the previous measures do not work and the person is in danger of hurting self or others.

Intermediate Responses

An unusual source of help when the usual measures listed do not work is described by Mintzer and colleagues (1993). Although their Behavioral Intensive Care Units are not widely available, some of the techniques used may be implemented in other settings.

This 3-week program involves intensive observation, behavior mapping, and development and implementation of a therapeutic regimen that may include redesign of the environment to which the individual will return. *Behavior mapping* involves notation of the frequency, intensity, and duration of the behavior of concern as well as the context in which it occurs.

An interesting element of this program is the careful titration of external (environmental) stimulus and demand. For the first 2 days in the unit, patients are given complete assistance with activities of daily living, including being fed their meals in their rooms. Verbal communication and cueing are kept to a minimum. For the third and fourth days, patients are allowed to participate in their own care if they do not become agitated over it, but they are not asked to do so. Verbal interaction is also increased if this does not increase agitation. This progresses to active interaction with staff and other patients and direct statements that patients are expected to participate in their own care. However, if agitation occurs, the levels of stimulus and demand are reduced and the progression slowed and reduced so that only one new stimulus or responsibility is introduced at a time (Mintzer et al., 1993). Throughout this process, particular attention is paid to what triggers outbursts and how the stimuli, demands, and their context can be modified to prevent new outbursts.

Longer-Term Responses

Behavior analyses are not unique to care of the person with Alzheimer's disease, but they do serve a useful purpose in such care. The purpose is to encourage caregivers to look behind the behavior; that is, to analyze the antecedents of the behavior. The steps in the process have been assigned various names, but the fundamental ideas are similar. The following may be considered a generic approach to behavior analysis:

1. Describe the problem in behavioral terms; that is, identify the behavior of concern and describe it in *objective, observable* terms (Teri & Logsdon, 1990). In the earlier example, for instance, Mae Jessup screamed and shook her fists at a staff member.
2. Identify probable antecedents of the behavior; in other words, seek a reason or reasons for the behavior. In doing so, consider the following questions and answers relating to the earlier example:

    Where?—in the restroom
    When?—after using the toilet
    Who?—new staff member
    What?—attempted to help adjust clothing

    After analyzing the entire context of the situation as well as the characteristics of the individuals involved, the probable triggers can be identified.

    Why?—invasion of privacy, embarrassment

    Often, the best source of information (although seldom suggested) is the person whose behavior is of some concern. The caregiver can ask, "What's the matter? Why are you upset? What do you want?" If the person can tell you, the analysis will be more accurate and the intervention more effective.
3. Design an individualized intervention plan that modifies or eliminates the identified antecedents of the behavior of concern. For example, the staff who worked with Mae Jessup decided to try several strategies to avoid upsetting her in the future. The strategies included reassigning her to the staff member with whom she was most

comfortable, asking the family to select dresses instead of trousers for her for a while to facilitate her rearranging her own clothing after toileting, offering to help instead of simply reaching out to adjust her clothing without permission, and taking her to the restroom at a time when no one else was using it.

4. Observe the results of the intervention, reevaluate the situation, and redesign the intervention if necessary.

Caregivers often need to evaluate their own responses to the behavior of concern to be sure that they are not inadvertently reinforcing and sustaining it rather than extinguishing it. This evaluation requires a considerable amount of self-knowledge and understanding as well as knowledge and understanding of the person with Alzheimer's disease.

GROUP-ORIENTED INTERVENTIONS

A variety of group-oriented interventions have been designed for different groups of people with cognitive impairment, but there is some uncertainty about their relative effectiveness. For example, one of the earliest, reality orientation, has fallen out of favor because it tends to emphasize deficits rather than accommodate them, yet reality orientation groups can still be found in many day centers and long-term care facilities. Certainly, there is nothing wrong with informing people what day it is or where they are, but the salience of these facts vis-à-vis the salience of information about their families or the next meal is questionable.

Critics of group approaches have suggested that research results have not been consistently supportive of their effectiveness in individuals with Alzheimer's disease (Kelly, 1995; Woods & McKiernan, 1995). At best, they say, groups may provide opportunities for stimulation and interpersonal interaction, particularly in impoverished environments. Another concern is that group interventions are often conducted by personnel who possess more enthusiasm than skill in facilitating groups of people with Alzheimer's disease. The latter concern can be relieved by providing adequate training for group leaders.

Other questions involve the function of the group. Much of the group work conducted with people with Alzheimer's disease has been activity focused, on the assumption that people with communication deficits may find activities a helpful channel through which they can express feelings (David, 1991). This focus on activities is in contrast to discussion-based mutual support groups, which emphasize the development of relationships and expression of feelings rather than the accomplishment of specific tasks. Can talk-based therapies be used effectively with people with Alzheimer's disease? The prevailing thinking seems to be that they are effective only in the earliest stages, but this is probably because we have not yet developed appropriate modifications for people in the later stages. In fact, there is some evidence that, with a skilled interviewer, individuals in the later stages can express their feelings and maintain a theme with help (Tappen & Williams-Burgess, 1996).

Value of Group Work

Why bring people together rather than working with them individually? Aside from the obvious efficiency of treating several people at one time, group experiences offer some therapeutic advantages over individual work for people with Alzheimer's disease.

Given an appropriate group membership, dynamics, and setting, group experience provides opportunities to develop new relationships and to reconnect with other people, especially people with similar concerns. When this happens, it can reduce the isolation often felt by people with Alzheimer's disease and increase their feeling of belonging, often lost when friends and acquaintances slip away and connections to people and organizations in the community are severed. In addition, groups can provide opportunities to share experiences and feelings with people who not only have similar concerns but may also be able to suggest ways to handle them (David, 1991). The benefits of a support group for people in the early stages of Alzheimer's disease were summarized nicely by a group member quoted by Yale (1994): "It helps to know you aren't alone . . . listening to how others deal with similar problems . . . it makes me feel better to know that there are people like me" (p. 1).

Groups are not the best modality for everyone, however. People with severe sensory impairment, visual or hearing, may gain more from individual approaches (Woods & McKiernan, 1995). Individual preferences also should be considered. Some people are not comfortable sharing personal information or discussing sensitive subjects in a group setting. Individuals with some computer skills may be more comfortable participating in an online chat group that is limited to people with Alzheimer's disease (McGowin, 1997).

Early-Stage Group Modalities

Support Groups   Support groups for people in the early stages of Alzheimer's disease often have a limited life span (e.g., 2–3 months) and are usually open only to people who are aware of their diagnosis, because their purpose is to enhance understanding of the disease and assist in the development of effective coping mechanisms (Yale, 1995).

The group leader's role is to provide structure and encourage constructive participation. The group leader also must be skilled in the communication techniques described earlier in the chapter. For example, if a group member has trouble remembering a word or explaining a complex situation, the group leader may ask if he or she wants help. The leader also must ensure that group members are tolerant of each other and respect each other's limits and limitations.

Because Alzheimer's disease is the common denominator in these support groups, issues surrounding living with the disease are the major themes of most discussions. The following is a list of common themes Yale (1994, 1995) noted in her support group:

- *Alzheimer's disease:* its cause, course, and current research
- *Diagnosis:* the experience of being tested, realizing the extent of the impairment
- *Changes in ability:* having problems with number tasks, getting lost, and other changes
- *Changes in lifestyle:* trying to expect less of oneself; having to depend on others for help; giving up work, driving a car, and other responsibilities
- *Family and friends:* concerns about people who do not understand or cannot bear to see the changes that are occurring
- *Uncertain future:* concerns about the progressing disease, needing more help in the future, making legal arrangements, living in the present

Activity-Oriented Groups   Activity-focused groups can accomplish much of what support groups do in terms of fostering relationships and increasing self-esteem, only in a less direct manner. People still unwilling to publicly recognize or discuss their diagnosis can be accommodated in these groups, many of which are referred to as "clubs" by the people who run them. If boredom and isolation are as much of a problem for people with Alzheimer's disease as some of their families indicate, activity groups can fulfill some important psychosocial needs.

Activity groups can encompass the range of activities described in Chapter 10. Their main purpose is to offer a comfortable social setting in which the person in the early stage can feel capable and accepted.

> The Wonderful Wednesday Club was sponsored by the local interfaith council to provide a social outlet for people with early-stage Alzheimer's disease and to provide a respite for their families. Members of the religious group took turns planning Wednesdays full of "wonderful" things to do. A factory tour during which people could see sweets being made and then sample some of them afterward was a favorite outing. Another favorite was a sing-along that followed watching a well-known choir rehearse. Trips to such places as the zoo and botanical gardens required a few more escorts to prevent people from getting lost but were equally popular and often attracted family members who could serve as escorts.

The activities selected need not be either elaborate or expensive to be therapeutic. They do need to be safe, enjoyable, and manageable for people whose cognitive processes are somewhat limited.

Middle- and Late-Stage Group Modalities

Although it has generally been assumed that people past the earliest stages of Alzheimer's disease cannot participate effectively in support groups, there is some evidence that they can benefit if given sufficient compensatory assistance by the group leader. David (1991) describes the challenges in leading such a group: communication deficits, perceptual problems, diminished insight, limited attention span, and impaired memory. Smaller numbers of participants and shorter meetings help to reduce the cognitive demands of group participation. The group leader may have to suggest subjects for discussion and assist individuals in their efforts to contribute to the group.

Several more elaborate aids may be used to enhance the sense of continuity of the group, particularly remembering what the group had discussed at previous sessions, which is threatened by poor memory. Portions of videotapes of previous meetings can be shown at the beginning of a meeting to remind group members of what transpired at earlier sessions. Instant replays can be used during meetings to review important points. The group leader or an assistant also can record key points on flip charts kept within view of group members. An even more elaborate (and potentially confusing) scheme would be to use separate flip charts for each group member to record that member's contributions during a session or from previous sessions (David, 1991).

Reminiscence Groups   Reminiscence and life review have been very popular modalities since Butler and his colleagues introduced the idea in 1963. Questions have arisen about the purposes and value of reminiscence. Is it simple recall of past events or is it a mechanism for increasing self-understanding? Does it encourage "living in the past" or is it a channel through which current problems can be solved by review of past successful and unsuccessful problem solving? Is it primarily a social activity or is it a form of therapy?

Although it has been difficult to separate the effects of reviewing the past from the interpersonal processes that accompany this sharing of memories, reminiscence and life review do appear to help people adapt to their current situations and may be a way to "exercise" remaining cognitive capacities (Parker, 1995). Reminiscence may be used in group settings to encourage individuals to interact with each other, to reduce feelings of isolation, and to increase self-esteem (Brody, 1993). However, reminiscence may not be useful for people in the late stages of Alzheimer's disease, when time confusion is more common—that is, when past and present events and people are easily confused (Feil, 1993).

The terms *reminiscence* and *life review* are sometimes used interchangeably. However, reminiscence refers to more casual sharing of memories, whereas life review refers to a structured, therapeutically oriented reflection of past experience, including the conflicts, regrets, and guilt that may have been suffered (Lashley, 1993). The latter type of life review may not be appropriate for people in the late stages of Alzheimer's disease. However, a less formal sharing of memories can be appropriate given sufficient compensatory assistance from the group facilitator. Responsibility for introducing subjects for discussion may need to be assumed by the group facilitator, although preferences and needs of group members need to be respected and used as a guide in making these choices.

A recurring topic in many reminiscence groups is the way holidays were celebrated in the past by group members. With a little prompting from the group facilitator and use of photographs or other props as additional stimuli, most group members can contribute something to the discussion.

> To evoke the memories of Christmases past, the group facilitator planned to decorate and bake cookies with members of the reminiscence group. As they became involved in these activities, group members began comparing notes on their favorite Christmas cookies and who made them in their families when they were children. The discussion expanded to the more general subject of the customs surrounding the celebration of Christmas and how they had changed over the years. The session ended with enthusiastic consumption of the products of their labors.

Topics for reminiscence are limited only by the imagination of the group and facilitator members: childhood games, school and work experiences, old movie stars, important historical events and people, and so forth. The level of complexity and difficulty of subjects introduced and requests made of members by the leader should be appropriate to the abilities of group members, of course.

Remotivation   Remotivation is another modality that has been used for many years. The purpose is to reignite the individual's interest in the world around him or her through a relatively structured group format. Remotivation is appropriate for people with moderate to severe levels of cognitive impairment. A typical remotivation group format would be as follows

> The group session always began the same way. As people came into the room, the facilitator would greet each one by name and ask the person a question or two about what had happened over the last week. As soon as everyone had arrived, the facilitator introduced the first topic, which was always something about the weather. Next, the events of the past week were briefly reviewed by the facilitator, who encouraged comments from the group. Then a sensory experience was introduced by the facilitator and group members were encouraged to actively participate in the experience (Brody, 1993).

For example, a beach experience included touching and smelling seaweed, passing around conch shells and holding them to one's ears to "hear the ocean," dipping hands in a bucket of sand, and tossing a beach ball to each other. Ocean sounds (e.g., waves, gulls, whales) were played on a tape and photographs of the sea passed around. At other sessions, slides were projected on the wall. With each of these sensory experiences, group members were encouraged to say what they felt, saw, heard, or smelled; if they liked it; what it reminded them of; and so forth.

The session always ended with recognition of each person's presence and participation in the group, reminders about the next meeting, and individual farewells.

Picture cards, word association games, drawing, and other education-oriented props may also be used. These activities are designed to involve every participant, stimulate as many senses as possible, and encourage group members to think and speak about the world around them.

Validation   As is true of most of the modalities described in this chapter, validation therapy may be used either individually or in a group setting. Developed by Naomi Feil, the approach has received increasing attention as the limitations of other approaches are recognized. The fundamental notion behind validation may be best summarized by using Feil's (1993) words: "When recent memory fails, older adults try to restore balance to their lives by retrieving earlier memories. When eyesight fails, they use the mind's eye to see. When hearing goes, they listen to sounds from the past" (p. 29).

Feil says that acknowledgment of painful feelings (e.g., fear, grief, anger) by a trusted listener will help reduce the pain for the person with Alzheimer's disease, whereas ignoring or suppressing feelings will only increase the pain. She does not recommend confronting confused older people about the inaccuracy of their perceptions or memories, however. Instead, she suggests encouraging them to talk about what they think is happening, rephrasing what they have said without questioning its validity. She also suggests asking them to talk about the worst example of what they are concerned about (e.g., somebody taking their money, knocking on their door at night) and to think about times when this problem did not occur (Feil, 1993).

In a group setting the validation approach emphasizes feelings (internal reality) rather than events or tasks (external reality). Topics are chosen to evoke expression and discussion of the internal reality. Being alone, missing loved ones (including those who have died), feeling bored or sad, and getting along with other people are a few examples of the kinds of topics that might be suggested by the group facilitator. Touch, music, and rhythmic movement also may be part of the validation group experience (Feil, 1993).

Validation therapy can be used with people in the late stages of Alzheimer's disease. Even people with limited verbal ability can participate actively in the music and rhythmic movement portions of the experience.

REFERENCES

Arkin, S. (1995). Trick or treat? The case for a rehabilitation approach to Alzheimer's. *American Journal of Alzheimer's Disease, 10*(5), 45.

Bayles, K.A., & Tomoeda, C.K. (1991). Caregiver report of prevalence and appearance order of linguistic symptoms in Alzheimer's patients. *Gerontologist, 31*(2), 210–216.

Biassou, N., Grossman, M., Onishi, K., Mickanin, J., Hughes, E., Robinson, K.M., & D'Esposito, M. (1995). Phonologic processing deficits in Alzheimer's disease. *Neurology, 45*, 2165–2169.

Bohling, H.R. (1991). Communication with Alzheimer's patients: An analysis of caregiver listening patterns. *International Journal of Aging and Human Development, 33*(4), 249–267.

Brody, C.M. (1993). Working with residents of a nursing home who have Alzheimer's disease. In C.M. Brody & V.G. Semel (Eds.), *Strategies for therapy with the elderly: Living with hope and meaning* (pp. 44–58). New York: Springer Publishing.

Butler, R.N. (1975). *Why survive? Being old in America.* New York: Harper & Row.

Clark, L.W., & Witte, K. (1991). Nature and efficacy of communication management in Alzheimer's disease. In R. Lubinski (Ed.), *Dementia and communication* (pp. 257–278). Philadelphia: Brian C. Decker.

Cohen-Mansfield, J., Marx, M.S., & Werner, P. (1992). Agitation in elderly persons: An integrative report of findings in a nursing home. *International Psychogeriatrics, 4*(Suppl. 2), 221–240.

David, P. (1991). Effectiveness of group work with the cognitively impaired older adult. *American Journal of Alzheimer's Care and Related Disorders and Research, 6*(4), 10–16.

Feil, N. (1993). *The validation breakthrough: Simple techniques for communicating with people with "Alzheimer's-type dementia."* Baltimore: Health Professions Press.

Hall, J. (1994, May/June). Only words. [Poem]. *Aging Today*, p. 13.

Jackson, M.E., Drugovich, M.L, Fretwell, M.D., Spector, W.D., Sternberg J., & Rosenstein, R.B. (1989). Prevalence and correlates of disruptive behavior in the nursing home. *Journal of Aging and Health, 1*(3), 349–369.

Kelly, J.S. (1995). Validation therapy: A case against. *Journal of Gerontological Nursing, 21*(4), 41–43.

Kemper, S., Anagnopoulos, C., Lyons, K., & Heberlein, W. (1994). Speech accommodations to dementia. *Journal of Gerontology: Psychological Sciences, 49*(5), 223–229.

Kolanowski, A. (1995). Aggressive behaviors in institutionalized elders: A theoretical framework. *American Journal of Alzheimer's Disease, 10*(2), 23–30.

Lashley, M.E. (1993). The painful side of reminiscence. *Geriatric Nursing, 14*(3), 138–141.

McGowin, D. (1997). *Living in the labyrinth: Coping with early stage Alzheimer's disease.* Paper presented at the 3rd Annual Alzheimer's Disease Educational Conference, Alzheimer's Association of Greater Palm Beach, West Palm Beach, Florida.

Mintzer, J.E., Lewis, L., Pennypaker, L., Simpson, W., Bachman, D., Wohlreich, G., Meeks, A., Hunt, S., & Sampson, R. (1993). Behavioral Intensive Care Unit (BICU): A new concept in the management of acute-agitated behavior in elderly demented patients. *Gerontologist, 33*(6), 801–806.

Parker, R.G. (1995). Reminiscence: A continuity theory framework. *Gerontologist, 35*(4), 515–525.

Spector, W.D., & Jackson, M.E. (1994). Correlates of disruptive behaviors in nursing homes: A reanalysis. *Journal of Aging and Health, 6*(2), 173–184.

Tappen, R.M., & Williams-Burgess, C. (1996, November). *Creating and maintaining therapeutic relationships in late stage Alzheimer's disease: What works, what doesn't.* Paper presented at the annual meeting of the Gerontological Society of America, Washington, DC.

Teri, L., & Logsdon R. (1990). Assessment and management of behavioral disturbances in Alzheimer's disease. *Comprehensive Therapy, 16*(5), 36–42.

Tomoeda, C.K., & Bayles, K.A. (1993). *Longitudinal effects of Alzheimer's disease on discourse production.* Alzheimer's Disease and Associated Disorders, 7(4), 223–236.

Woods, B., & McKiernan, F. (1995). Evaluating the impact of reminiscence on older people with dementia. In B.K. Haight & J. Webster (Eds.), *The art and science of reminiscing: Theory, research, methods and applications* (pp. 233–242). Washington, DC: Taylor & Francis.

Yale, R. (1994). *Early stage Alzheimer's patient support groups: Research, practice and training.* San Francisco: Special Projects Press.

Yale, R. (1995). *Developing support groups for individuals with early-stage Alzheimer's disease: Planning, implementation, and evaluation.* Baltimore: Health Professions Press.

Chapter 8

Medications

His doctor told him, "I wish I could tell you that it's cancer . . ."

Ben Haden (1989)

Probably every reader of this book knows that there is no cure for Alzheimer's disease but wishes that one existed. However, exciting breakthroughs are occurring in Alzheimer's disease research. Many of these discoveries suggest possible pharmacological treatments for Alzheimer's disease. Evidence to support this optimistic view appears in the news and the scientific literature almost weekly.

This chapter considers two groups of medications that are prescribed for people with Alzheimer's disease. The first group of drugs includes the cognition enhancers—drugs developed specifically for people with Alzheimer's disease for the purpose of helping them improve their cognitive function. The second group of drugs includes a variety of medications prescribed for the purpose of alleviating the symptoms of Alzheimer's disease, particularly anxiety, difficulty sleeping, depression, and psychotic symptoms. In the last section of the chapter some general principles related to giving medications to people with Alzheimer's disease are examined.

MEDICATIONS FOR THE TREATMENT OF COGNITIVE IMPAIRMENT

Although a variety of drugs are being tested in research studies, few have been approved for general use in the treatment of Alzheimer's disease. Few drugs have been found to be consistently effective in improving the memory and ability to learn or in halting the cognitive decline. Some promising developments have been announced, however, and several of these are mentioned in addition to the drugs that are already available.

Modification of the Amyloid Pathway

As of 1997 no drugs were available outside of clinical trials that modify the amyloid pathway (examined in Chapter 2) of Alzheimer's disease (Standaert & Young, 1996). However, there are several possible ways to prevent, modify, or reverse the amyloid cascade that is considered central to the development of the disease. The most direct approach would be manipulation of the amyloid precursor protein, a goal of much research. However, virtually any point in the process of development of β-amyloid protein and the eventual destruction of the nerve cell could be the focus of drug intervention. It may be possible, for example, to interfere with the production and accumulation of β-amyloid, reduce its toxicity, increase its solubility, or accelerate its breakdown (Whyte, Beyreuther, & Masters, 1994). Drugs with any or all of these capabilities may be available eventually to treat Alzheimer's disease.

Neurotransmitter Enhancers

The cholinergic theory (examined in Chapter 2) is the basis for a drug for Alzheimer's disease approved in 1993, tacrine hydrochloride. *Tacrine hydrochloride* (Cognex) enhances cholinergic activity by inhibiting acetylcholinesterase, an enzyme that breaks down acetylcholine (Farlow et al., 1992). The introduction of tacrine has been termed a "modest milestone" ("In Alzheimer's disease," 1994) because it helps some but not all people with Alzheimer's disease and because the improvement is usually modest although clinically observable (Schneider, 1994).

Tacrine has been shown to benefit about 30% of the people with mild to moderate Alzheimer's disease who participated in several research studies. Some were forced to discontinue the drug because of side effects. Approximately one half of the people who were able to take the drug showed statistically significant improvement on cognitive tests. Caregivers' clinical global impressions of change were also significant at both 6 and 12 weeks on the drug, but clinicians' ratings were only significant after 12 weeks (Farlow et al., 1992). In a longer study about one third of people who took the drug were rated as minimally improved while 40% experienced no change ("In Alzheimer's disease," 1994). In another study, 83% of the participants without the apo E4 allele (see Chapter 2) improved, whereas 60% of participants with the allele showed deterioration with tacrine treatment (Schneider & Forette, 1996). No evidence has been found that tacrine can reverse the effects of the disease or return individuals to their premorbid (i.e., before onset of the disease) level of function. It may slow or delay the decline, however, in people who respond well to the drug. Little information is available on its effect in people in advanced stages of Alzheimer's disease (McEvoy, 1996).

It has been suggested that there may be a specific subgroup of people with Alzheimer's disease with certain neuropathological and biochemical changes who respond favorably to tacrine (McEvoy, 1996; Small, 1992). Additional research is needed to identify the people who belong to this subgroup.

Because liver damage may occur with tacrine use, everyone who takes it should have weekly blood tests for the first 18 weeks and continue the tests at least quarterly thereafter. Almost one third of the people who took the drug also experienced gastrointestinal upsets. Patients and their families should be advised that it is important to follow the recommended dosage and schedule. Reducing or stopping the drug may cause cognitive decline and behavior disturbances and increasing the dosage may cause serious side effects. Anyone with a history of liver problems or gastric ulcer should be monitored closely or not take this drug at all ("In Alzheimer's disease," 1994).

Donepezil hydrochloride (Aricept) is a second-generation acetylcholinesterase inhibitor that has been found to be similar to tacrine in terms of its effectiveness but with fewer side effects. In one study, 30% of the participants taking donepezil hydrochloride showed improvement as compared with 16% of the participants taking a placebo. The advantage of donepezil hydrochloride over tacrine seems to be that it only needs to be taken once a day and that it is not toxic to the liver, as is tacrine (Clark & Arnold, 1997).

The action of tacrine and donepezil are directed toward prolonging the effect of acetylcholine by slowing its breakdown. *Physostigmine* (Antilirium) has a similar action. Some people with Alzheimer's disease demonstrate mild, transitory short-term memory improvement with this drug, but the benefit has been inconsistent at best (American Medical Association [AMA], 1993; Standaert & Young, 1996). A related drug, eptastigmine, has been found in an Italian study (Canal & Imbimbo, 1997) to be potentially helpful in approximately one third of the patients receiving it, when the correct dosage for the individual is found.

Physostigmine has been given alone and in combination with lecithin (McEvoy, 1996). *Lecithin* is a dietary precursor of choline (i.e, choline is derived from lecithin). Although it has not been found useful when given alone, it may have some benefit when given in combination with other drugs, including tacrine (Whyte et al., 1994). Another cholinergic agent, arecoline, may improve memory if optimal dose and stable levels of the drug can be maintained (Asthana et al., 1996).

Other neurotransmitters are affected in Alzheimer's disease. Monoamine oxidase (MAO) is an enzyme involved in the breakdown of several important neurotransmitters, including dopamine, norepinephrine, and serotonin. An inhibitor of MAO, *L-deprenyl* (Eldepryl) is used in Parkinson's disease and may have some benefit in treating Alzheimer's disease as well (McAllister & Powers, 1994; *Physicians' Desk Reference*, 1996), as could another MAO inhibitor, Lazabemide (Henriot, Kuhn, Ketler, & DePrada, 1994; Parkinson Study Group, 1996). It is possible that a combination of neurotransmitter enhancers will be used to treat Alzheimer's disease.

Nerve Growth Factor

Nerve growth factor is one member of a family of compounds called neurotrophic factors. It is thought to support nerve cell function and structural integrity. Although not considered to play a central role in the pathology of Alzheimer's disease, nerve growth factor has been found to exert a protective effect on cholinergic neurons. For example, spatial memory of aged animals is improved when nerve growth factor is injected into their brains (Fernandez, Gonzalez, Soto, Alvarez, & Quijano, 1996; Wilcock, 1993). Unfortunately, the only way to administer this drug has been by injection into the ventricles of the brain, a procedure too complicated to do on a regular basis at this writing. Propentofylline, a stimulator of nerve growth factor synthesis, may be useful for both vascular dementia and Alzheimer's disease (Mielke et al., 1996; Nakeshima, Nitta, & Hasegawa, 1993; Rother, Kittner, Rudolphi, Rossner, & Labs, 1996).

Metal Ions

Although their role in the process of neuronal destruction in Alzheimer's disease is not clear, both aluminum and iron accumulate in the plaques and tangles found in the brains of people with Alzheimer's disease. Chelating drugs (which combine with and bind the metals) such as *deferoxamine* can be used to remove the metal from the brain. More research is needed to demonstrate any real benefit from this process, however (Whyte et al., 1994).

Cognitive Enhancers

Ergoloid mesylates (Hydergine) is probably familiar to health care professionals who have worked with people with Alzheimer's disease. It has been prescribed to relieve the negative responses to decline in mental capacity (e.g., confusion, unsociability, depression, lack of self-care) in older people (McEvoy, 1996). Originally thought to act by dilating cerebral blood vessels, Hydergine is now classified as an enhancer of cerebral metabolism and neurotransmitter action. This drug has not demonstrated a significant improvement in memory and learning (McAllister & Powers, 1994), but has demonstrated a mild improvement in mood in people who take the drug (Whyte et al., 1994). It has been claimed that Hydergine slows the rate of cognitive decline, although most experts remain skeptical about its true benefits (AMA, 1993).

Another drug in this category, *acetyl-L-carnitine,* has been reported to affect both cholinergic activity and brain metabolism (Whyte et al., 1994).

Other Agents

Several other categories of drugs may influence the development and outcome of Alzheimer's disease. Anti-inflammatory drugs, such as steroids, antimalarials, and colchicine, may reduce the body's destructive response to this disease in the same way that they do for other inflammatory diseases such as arthritis (Aisen, 1996). Calcium channel blockers may reduce the rate of cognitive decline by slowing the progress of neuronal destruction (Whyte et al., 1994). Another group of compounds called nootropic agents may improve information storage and retrieval. Several hormones, such as estrogen and adrenocorticotropic hormone, and angiotensin-converting enzyme inhibitors are also considered potentially helpful.

MEDICATIONS FOR NONCOGNITIVE SYMPTOMS

The medications described in this section were not developed specifically for people with Alzheimer's disease but have been widely prescribed for such problems as anxiety, depression, insomnia, and psychosis.

Antianxiety Medications

Medications used to reduce anxiety are also known as the *minor tranquilizers*. They may be prescribed for a person with Alzheimer's disease who is experiencing extreme restlessness, agitation, or other signs of anxiety. Table 8.1 lists some common tranquilizers and their rate of onset and duration.

Once, diazepam (Valium) was often given in increasingly large doses until behavior was controlled. This approach is no longer used because of the drug's deleterious side effects, including oversedation, impaired cognitive function, and rebound agitation (Ashford & Zec, 1993). Newer drugs such as buspirone (BuSpar) seem to have fewer negative effects on cognitive function.

Relief may be experienced relatively quickly when these tranquilizers are administered. However, the drugs may accumulate in the body until they reach toxic levels, causing unsteadiness, oversedation, and speech difficulties. Other common side effects include drowsiness, lightheadedness, slowed reactions, and increased cognitive impair-

Table 8.1.   Common antianxiety drugs

Generic name	Brand name	Rate of onset	Duration of action
Alprazolam	Xanax	Intermediate	Short
Buspirone	BuSpar	Intermediate	Long
Chlordiazepoxide	Librium	Intermediate	Short
Clorazepate dipotassium	Tranxene	Fast	Long
Diazepam	Valium	Fast	Intermediate
Lorazepam	Ativan	Intermediate	Long
Oxazepam	Serax	Slow–intermediate	Short
Prazepam	Centrax	Slow	Long
Temazepam	Restoril	Slow–intermediate	Short
Triazolam	Halcion	Fast	Short

Excerpted from the *Alzheimer's Disease* Special Report, published by the Harvard Health Publications Group, © 1994, President and Fellows of Harvard College.

ment (Gregg, 1994). In fact, Baldessarini (1996b) noted that one of the most common causes of increased confusion in older people is the overuse of sedating drugs including what is generally considered a relatively small dose of a tranquilizer. Such side effects are more likely to occur when dosages and drug schedules are not adjusted to reflect the needs of older people. If any of these side effects occur, the caregiver should consult with the primary care provider to discuss the appropriate action to take. Stopping these drugs abruptly may cause severe withdrawal symptoms.

Antidepressant Medications

In general, physicians believe that antidepressants are an effective treatment for depression in people with Alzheimer's disease (Ashford & Zec, 1993). This belief does not negate the need for caution in prescribing these drugs and the value of using nonpharmacological measures first. A number of factors must be considered in selecting antidepressant medication. It is important to determine whether a person is suffering from an agitated (overactive) or a retarded (underactive) type of depression. Some antidepressants have a secondary tranquilizing, or sedating, effect that could be helpful for people with agitated-type depression but may be undesirable for people with retarded-type depression.

Of particular importance in treating people with Alzheimer's disease is the avoidance of medications that have even a moderate anticholinergic effect because this system is already disrupted by the disease (see Table 8.2) (Ashford & Zec, 1993). Common anticholinergic side effects include impaired memory and constipation.

Confusion or delirium, including memory problems, may occur in as many as 30% of people over age 50 when taking some of these drugs. These side effects are often

Table 8.2.   Common antidepressant drugs

Generic name	Brand name	Likelihood of side effects		
		Anticholinergic	Sedation	Orthostatic hypotension
Amitriptyline	Elavil, Endep, Etrafon, Limbitrol, Triavil	High	High	High
Amoxapine	Asendin	Low	Moderate	Moderate
Bupropion	Wellbutrin	Low	Low	Low
Clomipramine	Anafranil	High	High	High
Desipramine	Norpramin	Low	Low	Low
Doxepin	Sinequan, Adapin	Moderate–high	High	High
Fluoxetine	Prozac	Low	Low	Low
Imipramine	Tofranil	Moderate	Moderate	Moderate
Maprotiline	Ludiomil	Low	High	Low
Nortriptyline	Pamelor	Low	Low	Low
Paroxetine	Paxil	Low	Low	Low
Sertraline	Zoloft	Low	Low	Low
Trazodone	Desyrel	Low	High	Moderate
Trimipramine	Surmontil	Moderate	High	High

Excerpted from the *Alzheimer's Disease* Special Report, published by the Harvard Health Publications Group, © 1994, President and Fellows of Harvard College.

overlooked or assumed to be a result of the illness rather than a side effect of the drug, especially in older adults (Baldessarini, 1996a). The most serious side effects are heartbeat irregularities, hypotension, seizures, and coma (AMA, 1993). Table 8.2 lists the common antidepressant drugs and their anticholinergic, sedative, and orthostatic hypotension effects.

One group of antidepressants, the MAO inhibitors, can react with certain foods to cause a hypertensive crisis. This is of particular concern in people with Alzheimer's disease, who may not remember instructions about the dietary restrictions necessary to prevent these side effects.

Unlike the minor tranquilizers, which act rapidly, it may take several days or even weeks before the full benefit of an antidepressant is realized. The antidepressant drug trazodone (Desyrel) has a calming effect that is useful when anxiety accompanies the depression, but it may cause postural hypotension (a drop in blood pressure when the person stands up). Fluoxetine (Prozac) is a frequently used but controversial drug. Others that may be appropriate for people with Alzheimer's disease include desipramine (Norpramin), nortriptyline (Pamelor), and bupropion (Wellbutrin). Ashford and Zec recommend that physicians "start low and go slow" (1993, p. 600) when prescribing antidepressant drugs for people with Alzheimer's disease, advice that is appropriate for antipsychotic medications as well.

Antipsychotic Medications

The antipsychotic drugs are also called *neuroleptics* or the *major tranquilizers*. These powerful drugs must be used with caution in older people, especially those with Alzheimer's disease.

Despite the well-publicized drawbacks of using these drugs, there is still some concern about their continued overuse, especially in long-term care facilities (AMA, 1993). Baldessarini (1996b) observed that their use alone "does not constitute optimal care of psychotic patients" (p. 4117). In addition, antipsychotic medications—or any medication—should never be used merely to sedate a person who is an annoyance to staff. The use of drugs to control behavior that could be treated without drugs is called *chemical restraint* (as compared with mechanical restraint, which is the use of devices such as belts and straps to restrict a person's movement) and is restricted by both state and federal regulations.

In addition, antipsychotic drugs have many side effects, some of which occur at relatively low doses. These side effects may include blurred vision, dry mouth, urinary retention, constipation, oversedation, orthostatic hypotension, dizziness, and increased cognitive impairment. The oversedated patient may become silent, withdrawn, and immobile, with all of the negative consequences of immobility, or may attempt to remain mobile despite the effects of the drugs, which often leads to falls and serious fractures (AMA, 1993). Extrapyramidal symptoms that resemble Parkinson's disease may occur. These symptoms include slow movement, tremors, shuffling gait, drooling, and a mask-like expression. Paradoxical reactions may also occur. People taking these drugs may become more agitated and this, in turn, may lead to the prescription of more drugs if symptoms are misinterpreted (Gregg, 1994).

The so-called high-potency antipsychotic drugs, such as haloperidol (Haldol), are preferred for people with Alzheimer's disease because they have fewer anticholinergic effects. Unfortunately, they usually cause more extrapyramidal symptoms. Chlorpromazine (Thorazine) and thioridazine (Mellaril) are low-potency neuroleptics that cause high levels of sedation and anticholinergic side effects but fewer extrapyramidal effects (Ashford & Zec, 1993; Gregg, 1994). Table 8.3 lists the common high-, moderate-, and low-potency antipsychotic medications in use.

Sleep Medications

People with Alzheimer's disease often experience sleep disturbances. These problems are believed to be related to the disruption of circadian rhythms resulting from damage in the basal forebrain. A common pattern is napping during the day with difficulty getting to sleep and staying asleep at night.

As with anxiety, depression, and psychotic symptoms, nondrug treatments are preferable and should be attempted before resorting to medication. Some people with Alzheimer's disease are able to sleep well at night if they are kept busy during the day. Inclusion of some type of exercise is especially helpful. Caffeine (from coffee, tea, cola drinks, and chocolate) and nicotine (from cigarettes and other tobacco products) are stimulants that should be reduced or eliminated altogether in people who have difficulty sleeping (Ashford & Zec, 1993).

Because sleep medications may increase confusion and cause rebound insomnia (i.e., strong opposite reaction caused by withdrawal from drug) (AMA, 1993), they should be used only when absolutely necessary. Many of the medications mentioned in previous sections have a sedative effect that may be useful in alleviating sleep problems if they are given at bedtime. If necessary, triazolam (Halcion) or temazepam (Restoril) may be given (Ashford & Zec, 1993). All of the precautions examined in the following section must be kept in mind when prescribing these drugs to people with Alzheimer's disease.

GUIDELINES FOR THE SAFE USE OF MEDICATIONS IN PEOPLE WITH ALZHEIMER'S DISEASE

The majority of people with Alzheimer's disease are older adults who have some physiological vulnerability to medications as a result of both the aging process and compromised brain function. This double jeopardy makes it particularly important to exercise caution in prescribing and administering any medication to a person with Alzheimer's disease. This final section examines some of the effects of aging on the body's response to drugs and considers some precautions specific to giving medications to people with Alzheimer's disease.

Effects of Aging

Although there are some important exceptions, as a rule, older people, especially old-old people (people over age 80), require lower doses of medication than do younger people. Several reasons for this exist, including increased sensitivity to drugs, changes in the distribution of fat throughout the body, and slower clearance and elimination of many drugs.

Most drugs target a certain type of cell in the human body. These targeted cells have receptors on which the drugs act. As people grow older, most of these receptors become more sensitive (an exception is β-adrenergic receptors), which magnifies the effects of the drugs given. The result is that the same amount of medication given to an older person usually has a greater effect than it would on a younger person. For example, older people may obtain more relief from the same dose of an antinausea drug than do younger people. They are also more sensitive to the effects of anticoagulants and may

Table 8.3.   Common antipsychotic drugs

Generic name	Brand name	Likelihood of side effects		
		Sedation	Anticholinergic	Extrapyramidal
Low Potency				
Chlorpromazine	Thorazine	High	High	Low
Thioridazine	Mellaril	High	High	Low
Intermediate Potency				
Molindone	Moban	Moderate	Moderate	Moderate
Loxapine succinate	Loxitane	Moderate	Moderate	Moderate
Perphenazine	Trilafon	Moderate	Moderate	Moderate
High Potency				
Haloperidol	Haldol	Low	Low	High
Fluphenazine	Prolixin	Low	Low	High
Thiothixene	Navane	Low	Low	High
Trifluoperazine	Stelazine	Low	Low	High

Excerpted from the *Alzheimer's Disease* Special Report, published by the Harvard Health Publications Group, © 1994, President and Fellows of Harvard College.

need to be given smaller doses to prevent excessive bleeding (White, 1993). The primary disadvantage of this increased sensitivity is that older people may develop toxicity at what is generally considered a normal dose or blood level of a drug (Avorn & Gurwitz, 1990).

Another change that occurs as people age is that body fat is redistributed. The cushion of fat that lies under the skin decreases in the extremities (arms and legs). Drugs that are fat soluble are concentrated in the fatty tissues; water-soluble drugs are concentrated in lean areas. Changes in the distribution of fat in the body thus affect the action of both fat-soluble and water-soluble drugs.

Clearance and elimination of drugs also change with age. Most drugs are cleared out of the body through either the liver or the kidneys. As the body ages, the blood flow to the liver diminishes and the liver actually decreases in size. Some changes in kidney function also occur, although these are more variable from individual to individual. If clearance and eventual elimination of a drug is slowed, then the drug remains in the system longer. If given in the usual amounts the drug may accumulate to the point at which it becomes toxic to the older person (Avorn & Gurwitz, 1990; Resnick, 1997).

The sleep medication flurazepam (Dalmane) provides a good example of the differences in drug responses of younger and older people. The half-life (i.e., time to eliminate half of the drug from the body) of this sleep medication is 160 hours in older people compared with 74 hours in younger people. The longer half-life in older people is the result of slower clearance by the liver and differences in distribution of this fat-soluble drug. If an older person consumes an alcoholic beverage the day after taking this medication, he or she may experience an additive effect from flurazepam and the alcohol. One's ability to drive a car also may be impaired the day after taking this drug (*Physicians' Desk Reference*, 1996). Using a lower dose, a greater interval between doses, or both can ameliorate the problem (Avorn & Gurwitz, 1990). It might be better for older adults to avoid flurazepam altogether, if possible.

Many drugs, including the antidepressants and antipsychotics described earlier, can cause symptoms that are mistaken for dementia. Adding these side effects to an already compromised cognitive system can produce profound impairment and even premature placement in a long-term care facility when the source of the increased impairment is not recognized.

Adding to the complexity of selecting an appropriate drug is the fact that various drugs interact with each other in both beneficial and harmful ways. Some drugs block the action of other drugs, rendering them ineffective. Caffeine, for example, is a stimulant that can interfere with the effect of a sleep medication. Both haloperidol and chlorpromazine block the uptake of the antihypertensive medication guanethidine (Ismelin), reducing its effectiveness and thereby raising blood pressure.

Other drugs potentiate one another (i.e., make them more potent than they would be if taken alone). An interaction of particular interest in people with Alzheimer's disease is the effect of haloperidol on the levels of a group of antidepressants known as the tricyclics. When given in combination, haloperidol increases the blood levels of the tricyclics (Stockley, 1991). This interaction is a common cause of overmedication in people with Alzheimer's disease (Stockley, 1991).

The potential exists for *subclinical* side effects that may continue for years without being noted. The older person may experience some additional unsteadiness, a slight decrease in memory, or a mild depression that is mistaken for a sign of aging. Any of these effects can be a time bomb leading to serious and sometimes irreversible damage by the point they are noted (Avorn & Gurwitz, 1990). Well-informed, observant caregivers and geriatricians are most likely to note these changes before they become serious problems.

Another common problem is a kind of prescribing inertia that occurs once an older person is placed on a medication (Gurwitz, 1994). Often, there is great reluctance to take the person off the medication, even when the problem for which it was originally prescribed has been resolved. This inertia has occurred for years with the heart medicine digoxin. It may also happen with the drugs prescribed for noncognitive problems described in this chapter. These problems are not relatively rare, nor are they confined to people in long-term care facilities. A research study using a national probability sample found that almost one quarter of the community-dwelling people over age 65 had been prescribed drugs judged to be inappropriate on the basis of their being ineffective, more toxic than available alternatives, or likely to adversely affect the central nervous system in these people (Willcox, Himmelstein, & Woolhandler, 1994).

One solution to the inertia is a regular review of the continuing necessity of all medications, prescriptions, and over-the-counter drugs an individual is receiving. Another solution is the institution of *drug holidays*, during which the older person is taken off all but life-sustaining medications and observed carefully for any untoward effects. Drug holidays not only help identify prescriptions that are no longer needed but also reduce the overaccumulation of those drugs that will be restarted after the holiday is over. Drug holidays should be instituted only under professional supervision.

Precautions in Giving Medications

A number of ways in which both formal and informal caregivers can make the use of medications safer for the person with Alzheimer's disease are available (Alzheimer's Association, 1990).

Make Sure Caregivers Are Well-Informed   The well-informed caregiver can frequently prevent major problems by noting untoward effects early and bringing them to the attention of the prescribing physician. The caregiver should know the reason that

any medication was prescribed, any reactions that may occur with the drug, and how to respond to these reactions—particularly which reactions are serious enough to require immediate medical attention and whether discontinuing the drug would have serious consequences.

Keep the Physician Informed   Caregivers also should ensure that any physician who prescribes a medication for the person with Alzheimer's disease knows every drug that person is taking, including over-the-counter preparations such as cold medicines or allergy drugs. Even at home, it may be helpful to write down the time and date of any problem that occurs. In long-term care facilities, careful record keeping is required by law.

Develop a Routine   Most long-term care facilities have well-organized routines for giving medications. Although such formal systems are not needed at home, it is helpful to develop a consistent routine. Some people find plastic pill organizers helpful; others prefer a calendar on which to record medications. Providing reminders for the person with Alzheimer's disease may be necessary. Making medication administration part of a consistent routine is also helpful to the person whose capacity to process new information is limited.

Provide Supervision   Even people without memory problems sometimes forget to take their medications. At other times they are not sure they took them and take them twice by mistake. The person with Alzheimer's disease has even more trouble remembering, and therefore is more likely to take too much or too little medication by mistake if unsupervised. To ensure that all medications are taken and that none has been spit out and picked up by children or pets, the caregiver should observe the person taking the medication. If the person has difficulty swallowing pills, the medication may be crushed and placed in applesauce or similar food, or a liquid form may be obtained. Some medications cannot be crushed, so caregivers should consult a physician, pharmacist, or nurse before doing trying to do so.

Keep Medications in a Safe Place   To avoid potential overdoses, caregivers should lock up medications and not leave the person alone with medication containers.

Prepare for Emergencies   Caregivers should post the telephone number of the poison control center, nearest emergency room, and police and fire rescue or ambulance service by the telephone in case of an emergency, drug related or otherwise. It also may be helpful to know in advance what pharmacies are open on weekends and during holidays in case the person with Alzheimer's disease runs out of medication and to keep an up-to-date list of drugs and their dosages in case of an emergency.

REFERENCES

Aisen, P.S. (1996). Inflammation and Alzheimer's disease. *Molecular and Chemical Neuropathology*, 28(1), 83–88.

Alzheimer's Association. (1990). *Medication.* Chicago: Author.

American Medical Association. (1993). *Drug evaluation annual 1993.* Chicago: Author.

Ashford, J.W., & Zec, R.F. (1993). Pharmacological treatment in Alzheimer's disease. In R.W. Parks, R.F. Zec, & R.S. Wilson (Eds.), *Neuropsychology of Alzheimer's disease and other dementias.* New York: Oxford University Press.

Asthana, S., Greig, N.H., Holloway, H.W., Raffaele, K.C., Berardi, A., Schapiro, M.B., Rapoport, S.I., & Soncrant, T.T. (1996). Clinical pharmacokinetics of arecholine in subjects with Alzheimer's disease. *Clinical Pharmacology and Therapeutics, 60*(2), 276–282.

Avorn, J., & Gurwitz, J. (1990). Principles of pharmacology. In C.K. Cassel, D.E. Riesenberg, L.B. Sorenson, & J.R. Walsh (Eds.), *Geriatric medicine.* New York: Springer-Verlag.

Baldessarini, R.J. (1996a). Drugs and the treatment of psychiatric disorders: Depression and mania. In J.G. Hardman & L.E. Limbird (Eds.), *Goodman and Gilman's the pharmacological basis of therapeutics* (9th ed., pp. 431–459). New York: McGraw-Hill.

Baldessarini, R.J. (1996b). Drugs and the treatment of psychiatric disorders: Psychosis and anxiety. In J.G. Hardman & L.E. Limbird (Eds.), *Goodman and Gilman's the pharmacological basis of therapeutics* (9th ed., pp. 399–430). New York: McGraw-Hill.

Canal, N., & Imbimbo, B.P. (1996). Relationship between pharmacodynamic activity and cognitive effects of eptastigmine in patients with Alzheimer's disease. *Clinical Pharmacology and Therapeutics, 60*(2), 218–220.

Clark, C.M., & Arnold, S.E. (1997). Alzheimer's disease. In R.E. Rakel (Ed.), *Conn's current therapy* (pp. 872–877). Philadelphia: W.B. Saunders.

Farlow, M., Gracon, S.I., Hershey, L.A., Lewis, K.W., Sadowsky, C.H., & Dolan-Ureno, J. (1992). A controlled trial of tacrine in Alzheimer's disease. *Journal of the American Medical Association, 268*(18), 2523–2529.

Fernandez, C.I., Gonzalez, O., Soto, J., Alvarez, J., & Quijano, Z. (1996). Effects of chronic infusion of nerve growth factor (NGF) in AF64A-lesioned rats. *Molecular and Chemical Neuropathology, 28*(1), 175–179.

Gregg, D. (1994). *Alzheimer's disease.* Boston: Harvard Medical School Health Publications.

Gurwitz, J.H. (1994). Suboptimal medication use in the elderly: The tip of the iceberg. *Journal of the American Medical Association, 272*(4), 316–317.

Haden, B. (1989). Foreword. In R. Davis. *My journey into Alzheimer's disease* (p. 9). Wheaton, IL: Tyndale House.

Henriot, S., Kuhn, C., Ketler, R., & DePrada, M. (1994). Lazabemidl, a reversible and highly sensitive MAO-3 inhibitor: Preclinical and clinical findings. *Journal of Neural Transmission (Supplement), 41*, 321–325.

In Alzheimer's disease, a modest milestone. (1994). *American Journal of Nursing, 94*(3), 58–62.

McAllister, T.W., & Powers, R. (1994). Approaches to the treatment of dementing illness. In V.O.B. Emery & T.E. Oxman (Eds.), *Dementia: Presentations, differential diagnosis and nosology* (pp. 355–383). Baltimore: The Johns Hopkins University Press.

McEvoy, G.G. (1996). *American Hospital Formulary Service.* Bethesda, MD: American Society of Health-System Pharmacists.

Mielke, R., Kittner, B., Ghaemi, M., Kessler, J., Szelies, B., Herholz, K., & Heiss, W.D. (1996). Propentofylline improves regional cerebral glucose metabolism and neuropsychological performance in vascular dementia. *Journal of Neurological Science, 141*(1–2), 59–64.

Nakeshima, T., Nitta, A., & Hasegawa, T. (1993). Impairment of learning and memory and the accessory symptom in aged rat as senile dementia model. III: Oral administration of propentofylline produces recovery of reduced NGF content on the brain of aged rats. *Yakubutsu Seishin Koda, 13*, 89–95.

Parkinson Study Group. (1996). Effect of Lazabemide on the progression of disability in early Parkinson disease. *Annals of Neurology, 40*, 90–107.

Physicians' desk reference. (1996). Montvale, NJ: Medical Economics Data Production Co.

Resnick, N.M. (1997). Geriatric medicine. In L.M. Turney, S.J. McPhee, & M.A. Papadakis (Eds.), *Current medical diagnosis and treatment 1997* (pp. 48–68). Stamford, CT: Appleton & Lange.

Rother, M., Kittner, B., Rudolphi, K., Rossner, M., & Labs, M.H. (1996). HWA 285 (propento-fylline), a new compound for the treatment of both vascular dementia and dementia of the Alzheimer type. *Annals of the New York Academy of Science, 777,* 404–409.

Schneider, L.S. (1994). Tacrine development experience: Early clinical trials and enrichment and parallel designs. *Alzheimer Disease and Associated Disorders, 8*(Suppl. 2), S12–S21.

Schneider, L.S., & Forette, F. (1996). Alzheimer's disease symptomatic drugs: Tacrine. In S. Gauthier (Ed.), *Clinical diagnosis and management of Alzheimer's disease* (pp. 221–237). Boston: Butterworth-Heinemann.

Small, G.W. (1992). Tacrine for treating Alzheimer's disease [Editorial]. *Journal of the American Medical Association, 268*(18), 2564–2565.

Standaert, D.G., & Young, A.B. (1996). Treatment of central nervous system disorders. In J.G. Hardman & L.E. Limbird (Eds.), *Goodman and Gilman's the pharmacological basis of therapeutics* (9th ed., pp. 503–517). New York: McGraw-Hill.

Stockley, I.H. (1991). *Drug interactions: A sourcebook of drug interaction, their mechanisms, clinical importance and management.* Oxford, England: Blackwell Scientific Publications.

White, C. (1993). Medications and the elderly. In D.L. Carnevali & M. Patrick (Eds.), *Nursing management for the elderly* (pp. 171–191). Philadelphia: J.B. Lippincott.

Whyte, S., Beyreuther, K., & Masters, C.L. (1994). Rational therapeutic strategies in Alzheimer's disease. In D.B. Calne (Ed.), *Neurodegenerative diseases.* Philadelphia: W.B. Saunders.

Wilcock, G.K. (1993). *The management of Alzheimer's disease.* Petersfield, England: Wrightson Biomedical Publishing Ltd.

Willcox, S.M., Himmelstein, D.V., & Woolhandler, S. (1994). Inappropriate drug prescribing for the community-dwelling elderly. *Journal of the American Medical Association, 272,* 292–296.

Chapter 9

Rehabilitation in Activities of Daily Living

[L]ife was simpler . . . before I lost all the instructions.

McGowin (1993)

Much of our daily routine—getting up, dressing, having breakfast—seems automatic to us. These tasks are so overlearned that we can "do them in our sleep." A change in routine makes us conscious of them: the alarm did not go off, there is no milk for the coffee, the car will not start. When the task environment changes, the usually automatic routine becomes effortful. Adding the effects of Alzheimer's disease to a change in routine would make the tasks even more effortful. In the late stages of the disease, getting dressed and having breakfast become major accomplishments.

These ordinary activities each one of us does every day of our lives can be divided into two categories. The *basic* activities of daily living (ADLs) are those tasks most of us do every day with little thought: bathing, dressing, grooming, eating, using the toilet. The *instrumental*, or independent, activities of daily living (IADLs) are just as ordinary but more complex: shopping, cleaning, doing laundry, making telephone calls, writing checks, driving the car, taking a bus to work.

Difficulty with some of the IADLs—in particular, balancing a checkbook and driving a car—appears relatively early in Alzheimer's disease. Problems with carrying out the basic ADLs appear later and progress from the minor decision-making deficits, such as selecting the right clothes, to profound difficulty in carrying out any tasks. It is important to keep in mind that the major source of difficulty with IADLs and ADLs lies with the thinking required, not with the physical performance requirements of the task (Thralow & Reuter, 1993). Physical impairment can, of course, occur in addition to the cognitive impairment that interferes with performance of IADLs and ADLs.

A story is told by people who care for individuals with Alzheimer's disease that is worth repeating:

> Bessie found her husband, Robert, sitting backward and fully clothed on the toilet. He was flushing the toilet again and again and muttering "Damn it, damn it."
>
> "Robert, what are you doing?" she asked him.
>
> "I can't get this darn thing out of second gear!"

Robert's confusion of toilet and automobile exemplifies the kind of cognitive problem that interferes with carrying out ADLs.

This chapter examines rehabilitation in ADLs and IADLs for people with Alzheimer's disease. Following a discussion of the cognitive processing underlying the performance of the tasks of everyday life, and the processing failures that can result from the degenerative effects of Alzheimer's disease, the chapter describes a rehabilitative approach to maximizing function and maintaining the dignity of people with Alzheimer's disease. Each of the most important IADLs and ADLs is described, along with some general principles, including the use of graded assistance with basic ADLs.

TASKS OF EVERYDAY LIFE

A Theoretical Perspective

A simple task such as preparing toast and coffee for breakfast actually involves a number of separate steps, each of which requires some cognitive processing. For example, making coffee requires either pouring hot water and instant coffee into a cup or adding coffee and water to a coffeemaker, turning it on, and later pouring it into a cup. These are the individual steps or details of a task that cognitive psychologists believe are processed within separate *cognitive subsystems* (see Figure 9.1). These cognitive subsystems are organized into larger *schemata* that integrate the separate tasks into familiar routines, such as driving a car or making coffee. These schemata are relatively automatic. However, the *supervisory attentional system* is not. The supervisory attentional system is needed to oversee the selection and use of the cognitive subsystems and schemata (an example can be found in Figure 9.2). When something happens that makes it necessary to alter the routine (e.g., the power goes out while preparing breakfast, the car stalls in heavy traffic), the supervisory attentional system inhibits or changes the automatic routines of the schemata and their cognitive subsystems in order to respond appropriately to the situation (Tupper & Cicerone, 1991). This inhibition or change is generally thought to occur in the frontal lobes.

Processing Failures

Any level of cognitive processing can be faulty or damaged by brain injury or a degenerative disease such as Alzheimer's disease. A number of different kinds of failures can occur, and careful observation of the person as he or she carries out a task is needed to identify the type. Tupper and Cicerone (1991) noted the following common types of failure:

> *Selection*—an inappropriate action is substituted for the correct one (e.g., the person sits on the toilet instead of getting into the shower, the person puts on a coat and hat instead of getting ready for bed).

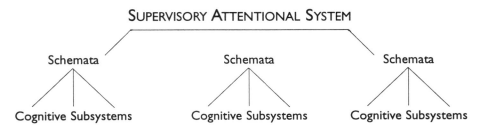

Figure 9.1. Hierarchical levels of cognitive processing. (Adapted from Tupper & Cicerone, 1991.)

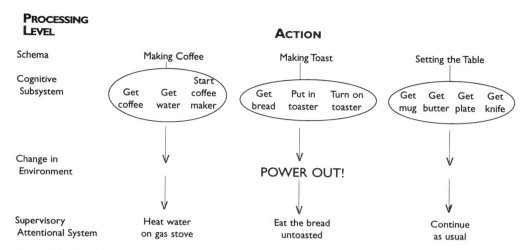

Figure 9.2. Cognitive processing of a routine task: preparing toast and coffee for breakfast.

Storage failure—the person forgets what he or she meant to do (e.g., the person goes to the kitchen but cannot remember what he or she wanted; the person places his or her glasses in a desk drawer and then cannot remember where they are).

Discrimination failure—the wrong person or object is chosen during completion of a task (e.g., the person pours dishwasher detergent into the coffeemaker instead of coffee, or the person squeezes hair gel instead of toothpaste on a toothbrush).

Test failure—task performance is terminated too soon or continued too long (e.g., the person washes only the front and not the back, the person begins combing his or her hair and then forgets to stop).

It is worth noting that both storage and selection failures are common in people with normal cognitive function. Once the type of failure is identified, intervention can be targeted to the specific problem.

Two other factors that contribute to processing failures are distraction and multitasking. Television, radio, other people's conversations, and similar *distractions* can draw the person's attention away from the task at hand. Distraction can become a serious problem in the later stages of Alzheimer's disease. Reducing or eliminating any type of distraction (e.g., moving to a quieter room, closing the door, turning off the television) is often a major factor in assisting the person to carry out a task to completion.

Attempting more than one task at a time (*multitasking*) also increases the likelihood of failure. It places too great a demand on compromised function by calling for attention to two or more tasks when the person already has difficulty attending to even one. Multitasking also multiplies the complexity of the demand, frequently beyond the capacity of the individual. Caregivers often find, for example, that telling the person with Alzheimer's disease to do one step at a time makes it easier to accomplish a multistep task. For example, rather than ask the person to help prepare lunch, the caregiver should divide the task into simpler steps (e.g., wash the lettuce, peel the carrots, take out the bread).

A Rehabilitative Approach

The purpose of a rehabilitative approach is to help the person with Alzheimer's disease maintain or regain as much independence as possible, for as long as possible, without endangering the health and safety of the person or other people. This approach is based on the belief that independent function provides a sense of control and accomplishment, which the person experiences less and less as the disease progresses. It also helps increase self-esteem and reduce the burden on the caregiver. Much of this section is based on the concepts of excess disability, enablement, and procedural memory, examined in Chapters 1 and 4.

In order to maintain or regain as much function as possible, the person with Alzheimer's disease should be provided with only as much assistance as is needed. Caregivers in a hurry may do much more for the person than is necessary. A common example is nursing assistants feeding residents of nursing facilities, even when the residents can feed themselves. Even family members may do this, especially if they become impatient with the slow and frequently error-laden efforts of the person. Family caregivers sometimes provide too much help out of a misguided attempt to shield the person from evidence of his or her deficits.

Tupper and Cicerone (1991) suggested a general framework for remediation after brain injury that is also appropriate for a rehabilitative approach with people with Alzheimer's disease. They divided the universe of intervention-oriented activities into three categories: 1) activities that create a facilitative environment, 2) activities that provide instrumental assistance and information, and 3) activities that increase the person's awareness of his or her capabilities and the application of the skills learned to real-life situations (metacognitive approach).

Facilitative activities are those that establish a supportive, therapeutic environment in which the person can achieve his or her highest possible level of functioning. These activities include actively engaging the person in the rehabilitative effort, providing feedback on the person's performance, and encouraging efforts to improve performance. Praise is an important part of this approach. Some experts also recommend using a concrete reward, such as cookies or a drink of juice, when working with people in the later stages of Alzheimer's disease (Beck, Heacock, Rapp, & Mercer, 1993). A particularly important aspect of treatment of people with Alzheimer's disease is to limit their frustration to tolerable levels. This is a fundamental principle behind the graded assistance approach that is described in detail in the section on the basic ADLs (p. 127).

Frequently overlooked when treating the person with Alzheimer's disease is the need to develop goals collaboratively. Many caregivers assume that the person cannot comprehend goals and, as a consequence, do not discuss them at all with him or her. This is unfortunate because it eliminates a major source of motivation. As indicated in Chapter 8, using simple terms facilitates communication of some fairly complex ideas. Even people in the advanced stages of Alzheimer's disease can understand the idea of working toward "walking better" or "feeding yourself." Responding to the emotional highs and lows of success and failure in task performance is another important part of facilitating rehabilitation in the ADLs.

Instrumental treatment actions (not to be confused with IADLs) are the core of the rehabilitative approach. They involve specific training designed to help the person maintain or regain function. As the person practices the task under the guidance of the caregiver, the caregiver assesses the types of deficits the person has, provides instruction on correct performance of the task (again, in simple terms), carefully monitors the person's success in performing the task, and provides assistance as needed to prevent discouragement. Research indicates that individuals with Alzheimer's disease benefit more from consistent rather than variable practice (Dick et al., 1996). Practice in using the same movement patterns, rather than changing the way a task is carried out, is most likely to help them improve and maintain their ability to perform the basic ADLs.

The caregiver may demonstrate the correct behavior so that the person can imitate it. Pacing may be important if the person is trying to complete the task too quickly. The caregiver may also provide simple explanations of why the person's accustomed way of performing the task must be modified.

Metacognitive activities are those that increase the person's awareness of his or her performance and help the person understand how to apply the learning to the daily routine. Gentle correction of incorrect or inappropriate behavior is helpful to people with Alzheimer's disease, especially to those who seem to be unaware of their increasing deficits.

It is also helpful to point out how the person can use improved skills outside of the treatment session. For example, the caregiver can say, "When your son comes tomorrow, you can show him the way to the auditorium now that you've learned how to get there," or "Now you can pick out your own clothes for church tomorrow." However, the ability of the individual with Alzheimer's disease to transfer learning from one situation to another may be limited.

INSTRUMENTAL ACTIVITIES OF DAILY LIVING

Independent performance of IADLs is a hallmark of the competent adult. Relinquishing any one of these activities is often a painful experience for the person with physical or cognitive impairment. It may also be harder for families of people with cognitive impairment to recognize the need to give up these hallmarks of adulthood because the person is still physically capable of performing such tasks, although he or she is cognitively unable to do them well or safely.

Employment

As retirement age moves upward from 65, more people may demonstrate the earliest signs of Alzheimer's disease while still employed. Alzheimer's disease strikes people in executive positions as well as those in menial positions. Surgeons, judges, and statesmen may develop Alzheimer's disease. Diminishing competence is dangerous in many of these positions. For some people, such as airline pilots, rigorous testing programs will detect cognitive losses, and retirement will be mandatory. For others, such as surgeons, teachers, or other professionals, whose work is open to the scrutiny of colleagues and the public, steps may be taken to remove them from their positions if they do not remove themselves.

In those jobs that require more physical ability than problem-solving or reasoning ability, people with Alzheimer's disease may be able to maintain employment longer. These positions might include house cleaning, lifting and moving goods, doorman and watchman positions, and serving meals in a cafeteria line. Eventually, however, the disease interferes with even these jobs. Inability to use public transportation to get to work, inability to learn new job skills, problems finding one's way around the facility, and, later, difficulty recognizing co-workers or customers eventually leads to dismissal if the individual does not leave first.

Many people with early-stage Alzheimer's disease try to hide their deficits in situations such as the workplace. They become guarded and avoid situations in which their deficits are apparent. In general, the literature on Alzheimer's disease has indicated that many people with Alzheimer's disease are not aware of their deficits. It is likely, however, that the guardedness that they develop as a defense mechanism has been mistaken for denial or lack of awareness.

Being forced to leave one's job can be a source of great guilt and shame (McGowin, 1993). Work is an important part of many people's lives and identities. In fact, many people in the middle stages of Alzheimer's disease who attend day programs refer to the program as their "work," just one small indication of the centrality of work in the lives of most adults. For these reasons, people in the early stages of Alzheimer's disease may try to maintain their position in the workplace beyond the limits of their ability to do so.

The caregiver who must confront their resistance needs to do so with sensitivity and understanding as well as firmness. For some individuals, advice from a physician to stop working may be the most acceptable way to leave. Approaching the need to stop working as "time to retire" may make relinquishing work acceptable for the person with Alzheimer's disease. Many people with Alzheimer's disease are actually relieved that the decision has been made for them and that the charade is over. In any case, employment is rarely an option beyond the early stages of the disease.

Driving

Giving up work is an anticipated event of the later years. Giving up driving, however, is not expected until much later, if at all. Relinquishing driving symbolizes the end of independence and control. The feared results are dependence, isolation, and helplessness (Shemon & Christensen, 1991).

Like many of the skills needed in the workplace, safe driving requires a complex set of abilities: judgment; attention; adequate reaction time; good vision and hearing; and some physical agility of the head, arms, and legs. Age alone can diminish some of these abilities. Many older drivers voluntarily restrict their driving to daytime hours and neighborhood streets to accommodate these changes (Marottoli et al., 1993).

The literature contains some evidence that people with Alzheimer's disease are involved in more accidents than normal, perhaps as much as twice as many accidents (Tuokko, 1992). In the early stages of the disease some family caregivers ride with the person in order to help him or her drive more safely. The family member can remind the person with Alzheimer's disease to check the rearview mirror, stop at a stop sign, and avoid many of the potential mishaps without taking driving privileges away altogether. Driving tests of people with Alzheimer's disease indicate that they do have problems in a number of areas: understanding road signs, staying in the proper lane, using signals and checking blind spots, coming to complete stops at stop signs, and using the gas and brake pedals correctly (Shemon & Christensen, 1991).

Becoming lost while driving is another problem frequently reported by people with Alzheimer's disease and their families. People with Alzheimer's disease often describe driving around for hours until they either figure out how to reach home or finally ask for directions. Drawing simple maps of the route to be taken and writing out directions for getting home may be helpful to people in the early stages of Alzheimer's disease.

Some experts believe that people with Alzheimer's disease should discontinue driving as soon as the disease is diagnosed. However, as awareness of the disease increases and diagnoses are made earlier, this rule may be too strict. People in the earliest stages of Alzheimer's disease may be able to safely navigate familiar routes for quite some time. Those who have been careful and competent drivers may represent better risks than those who were always poor drivers.

When the person with Alzheimer's disease shows poor judgment, inattentiveness, slow or inappropriate reaction, or reduced physical agility, he or she should no longer drive (Gregg, 1994). In some areas of the United States written and skill-based driving tests may be available at memory disorder centers or rehabilitation centers. The results of a study on driving ability in people with Alzheimer's disease suggest that those with a Mini-Mental Examination score of 22 or less should be evaluated for their ability to continue driving (Shua-Haim & Gross, 1996). Official motor vehicle tests can also be considered, but the personnel of these offices are generally not prepared to deal with people with Alzheimer's disease.

How does one broach the subject of giving up driving? Suggesting that the car is unsafe may be more acceptable to the person than the suggestion that he or she is an unsafe driver. Often, families are concerned about the person's reaction to confrontations over issues such as driving and welcome the support and intervention of professionals in this matter. Gregg (1994) suggests obtaining a written prescription from the physician that simply says DO NOT DRIVE. People who never cared much about driving may stop driving willingly. Others become frightened after a mishap or close call and are also willing to stop. Some families find that their loved one is willing to stop driving but wants to retain a driver's license, which can be used as a means of identification and is symbolic of adulthood and independence, even if it is not used.

Many people with Alzheimer's disease are not willing to stop driving, however, and this presents a dilemma for family members, who feel badly about the number of things the person has already had to relinquish.

Sometimes greater resistance requires stronger measures. Taking the keys away may not be enough, especially if the person can find them again. Some families have resorted to antitheft devices or temporarily disabling the car by pulling battery or distributor wires. Selling the car removes the possibility of driving but may leave the family without transportation. Whatever method is selected, identification of alternate means of transportation is essential to the plan.

Finances

Both large and small issues arise regarding the question of managing finances. They range from keeping pocket change to adjusting wills and trusts to provide for the person with Alzheimer's disease if the caregiver should die first. The following are a few examples:

Jack always kept change in his pants pockets. He liked to walk around with his hands in his pockets, jingling the change just a little when he talked with people. He had no objection to his wife taking over the checkbook and managing their bank accounts but became enraged when she tried to take away his wallet and change. When she returned his wallet with $10 and an expired driver's license in it and left change on the dresser for him every morning, Jack was content with the arrangement.

Sarah left her church of 25 years with the intention of joining a new religious group in town. Her daughter became concerned when she saw that Sarah had written several checks in large amounts to this group. Sarah became angry when her daughter questioned the size of the checks, saying it was her money and she could do anything she wanted with it. Sarah also loaned her car to several members of this new group. Her daughter worried about this, too, but did not want to interfere because her mother enjoyed the company of the people so much.

The problem resolved itself. Sarah looked out her window one morning and discovered that her car was gone. She reported the missing car to the police, who found it and brought the members of the religious group in for questioning. After this unsettling experience, the group decided that Sarah could not join them and left her alone.

In the early stages of Alzheimer's disease Ruby's husband hid cash all over the house. Apparently he would forget where he had hidden it, because he constantly asked Ruby for money and never retrieved any of the hidden cash. "Even now," said Ruby, "after all these years, I am still finding money in the house. Just the other day, I found $20 in a book he used to read."

Like working and driving a car, controlling one's finances and having some money in one's wallet are symbols of independence and autonomy. Relinquishing control may be difficult. For people who pride themselves on their financial acumen, giving up control over money may be especially difficult. The decisions about when a family member must intercede and how to do it are similar to those related to driving a car. When it becomes apparent that the person is no longer exercising good judgment or is making serious mistakes, such as forgetting to pay bills or overdrawing the checking account on a regular basis, it is time to intercede.

Tact and sensitivity to what is especially important to this individual are essential to this endeavor. A responsible family member (or other party if no family member is available) must be allowed access to all accounts. In some cases families instruct the bank not to allow the person to withdraw more than a limited amount of money. If this arrangement is made, it is important to inform the person so that he or she is not unnecessarily exposed to the embarrassment of the bank's refusal. A durable power of attorney may be helpful to the individual who manages the finances of the person with Alzheimer's disease (see Chapter 15).

Household Maintenance

Failure to maintain the household property may be of greater significance to the older woman with Alzheimer's disease than to many of the men of a generation in which men were not actively involved in housework. However, men who took pride in their home workshops or weekend cooking may eventually face some restrictions as well.

Health and safety hazards are the primary concern, with damage to valuable property a secondary concern. Household tools, whether they are sharp kitchen knives or rotary saws in the workshop, at some point become dangerous for the person to use and must be locked away. Appliances are another common hazard. Many fires have resulted from food left cooking for hours, forgotten when the person was distracted. Removing knobs or unplugging an electric stove may prevent a fire when the person is unattended. Many family caregivers feel that microwave ovens are safer, but fires can occur in them as well, for example, when paper is placed in the microwave. Incorrect use of washers and dryers is more likely to damage the clothes or the machine than to cause bodily harm. Washing clothes by hand may be an appropriate solution for the person with Alzheimer's disease.

In most cases part of the job of household maintenance can be done safely by the person with Alzheimer's disease. Washing fruit and vegetables, for example, involves no risk of injury. Sweeping and mopping are also low-risk tasks. Outdoors, watering plants and raking leaves are lower risk than running the lawn mower. Substituting these safer activities allows the person to remain involved in productive activities long after impairment has reduced or eliminated similar opportunities outside the home.

BASIC ACTIVITIES OF DAILY LIVING

The basic ADLs are important personal activities—toileting, bathing, eating, dressing—with which the person with Alzheimer's disease will need some help in the later stages of the disease. Graded assistance, a general approach to helping a person with dementia with the basic ADLs, is described first. Then some specific considerations for each of the basic ADLs are discussed.

Graded Assistance

The idea behind the graded assistance approach is to provide only as much help as the person needs to complete a task—not more, not less. If the caregiver is providing rehabilitative skill training, the person will be asked to try to complete the task before help is offered. The type of assistance offered is carefully graded: just a verbal cue to help the person get started, a nonverbal demonstration of what needs to be done, some physical guidance of the hand or other body part, or full assistance (i.e., doing the task for the person). Table 9.1 shows how graded assistance would work for a simple task such as drinking from a cup.

A *task analysis* is necessary before beginning to retrain the person. As simple as using a spoon or putting on socks may seem, each task is composed of a number of separate actions. Breaking down the task into these component steps helps the caregiver assess the portions with which the person has some difficulty. For example, brushing the teeth involves picking up the toothbrush, putting toothpaste on the brush, bringing the toothbrush to one's mouth, brushing (all the teeth on both sides, not just the ones in front), rinsing, spitting out the rinse water, rinsing off the toothbrush, and replacing it in the holder (Tappen, 1994a). A breakdown of many of the basic ADLs into component steps can be found in the Refined ADL Assessment Scale in the appendix to this chapter.

Table 9.1.   Graded assistance

	Assistance given	Example
No help needed	Unassisted	Person picks up cup and takes a drink from it by him- or herself.
Least amount of help needed	Verbal prompt	"Sid, pick up your cup."
	Demonstration (nonverbal prompt)	Caregiver reaches out hand as if to pick up a cup.
	Physical guidance	Caregiver moves person's hand toward cup or picks up cup and hands it to person.
	Physical assistance	Caregiver puts person's hands around the cup and steadies the cup.
Greatest amount of help needed	Complete assistance	Caregiver picks up cup and brings it to person's mouth for him or her to drink.

Effectiveness of graded assistance is based on the idea that excess disability is common in people in the advanced stages of Alzheimer's disease. Research has shown that people with Alzheimer's disease can do more for themselves when given carefully graded assistance than when they are given the all-or-nothing assistance typically offered in long-term care facilities (Osborn & Marshall, 1993). Intensive training in the basic ADLs using graded assistance can help them perform these tasks more independently (Tappen, 1994b).

Dressing

Dressing involves selecting appropriate garments and putting them on in the proper order (use of sequencing and motor skills). Selection is a decision-making process based on information about the season, weather, and occasion. Color and styles also should be considered in order to be socially acceptable: pajamas are not worn on the street, a sweater is too warm when the temperature tops 80°, orange and purple do not go well together, an old T-shirt does not go well with a silk skirt. People with Alzheimer's disease may try any or all of these combinations unless they receive guidance in making their selections.

Out-of-season clothing can be stored in a different closet to avoid mistakes (Namazi & Johnson, 1992). Once clothes have been chosen, they need to be put on correctly and in the right order. For example, underwear does not go on over trousers, shirts need to be buttoned correctly, and zippers on pants need to be pulled all the way up.

If selection is the main problem, the caregiver can lay out the appropriate clothes for the person's approval. Clothes are placed face down so that they do not have to be turned around before putting them on, and are placed in the order in which they should be put on. Developing a consistent routine that reflects the way the person dressed in the past may be helpful. For example, if the individual always showered and dressed before having breakfast, then this sequence should be continued. Using the same order for putting on clothes every day is also helpful in maintaining consistency. Keeping distractions to a minimum and allowing plenty of time to get dressed (rushing the person is usually counterproductive) also facilitate completion of this task (Vogelpohl, Beck, Heacock, & Mercer, 1996).

Different problems with dressing may arise as the disease progresses:

> My brother refused to change his underwear. He wore the same briefs for 2 weeks before he finally changed them.

> My wife put on too many bras. And panty hose. She would put on one pair after the other and scream at me if I tried to take them off.

> Dad wouldn't remove his cowboy boots. He even wanted to wear them to bed. I think it was because he was afraid he couldn't get them back on if he took them off.

> Mom wore the same housecoat day after day. I couldn't get her to wear any other clothes.

These dressing problems become behavior problems for the caregiver when the person resists their correction. They should be handled in the same manner as any other behaviors of concern to the caregiver (see Chapter 7).

As the dementia progresses, the person will experience difficulty with putting on whatever clothes are chosen. Too much help or deep discouragement about the progressive decline can lead to excess disability. Rehabilitative training using graded assistance may help the person do as much for him- or herself as possible.

Unless they are too ill to get dressed, people in long-term care facilities should dress in daytime clothes every day as they would at home because they are residents, not patients. Names can be placed inside a garment to avoid mixups but should not be written across the back of a sweater or shirt like a camp shirt or prison garb. Clothing protectors (bibs) may be necessary to protect clothing at mealtimes, although large dinner napkins would be more dignified. If clothing protectors are used, they should be removed immediately after the meal to maintain the person's dignity and self-respect.

Eating

Eating is important psychologically, socially, and physiologically. Eating problems early in the disease are usually minimal. Sometimes people in the early stages have difficulty with making nutritionally well-balanced food selections or with remembering dietary restrictions. Appetite problems may be the result of other factors. Depression, medications, and other medical problems can cause weight loss that is too easily ascribed to Alzheimer's disease. The reasons for loss of appetite and weight loss should be investigated thoroughly.

As the disease progresses, however, maintaining good nutrition becomes more of a problem. If living alone or remaining alone during the day, the person may either forget to eat or forget that he or she has already eaten and eat a second time, sometimes accusing others of starving him or her. Food may spoil unnoticed and be consumed anyway, occasionally leading to accusations of being poisoned. The person may eat only "junk food": Cookies, ice cream, and potato chips are easy to buy and eat but are nutritionally inadequate (Hall, 1994).

A shortened attention span, easy distractibility, and perceptual problems seem to cause problems at mealtimes. The person may get up and wander off without finishing the meal, play with the utensils instead of eating, or eat from only one section of the plate, leaving the rest untouched. Eating may take twice as long as it once did (Hall, 1994). In fact, it is not unusual for a person in the late stages of Alzheimer's disease to take a full hour to finish a meal. In the late stages of the disease the person may mistake inedible items, such as styrofoam cups or bars of soap, for food. If upset or unhappy, he or she may spit out the food or throw it at the caregiver.

Weight loss is common in the later stages of the disease, but the reason for it is unclear. It may be caused by inadequate intake (Holzapfel et al., 1996) or by the high expenditure of energy that occurs with pacing. It may be necessary to supplement meals with puddings, ice cream, milkshakes, or commercially prepared supplements that appeal to the common fondness for sweet foods to reverse the weight loss. Serving the main meal at noon may also help because there seems to be less fatigue at this hour.

With estimates that half of all residents of long-term care facilities need help with eating, it is not surprising that providing adequate nutrition and helping people maintain as much independence as possible are major concerns. Nursing assistants, who do most of the feeding, have been noted to use an all-or-nothing approach to assistance: They either feed the person or leave the person to fend for him- or herself (Osborn & Marshall, 1993). Typically, they provide few prompts except "open your mouth" or simply "eat" (Van Ort & Phillips, 1992). An unfortunate tendency to mix foods together and to try

to spoon in meat-vegetable-potato mixtures mashed together may destroy fragile appetites. In some instances, staff will even blenderize all of the foods together, creating a
"gruel-like mixture" that is easily fed to residents but is rarely appetizing (Phillips &
Van Ort, 1995, p. 251). Nursing assistants are also often in a hurry. Add to this the
noisiness of a large dining room, a medication nurse crushing pills with a steady pounding
that echoes throughout the room, and a radio or television for background sound, and
the person with Alzheimer's disease faces too many distractions to concentrate on eating
(Durnbaugh, Haley, & Roberts, 1996).

A better approach would be to group people in small clusters of three or four in
quiet areas for their meals. This approach provides some human company but fewer
distractions. Medication administration and other tests or treatments should be undertaken before or after meals, not during them. Televisions should be turned off (Van Ort
& Phillips, 1995). Plate guards (i.e., metal rims that are put on plates to keep the food
from being pushed off) and built-up handles on forks or spoons can help people with
clumsy fingers pick up the food. Plates can also be placed on mats so that they do not
slip easily. Foods that can be picked up and eaten by hand allow self-feeding without
using utensils. Examples are cut-up fruit, sandwiches, and crackers. Straws and spouted
cups may prevent spills. Hot liquids should be allowed to cool a little before serving
them.

Favorite foods can be served to avoid futile arguments as long as nutritional needs
are satisfied. Smaller meals served more often may help when appetites are poor, as will
small bites of food. Small bites of food also help to prevent choking, a common problem
that frightens many family caregivers. Ensuring that the person sits upright (not reclin-
ing) during a meal also helps to prevent choking. Syringes are not recommended for
feeding people because they may force the food too far back in the throat, where it can
be aspirated into the lungs.

A little creativity and imagination can go a long way toward making mealtimes
more pleasant for the person and caregiver alike.

Bathing and Grooming

As with eating, the bathing and grooming problems that appear in the early stages of
Alzheimer's disease are primarily caused by forgetting and distractibility. The person
with early-stage Alzheimer's disease generally manages these tasks alone but may need
an occasional reminder, for example, to brush teeth or use deodorant.

As the disease progresses, these personal care tasks may be completed more haphazardly than in an earlier stage. Shampoo may be left in the hair, or feet may not be
washed. Frequently, family caregivers do not realize at first that part of the daily cleaning
and grooming routine is being skipped and may react with shock or dismay that they
did not notice what was happening. The dilemma for caregivers is when to intervene,
when to enter into the individual's personal space and "intrude" in these private matters.
Even spouses may find it difficult to inquire into their husband's or wife's personal
hygiene habits. Changing soiled or wet underclothes may be the most difficult of all
personal care tasks for family members. In a novel about the pain and pleasure of caring
for a family member with Alzheimer's disease, Sawako Ariyoshi (1987, pp. 133–134)
describes this dilemma and its consequences vividly. The individual with Alzheimer's
disease is Akiko's father-in-law.

> Trying to help his wife give his father a pill, Akiko's husband "was suddenly
> assailed by a foul odor, smelling like poison gas," coming from his father's mouth.

Akiko told her husband that she had been aware of this odor but hadn't done any thing about it. "I think it comes from his dentures, because I haven't seen him clean them once. I can't bear the thought of touching them, so I've left them alone. Come to think of it, though, it's terribly unhygienic to leave them like that."

Knowing she could no longer ignore the odors and what they signified, Akiko thrust her hand into her father-in-law's mouth and pulled out his dentures.

Akiko and her husband screamed when assailed with the "powerful stench, stronger than that of faeces," that "made them think of the putrefying odor of Dream Island, the gargantuan garbage dump" in their city. Stifling the urge to vomit, Akiko washed the dentures in the kitchen sink. She knew that remembering to clean the dentures had become her responsibility.

As cognitive processes decline, observation is needed to identify the areas being missed. Reminders to "wash your back," "rinse your hands," or "use toothpaste" become necessary. Finally, actual assistance becomes necessary and should be provided using the graded assistance procedures described earlier.

Grooming should not be neglected because the person has dementia. Aftershave lotions and a fashionable haircut feel as good to an older man with dementia as they do to an older man without dementia. Lipstick and nail polish please older women with Alzheimer's disease in the same way that they please older women without Alzheimer's disease. Compliments about how one looks bring smiles at any age as long as the person can comprehend the words or relate to the positive tone of voice.

Refusals are probably the biggest problem in helping the person with bathing and grooming. Even paid caregivers find the blood-curdling screams of a person put unwillingly into a shower somewhat unsettling. Why showers and baths frighten some people with Alzheimer's disease is still unexplained. The fear may be related to the invasion of privacy that occurs in removing one's clothes in front of others, whether family or stranger. It is also possible that the hard, cold walls and echoes of a shower or bathroom frighten the person.

Whatever the reason, baths and showers are better accepted when given by a trusted person, making continuity of assignment important in long-term care facilities. Changing the time of the bath or substituting a sponge bath may also help counter strenuous resistance to a bathing routine. Simply handing the person a warm washcloth soaked in a cleansing solution rather than forcing entry into a shower or tub may be sufficient. In the drive to keep people clean, the soothing effect of warm water and a gentle touch can be forgotten. Perhaps if this approach to bathing were taken, there would be less resistance. An example of an individualized bathing routine may be found in Table 9.2.

Toileting

Helping a person with toileting needs also requires invasion of personal space and privacy. It is difficult for some family caregivers to handle urine- and feces-soiled clothing and bodies. Some family members find it easier to manage these tasks if they do it with a little humor and recognition that elimination is a natural function:

We were finding puddles all over the house. You had to watch where you stepped. So we bought her incontinence pants, the ones you can pull down like regular underclothes.

> He started using the wastebasket to urinate, especially at night when he couldn't find the bathroom. But I don't complain. It's better than doing it on my carpet.

Incontinence (inability to control the discharge of urine or feces) may be caused by physical problems that can be improved with the use of medication, exercise, or surgery. For this reason, a thorough medical evaluation of the causes of incontinence is recommended before instituting behavioral treatment.

Incontinence may also be related to Alzheimer's disease: inability to find the bathroom or to remember what to do after finding it; inattentiveness to body signals; and reduced concern about social strictures against voiding or defecating outside designated areas. Problems with incontinence usually appear relatively late in Alzheimer's disease (earlier with vascular dementias) and make a considerable contribution to the heavy workload of caregivers.

Reminders and regular trips to the toilet may be all that is required to maintain continence long into the disease process. Knowing when the person usually urinates and has bowel movements makes these reminders and trips to the bathroom more effective in the later stages. It is also important to encourage the person to drink lots of fluids (the equivalent of eight glasses of water a day, if possible), to eat a high-fiber diet and drink prune juice if constipation is a problem, and to keep active (Karam & Nies, 1994). Maintaining mobility actually has been found to reduce incontinence; a person who cannot walk well often cannot reach the bathroom in time (Jirovec, 1991). Treating bladder infections rapidly and effectively is also important because they greatly increase the urgency to void.

The *prompted voiding* approach has been used with some success in people with Alzheimer's disease. Prompted voiding involves a carefully spelled-out routine designed to recapture previously learned toilet habits and encourage their continuance. With this procedure, the person who is incontinent is checked regularly by the caregiver. The caregiver asks the person if he or she is wet or dry. Then the person is prompted to try to use the toilet. This routine is usually conducted every 2 hours during waking hours, although the hours can and should be adjusted to individual toileting needs. The time can be stretched to 3–4 hours after success with the every-2-hour schedule (Urinary

Table 9.2.   Example of a personalized bathing routine for an individual with dementia

1. Shower me in a PVC pipe stand-up walker (Ultimate Walker), so I can stand.
2. Place beach shoes on my feet to improve traction and safety.
3. When you want me to move from place to place (when using the walker and when not) extend your arms and have me hold your hands to guide me.
4. Give me a wash rag to hold onto. I may follow your directions to wash myself or to wash the wall. I enjoy both.
5. I like having my hair and head washed, massaged, and scrubbed.
6. It requires two people to dress and undress me, as one person needs to loosely hold onto my hands while the other dresses me.
7. If you are comfortable with it, I like very much to be hugged and for you to allow me to touch you. I usually do this on your face, arms, upper body.
8. When drying, give me a towel to hold onto. This helps me to avoid grabbing onto you during drying.
9. I do better if my shower is given by someone I know and who knows me well, so please attach my shower to my primary care aide and not a day of the week.

From Rader, J., Lavell, M., Hoeffer, B., & McKenzie, D. (1996). Maintaining cleanliness: An individualized approach. *Journal of Gerontological Nursing, 22*(3), 32–38; reprinted by permission.

Incontinence Guidelines Panel, 1992). If the person is clean and dry when checked, the caregiver says so and praises the person for this success (Urinary Incontinence Guidelines Panel, 1992). Rewards such as an extra snack or a walk outside may also be offered if verbal praise does not seem to be sufficient. For most people, being clean and dry is a reward in itself. It is important not to withhold food or pleasurable activities because the person is incontinent. This may be construed as punishment.

The prompted voiding procedure is simple, but carrying it out is time consuming. Consistency and persistence over time (months, not days or weeks) are essential to success. Family members may be more motivated to do this because they are responsible for only one person. Staff of long-term care facilities unfortunately find it easier simply to change the person's incontinence pads or pants than to follow the strict routine for taking the person to the bathroom and helping them to toilet (Schnelle et al., 1993).

When all else fails, incontinence pads and pants save the person from embarrassment and protect the immediate environment from constant soiling and wetting. Several concerns about their use have been expressed. The first is that they encourage incontinence—there is no need to reach the bathroom, and nursing assistants may encourage the person to "just go where you are." Second, they are often left on for hours after becoming wet or soiled, thereby becoming precipitants of skin breakdown and infection. Third, when wet they become heavy and fall off when the person stands up. Finally, they are expensive in terms of both money and human dignity, especially when they are called diapers.

Clearly, there is far more to assistance with ADLs than "lending a hand" to help the person wash or put on a coat. A rehabilitative approach utilizing the lessons learned from research and from clinical observation will help the individual with Alzheimer's disease maintain as much independent function as possible for as long as possible.

REFERENCES

Ariyoshi, S. (1987). *The twilight years.* Tokyo: Kodansha International.

Beck, C., Heacock, P., Rapp, C.G., & Mercer, S.O. (1993). Assisting cognitively impaired elders with activities of daily living. *American Journal of Alzheimer's Care and Related Disorders and Research, 8*(6), 11–20.

Dick, M.B., Shankle, R.W., Beth, R.E., Dick-Muehlke, C., Cotman, C.W., & Kean, M.L. (1996). Acquisition and long-term retention of a gross motor skill in Alzheimer's disease patients under constant and varied practice conditions. *Journal of Gerontology: Psychological Sciences, 52B*(2), 103–111.

Durnbaugh, T., Haley, B., & Roberts, S. (1996). Assessing problem feeding behaviors in mid-stage Alzheimer's disease. *Geriatric Nursing, 17*(2), 63–67.

Gregg, D. (1994). *Alzheimer's disease.* Boston: Harvard Medical School Health Publications.

Hall, G.R. (1994). Chronic dementia: Challenges in feeding a patient. *Journal of Gerontological Nursing, 20*(4), 21–30.

Holtzapfel, S.K., Ramirez, R.F., Layton, M.S., Smith, I.W., Sagl-Massey, K., & DuBose, J.Z. (1996). Feeder position and food and fluid consumed by nursing home residents. *Journal of Gerontological Nursing, 22*(4), 6–12.

Jirovec, M.M. (1991). The impact of daily exercise on the mobility, balance and urine control of cognitively impaired nursing home residents. *International Journal of Nursing Studies, 28*, 145–151.

Karam, S.E., & Nies, D.M. (1994). Student/staff collaboration: A pilot bowel management program. *Journal of Gerontological Nursing, 20*(3), 32–40.

Marottoli, R.A., Ostfeld, A.M., Merrill, S.S., Perlman, G.D., Foley, D.J., & Cooney, L.M. (1993). Driving cessation and changes in mileage driven among elderly individuals. *Journal of Gerontology: Social Sciences, 48*(5), s255–s260.

McGowin, D.F. (1993). *Living in the labyrinth: A personal journey through the maze of Alzheimer's*. San Francisco: Elder Books.

Namazi, K.H., & Johnson, B.D. (1992). Dressing independently: A closet modification model for Alzheimer's disease patients. *American Journal of Alzheimer's Care and Related Disorders and Research, 7*(1), 22–28.

Osborn, C.L., & Marshall, M.J. (1993). Self-feeding performance in nursing home residents. *Journal of Gerontological Nursing, 19*(3), 7–14.

Phillips, L.R., & Van Ort, S. (1995). Issues in conducting intervention research in long-term care settings. *Nursing Outlook, 43*, 249–253.

Rader, J., Lavell, M., Hoeffer, B., & McKenzie, D. (1996). Maintaining cleanliness: An individualized approach. *Journal of Gerontological Nursing, 22*(3), 32–38.

Schnelle, J.F., Newman, D., White, M., Abbey, J., Wallston, K.A., Fogarty, T., & Ory, M. (1993). Maintaining continence in nursing home residents through the application of industrial quality control. *Gerontologist, 33*(1), 114–121.

Shua-Haim, J.R., & Gross, J.S. (1996). A simulated driving evaluation for patients with Alzheimer's disease. *American Journal of Alzheimer's Disease, 11*(3), 2–7.

Shemon, K., & Christensen, R. (1991). Automobile driving and dementia. *American Journal of Alzheimer's Care and Related Disorders and Research, 6*(5), 3–8.

Tappen, R.M. (1994a). Development of the Refined ADL Assessment Scale for patients with Alzheimer's and related disorders. *Journal of Gerontological Nursing, 20*(6), 36–42.

Tappen, R.M. (1994b). The effect of skill training on functional abilities of nursing home residents with dementia. *Research in Nursing and Health, 17*, 159–165.

Thralow, J.U., & Rueter, M.J. (1993). Activities of daily living and cognitive levels of function in dementia. *American Journal of Alzheimer's Care and Related Disorders and Research, 8*(5), 14–19.

Tuokko, H. (1992). Psychological evaluation and management of the Alzheimer's patient. In R.W. Parks, R.F. Zec, & R.S. Wilson (Eds.), *Neuropsychology of Alzheimer's disease and other dementias*. New York: Oxford University Press.

Tupper, D.E., & Cicerone, K.D. (1991). *The neuropsychology of everyday life: Issues in development and rehabilitation*. Boston: Kluwer Academic Publishers.

Urinary Incontinence Guidelines Panel. (1992). *Urinary incontinence in adults: Clinical practice guideline* (AHCPR Publication No. 92-0038). Rockville, MD: Agency for Health Care Policy and Research.

Van Ort, S., & Phillips, L. (1992). Feeding nursing home residents with Alzheimer's disease. *Geriatric Nursing, 13*, 249–253.

Van Ort, S., & Phillips, L.R. (1995). Nursing interventions to promote functional feeding. *Journal of Gerontological Nursing, 21*(10), 6–13.

Vogelpohl, T.S., Beck, C.K., Heacock, P., & Mercer S.O. (1996). "I can do it!" dressing: Promoting independence through individualized strategies. *Journal of Gerontological Nursing, 22*(3), 39–42.

Directions

Administration of this test requires carrying out the prompts and assistance as needed and the rating and timing of each sequence.

Place a check mark in the box indicating the highest degree of assistance needed to complete each component of the task:

Unassisted: Done without further action on the part of the rater after initial prompt

Verbal Prompt: Spoken directions only from rater

Nonverbal Prompt: Gestured direction in addition to spoken directions from rater

Physical Guiding: Rater actually provides some assistance but respondent is able to participate in carrying out the step

Full Assist, Attempted: Respondent attempts but is unable to contribute to carrying out the step; rater provides full assistance

Full Assist, No Attempt: Respondent makes no attempt and is unable to contribute to carrying out the step; rater provides full assistance

N/A: Component not applicable

A maximum of five verbal or nonverbal prompts or attempts to physically guide are allowed before scoring.

The test should be given as a part of the regular routine. The respondent should have his or her glasses and hearing aid in place if needed and be fully awake before beginning.

Comments regarding spilling of water or food, any agitation, or refusal to participate may be noted at the bottom of the page.

Subscale scores are attained by summing the rating for each item (i.e., toileting, washing, grooming, dressing, eating) within that subscale.

A. Entering Bathroom

Given: Person sitting at edge of bed or in chair or wheelchair; obstacles to standing (rails, footrests, etc.) removed; door to bathroom is shut
Initial cue: "It's time to go to the bathroom."

	Unassisted 6	Verbal Prompt 5	Nonverbal Prompt 4	Physical Guiding 3	Full Assist, Attempted 2	Full Assist, No Attempt 1	N/A 0
Assume standing position							
Gain balance							
Turn toward bathroom							
Walk to bathroom							
Place hand on doorknob							
Turn doorknob							
Open door							
Remove hand from doorknob							
Walk to toilet							

Time to complete this action_____minutes.

B. Toileting (Defecating)

Given: Person facing toilet, adult diaper or underclothes in place
Initial cue: "Now, use the toilet."

	Unassisted 6	Verbal Prompt 5	Nonverbal Prompt 4	Physical Guiding 3	Full Assist, Attempted 2	Full Assist, No Attempt 1	N/A 0
Turn around and back up to toilet							
Pull down underwear or adult incontinence pads, pants							
Sit on toilet							
Void/defecate							
Wipe self							
Drop toilet paper							
Stand up							
Turn around toward toilet							
Pull up underwear							
Pull pants up or pull skirt down							
Rearrange clothing							
	Time to complete this action_____minutes (subtract time on toilet).						

C. Wash Hands

Given: Person standing or sitting at wheelchair-height sink
Initial cue: "Now, wash your hands."

	Unassisted 6	Verbal Prompt 5	Nonverbal Prompt 4	Physical Guiding 3	Full Assist, Attempted 2	Full Assist, No Attempt 1	N/A 0
Walk to sink							
Turn on water							
Get soap							
Place both hands in water							
Put soap on hands							
Put soap down							
Rub hands together							
Rinse hands							
Turn off water							
Get paper towel							
Dry hands							
Drop towel in wastebasket							
Leave bathroom							

Time to complete this action_____minutes.

D. Wash Face

Given: Basin of water (or running water at sink), bar of soap, washcloth, and handtowel
Initial cue: "Now, wash your face."

	Unassisted 6	Verbal Prompt 5	Nonverbal Prompt 4	Physical Guiding 3	Full Assist, Attempted 2	Full Assist, No Attempt 1	N/A 0
Reach for washcloth							
Take cloth in hand							
Put cloth in water							
Squeeze water from cloth							
Take soap in hand							
Rub soap on wet cloth							
Put soap down (release)							
Place cloth on face							
Wipe cloth over face							
End washing action							
Place cloth under water							
Squeeze water and soap from cloth							
Put cloth back on face							
Wipe cloth over face							
End rinsing action							
Put cloth down							
Reach for towel							
Grasp towel							
Wipe towel over face							
End drying action							
Put towel down							

Time to complete this action_____minutes.

E. Brush Teeth

Given: Brush, basin for water, and paper towel on tray or table
Initial cue: "Now, brush your teeth."

	Unassisted 6	Verbal Prompt 5	Nonverbal Prompt 4	Physical Guiding 3	Full Assist, Attempted 2	Full Assist, No Attempt 1	N/A 0
Locate toothpaste							
Pick up toothpaste tube							
Unscrew cap							
Put cap down							
Pick up toothbrush							
Dip brush in water							
Move toothbrush under toothpaste tube							
Squeeze toothpaste onto brush							
Put toothpaste down							
Place brush in mouth							
Brush upper and lower teeth							
Remove toothbrush from mouth							
Rinse mouth							
Spit rinse water out in basin							
Rinse toothbrush in water							
Put toothbrush down							
Pick up toothpaste tube and cap							
Put cap on tube							
Put tube down							

Time to complete this action_____minutes.

F.   Brush Teeth (Denture Version)

Given: Toothbrush, toothpaste with cap, basin of water
Initial cue: "Now, clean your dentures."

	Unassisted 6	Verbal Prompt 5	Nonverbal Prompt 4	Physical Guiding 3	Full Assist, Attempted 2	Full Assist, No Attempt 1	N/A 0
Remove dentures from mouth							
Place dentures in basin							
Locate toothpaste							
Pick up toothpaste tube							
Unscrew cap							
Put cap down							
Pick up toothbrush							
Dip brush in water							
Move toothbrush under toothpaste tube							
Squeeze toothpaste onto brush							
Put toothpaste down							
Pick up denture							
Brush denture							
Rinse denture							
Repeat for second denture							
Rinse toothbrush in water							
Put toothbrush down							
Put denture(s) back in mouth							
Pick up toothpaste tube and cap							
Put cap on tube							
Put tube down							

Time to complete this action_____minutes.

G. Comb Hair

Given: Comb or brush and mirror on table; loose (unpinned) hair
Initial cue: "Now, comb your hair."

	Unassisted 6	Verbal Prompt 5	Nonverbal Prompt 4	Physical Guiding 3	Full Assist, Attempted 2	Full Assist, No Attempt 1	N/A 0
Locate comb							
Grasp comb on nontooth side							
Place comb on hair							
Comb left side							
Comb right side							
Comb top							
Comb back							
Check in mirror							
End combing action							
Put comb down							

Time to complete this action_____minutes.

H. Dressing—Pants

Given: Elastic-waist underclothes and front- or side-zipper pants
Initial cue: "Now, put on your underclothes and pants."

	Unassisted 6	Verbal Prompt 5	Nonverbal Prompt 4	Physical Guiding 3	Full Assist, Attempted 2	Full Assist, No Attempt 1	N/A 0
Gain standing balance							
Hold underclothes open							
Step into underclothes							
Pull up							
Hold outer pants open							
Step into pants							
Pull up							
Locate zipper							
Pull up							
Locate button							
Button pants					.		

Time to complete this action_____minutes.

I. Dressing—Shirt/Blouse

Given: Shirt or blouse with large front buttons
Initial cue: "Now, put on your shirt/blouse."

	Unassisted 6	Verbal Prompt 5	Nonverbal Prompt 4	Physical Guiding 3	Full Assist, Attempted 2	Full Assist, No Attempt 1	N/A 0
Take front opening of shirt/blouse with one hand							
Insert other hand into correct sleeve							
Pull shirt/blouse to center of chest							
Grasp other side of shirt/blouse							
Insert other arm into sleeve							
Pull sleeve over arm							
Pull both sides together at center							
Button shirt/blouse							

Time to complete this action_____minutes.

J. Dressing—Shoes

Given: Pair of shoes, socks or stockings already on
Initial cue: "Now, put on your shoes."

	Unassisted 6	Verbal Prompt 5	Nonverbal Prompt 4	Physical Guiding 3	Full Assist, Attempted 2	Full Assist, No Attempt 1	N/A 0
Locate shoe							
Pick up shoe							
Match shoe to correct foot							
Put foot in shoe							
Pull shoe onto foot							
Repeat for other foot							

Time to complete this action_____minutes.

K. Cutting Food

Given: Knife, fork, meat
Initial cue: "Now, cut your meat."

	Unassisted 6	Verbal Prompt 5	Nonverbal Prompt 4	Physical Guiding 3	Full Assist, Attempted 2	Full Assist, No Attempt 1	N/A 0
Pick up fork at handle end							
Hold fork							
Press fork into meat							
Pick up knife at handle end							
Move knife across meat while exerting downward pressure							
Put knife and fork down							

Time to complete this action_____minutes.

L. Using a Fork

Given: Solid food and fork on plate
Initial cue: "Now, use your fork and eat."

	Unassisted 6	Verbal Prompt 5	Nonverbal Prompt 4	Physical Guiding 3	Full Assist, Attempted 2	Full Assist, No Attempt 1	N/A 0
Pick up fork at handle end							
Hold fork							
Press fork into cut food							
Lift fork and food to mouth							
Place food on fork into mouth							
Remove fork from food							
Chew food							
Swallow food							
Repeat action							

Time to complete this action_____minutes.

M. Using a Spoon

Given: Soft food (pudding, ice cream) and spoon
Initial cue: "Now, use your spoon to eat the [pudding, ice cream]."

	Unassisted 6	Verbal Prompt 5	Nonverbal Prompt 4	Physical Guiding 3	Full Assist, Attempted 2	Full Assist, No Attempt 1	N/A 0
Pick up spoon at handle end							
Hold spoon							
Push spoon under soft mass							
Lift spoon and food to mouth							
Place food on spoon into mouth							
Hold food in mouth							
Pull spoon out of mouth							
Swallow food							
Repeat action							

Time to complete this action_____minutes.

N. Drinking from Glass or Cup

Given: Glass or cup without handle, 3/4 filled with water or juice
Initial cue: "Now, drink the [water, juice]."

	Unassisted 6	Verbal Prompt 5	Nonverbal Prompt 4	Physical Guiding 3	Full Assist, Attempted 2	Full Assist, No Attempt 1	N/A 0
Extend arm and hand toward glass/cup							
Close hand around glass/cup							
Lift glass/cup to mouth							
Tilt glass/cup up until liquid enters mouth							
Swallow liquid							
Tilt glass/cup down							
Return glass/cup to table or repeat action							

Time to complete this action_____minutes.

O. Using a Napkin

Given: Paper napkin
Initial cue: "Now, use your napkin to wipe your mouth."

	Unassisted 6	Verbal Prompt 5	Nonverbal Prompt 4	Physical Guiding 3	Full Assist, Attempted 2	Full Assist, No Attempt 1	N/A 0
Reach for napkin							
Grasp napkin							
Move hand and napkin to mouth							
Pat/wipe mouth							
Put napkin down							

Time to complete this action_____minutes.

Time to complete meal_____minutes.

Chapter 10

Therapeutic Recreation

"Life" exists in the activities of being and doing.

C.R. Hellen (1992)

The web of activities that forms the framework of most of our lives is weakened and gradually destroyed by Alzheimer's disease. Disconnection from the mainstream of life occurs as the person with the disease loses the ability to participate unless efforts are made to reconnect the person to a modified set of activities and relationships (Hellen, 1992).

Any activity termed "recreation" may appear frivolous, but recreation, in the broadest sense, is not a trivial human activity. Its loss may lead to depression, diminished function, even death as the person is deprived of this form of nourishment for the body, mind, and spirit (Whitcomb, 1993).

When an individual is no longer capable of planning and initiating recreational activities alone, this becomes the responsibility of the formal and informal caregivers. Some evidence suggests that the individuals least able to do this for themselves are the ones for whom the least effort is made by others. In some facilities, for example, people with the greatest cognitive impairment may not participate in any activities at all. This occurs despite the fact that the Omnibus Budget Reconciliation Act of 1993 (OBRA; PL 103-66) requires that facilities provide activities for all of their residents and that participation in various activities has been shown to be therapeutic in terms of improving flexibility, ambulation, mental status, mood, and function (Voelkl, Fries, & Galecki, 1995).

ASPECTS OF THERAPEUTIC RECREATION

Nourishment of Body, Mind, and Spirit

The variety of recreational activities in which even a person with advanced Alzheimer's disease can participate indicates the potential benefits. *Physical activities* can increase a person's flexibility, strength, balance, and endurance. Improvement in any or all of these attributes helps the person remain functionally independent for as long as possible. Regular exercise reduces blood pressure, improves mood, and may even improve function. *Social activities* provide opportunities to increase morale and self-esteem and reduce withdrawal, loneliness, and depression. *Psychotherapeutic* and *cognitively oriented activities* can reduce anxiety and stimulate thinking. Continuation of *religious* and *cultural activities* connects the person with his or her own belief system (Vecchione, 1994). All of these activities offer the possibility of enjoyment and improved quality of life, elements often missing from the lives of people with Alzheimer's disease.

Levels of Involvement

An individual's involvement in an activity varies with the degree of impairment, motivation, and the type of activity chosen. Cognitively intact older people can choose and undertake their own activities. All they may need or want would be ideas for new activities, some guidance in learning new activities, and opportunities to participate in them. People with cognitive impairment, however, need more assistance, ranging from the generation of ideas to considerable help as well as supervision when carrying out the activity (Zgola, 1987).

Modifications

Clearly, some modifications for people with Alzheimer's disease and related diseases must be made to many ordinary activities. Modifications are made for several reasons: to encourage participation, to make active participation possible, to prevent failure, and to ensure safety. Although some experts propose providing "failure-free" activities, it is really more important to keep frustration within tolerable limits than to attempt to eliminate failure altogether.

Modifications may take one or all of several forms:

- *Selecting appropriate activities:* choosing activities the person is capable of carrying out and enjoying
- *Reducing demand:* changing the activity so that it is easier to do (e.g., reducing the distance from the bowling pins, allowing the person to sit instead of stand)
- *Adding assistance:* as with the activities of daily living (ADLs; see Chapter 9), providing graded assistance to make more activities available to the person with Alzheimer's disease
- *Altering equipment and materials:* substituting easier-to-use equipment and materials (e.g., larger scissors, larger type for reading, softer balls to play catch)
- *Simplifying directions:* reducing the complexity of games and other activities (e.g., letting the person turn over cards one by one in solitaire, ignoring penalties for stepping over a foul line, assembling ingredients for baking brownies)
- *Increasing supervision:* doing activities normally done alone with a companion or with someone in the room to ensure safety (e.g., walking with a companion instead of alone, having someone in the kitchen when using the stove)

The most common problems encountered in making these modifications are making the activity too childish or a meaningless shell with no therapeutic value. The following is an example of the latter:

> Papier mache work requires planning, manual dexterity, and a modicum of artistic talent but is forgiving in the sense that mistakes can be corrected and primitive forms can be attractive. The activity therapist assigned to the Alzheimer's special care unit of a large nursing facility thought that the residents would enjoy creating figures for a holiday display if some assistance was provided.
>
> Most of the residents took on their task with some enthusiasm. As they worked, a few reminisced about past holidays and how they had celebrated them. The results, however, were disappointing to the activity therapist. To compensate, she began giving the residents more directions about how the figures should look and how to achieve that look. When this did not result in any appreciable improvements, she began "helping" them. She reshaped most

of the figures and repainted virtually all of them. The residents realized that she was doing a much better job than they had done, so they sat back and watched her finish the figures.

The secondary goal of preparing a holiday display had been accomplished, but the primary goal of involving the residents in a satisfying and meaningful activity had been abandoned. The result was that the residents themselves experienced yet another episode in which their own shortcomings were made evident.

ACTIVITIES FOR PEOPLE WITH ALZHEIMER'S DISEASE

Recreational activities may be primarily physical, social, psychological, or cognitive in nature and many combine two or more of these aspects. Activities may be carried out individually, in small groups, or in large groups. The physical activities may involve primarily large motor tasks (i.e., use of primarily large muscle groups—walking, throwing a ball) or small motor tasks (i.e., use of primarily small muscle groups—writing, painting). Even when an individual is extensively impaired, there is a wide variety of activities from which to choose. A number of these are examined in this section.

Long-term care facilities have been required to provide recreational activities for their residents since the 1970s. Most facilities provide *general recreational activities* such as entertainment, bingo, and occasional outings, primarily geared toward residents who are cognitively intact. The main purpose of these general activities is to provide some social outlets for residents (Connolly & Gabarini, 1995).

Recreational therapy, by way of contrast, is a higher level of activity designed to improve the resident's condition in some way. Selection should be based on assessment of the individual's needs and capabilities. In this section, therapeutic activities are emphasized.

Music

A number of research studies have been undertaken on the effects of music in people with Alzheimer's disease, many with positive results. One small study, for example, found that 15 minutes of calming music reduced agitation during and after the music session (Tabloski, McKinnon-Howe, & Remington, 1995). Music can be used to reduce tension, communicate nonverbally, and create a comfortable atmosphere for social visits. It also can be used to evoke memories and stimulate movement, especially dancing and exercise (Whitcomb, 1993).

Whitcomb (1993) theorizes that listening to music activates the "musical brain," acting like a battery charger for the neural circuits damaged by Alzheimer's disease. She describes an awakening phenomenon that is often observed in people with the disease when music is played.

The beneficial effect of music on people with Alzheimer's disease can be explained in other ways. For example, a high level of verbal ability is not necessary to enjoy music. Furthermore, the rhythms evident in most music may contribute to *resynchronization*. In other words, rhythmic actions are thought to integrate the timing of motor actions such as stepping, walking, or swinging arms by influencing the central timing mechanisms in the brain (Shepherd, 1988). The latter theory supports the use of music during exercise and other physical activities.

Fortunately, it is not necessary to be a musician to use music in a therapeutic manner. Although live music is more engaging than prerecorded music, especially when the music makers talk, smile, and otherwise relate to their audience, prerecorded music has the advantage of immediate, continuous availability and portability. Battery-operated tape recorders and compact disc players can be taken right to the bedside of the person with severe illness or disability. Clock radios can be set to play for 30–40 minutes to help the individual fall asleep at night. Larger recorders and compact disc players can also be used to play music for a group, as background for meditation, religious services, exercise, or dancing, for example. The versatility of music is reflected in its multiple uses, particularly in its value for both calming and stimulating people.

Calming Music   Certain types of music may be thought of as "nonpharmacological sedatives," ones with minimal side effects, especially when compared with some of the powerful drugs that are often prescribed for people with Alzheimer's disease. ("Haldol or Haydn?" quips one group of researchers [Tabloski et al., 1995].) Tabloski et al. suggest that music could be "prescribed" and its effect evaluated before sedative drugs are used for restlessness, insomnia, or agitation.

The way in which music is selected and administered for its calming effect is important. The following guidelines are designed to maximize music's calming effect (Tabloski et al., 1995; Whitcomb, 1993):

- Select music with a slow tempo, soft dynamic level, and repetitive themes. Consider using music with a tempo of less than 72 beats per minute, the average rate of the heart at rest.
- Consider the individual's preferences, if known, or ask the individual and his or her family if they are not known.
- Administer music therapy before agitation intensifies.
- Adjust the volume of the music so that it is easily heard but is not too loud, which can increase anxiety and restlessness.
- Eliminate competing sounds (e.g., conversation, alarms, telephones, televisions, traffic).
- Use touch, especially light massage, to enhance the calming effect.
- Observe the individual's response and make adjustments accordingly.
- Ask the individual if he or she is enjoying the session.

The use of music for its calming effect may become a regular part of the individual's schedule at home or plan of care in a long-term care facility.

Music that is significant to the individual may, in some cases, be a good choice for reducing anxiety or restlessness. However, personal meaning may be more important when using music for stimulation.

Stimulating Music   Music can be used to stimulate as well as to calm. In this instance, we are tapping the "awakening" effects of music that Whitcomb (1993) described. In particular, music can be used to evoke memories and to encourage activity.

- Holiday music reminds people of the season and stimulates memories of past holidays.
- Religious music connects people with their spiritual side.
- Ethnic music strengthens bonds with people's families and cultural heritage.
- Music from childhood reminds people of earlier experiences and links them with their extended family.
- Love songs from adolescent and young adult years reconnect people with memories of those strong emotions and intimate relationships.

- Lively music with a strong beat and fast tempo stimulates foot tapping, hand clapping, rhythmic moving, dancing, and singing. Dancing is excellent exercise, and most of these musical activities may be social activities as well.

The Arts

The arts provide additional avenues of expression for people in the early stages of Alzheimer's disease. Painting, sculpture, crochet, embroidery, music, poetry, and crafts of all kinds are enjoyable activities so long as the person is capable of them. Expression, not perfection, is the goal.

Many facilities fail to provide as many male-oriented arts and crafts activities as they do female-oriented activities, a real mistake in helping male residents find outlets for their creative energies. Drawing or tracing geometric shapes, practicing one's signature or using stamp pads may appeal to some men. Dowling (1995) observed that painting is especially engaging: "[T]hen, the paints came. When folks first touched brush to paint, then to paper, a magic started to flow. . . . Smiles . . . spontaneous singing . . . rapt attention . . . reminiscing" (p. 123). Dowling also noted that fingerpainting and string art were "nearly disastrous" (p. 126), not only because people were less interested in them but also because many were distressed by the messiness of these particular activities.

Enjoyment of others' work is another way to participate in the arts. Poetry readings, art exhibitions, and crafts fairs may be appreciated in the early to middle stages of Alzheimer's disease because they require only social skills and some attentiveness for participation.

Games

Games can be used to stimulate thinking, encourage social interaction, and increase physical activity. The temptation to suggest childish games seems to be almost irresistible for some activity personnel, but this should be avoided because it risks turning off potential participants and demeans those who do agree to participate. Hide-and-Go-Seek or King of the Mountain are children's games that adults rarely, if ever, play unless they are with children. Horseshoes and bowling are adult games. Many people with Alzheimer's disease are quite sensitive to being treated like children and will express this by saying such things as, "Isn't this a child's game?" or by refusing to participate. Having fun or being silly is not precluded, however. Within such a context, adult materials and games should be used and modified as needed. Probably the best measure of appropriateness is to ask, "How would I feel if I were asked to do this?" and "How would my (significant other/mother/father) feel if asked to do this?" An honest response should help distinguish being lighthearted from being childish.

It is not necessary to avoid a game that might challenge the individual's memory. Successes should outnumber failures, and frustration should not become too great. Taking instant photographs of one another; listening to and guessing the sources on a sound effects record; passing around a working microphone; and inspecting and discussing a seashell, hat, or other type of collection are low-frustration, adult-level activities. The following are some games suggested by Hellen (1992):

Who's Who: pictures or quotes from famous people
Letter Games: words that begin with a particular letter
Word Games: opposites, rhymes, fill in the blanks, familiar sayings
Geography: familiar and fascinating places

Shopping: pick a favorite item from a catalog, guess costs
Adapted Games: bingo, Scrabble, checkers, dominos, solitaire

The more "automatic" the response, the more likely that individuals with severe impairment will be able to participate in these games. Dowling (1995) suggests using action phrases such as "A new broom sweeps . . . [clean]" or "Haste makes . . . [waste]" and four-word phrases such as "the more, . . . [the merrier]" and "cold hands, . . . [warm heart]" (pp. 34, 38). People with severe language impairment will experience difficulty even with these phrases but may still enjoy being part of a group that is playing the game as long as answers are spontaneous and no one is called on for an answer.

These games are but a sample of the many that can be played. Most are suitable for groups of people. In fact, the mistakes of others may cause participants to feel more comfortable with attempts to guess the right answer. The level of difficulty of these games and the way in which the group facilitator responds to mistakes are crucial factors in determining the therapeutic or nontherapeutic outcomes of participation.

Exercise

From the 1920s to the 1960s conventional wisdom held that any exercise more vigorous than walking was ill-advised for adults. The idea behind this attitude was that the body would wear out more quickly if overused (Holloszy, 1993). In the 1990s we are more aware of the deleterious effects of inactivity, especially on older adults. The potential therapeutic power of exercise is increasingly recognized as applying to people with Alzheimer's disease as well as to older people in general. If it is possible to do so, some physical activity should be provided three times a day; early evening activity helps minimize the effects of sundowning (A. Ortigara, personal communication, November 1996). We now know that exercise is beneficial throughout life if it is done correctly. The potential benefits for people with Alzheimer's disease are improved health, physical function, cognition, and mood. Some of these outcomes have been supported by research, whereas others remain to be tested.

Effect of Alzheimer's Disease on Physical Function   Although there are subtle effects earlier in the course of the disease, most of the noticeable changes in motor ability occur in the later stages: the individual begins to take smaller steps, walks more deliberately, and needs help ascending and descending stairs. At Reisberg's Stage 7 (see Chapter 1 for an explanation of Reisberg's stages), the individual also may begin to tilt forward, backward, or laterally and may develop an abnormal gait (Sclan & Reisberg, 1992). Eventually, the individual is unable to walk or even hold up his or her head (American Psychiatric Association, 1994; Berg, 1984; Traber & Gispen, 1985).

Problems with spatial orientation also affect motor ability. As people age, they begin to depend more on visual input rather than on somatic signals to determine their position in space and maintain their balance (Whipple, Wolfson, Derby, Singh, & Tobin, 1993). Alzheimer's disease eventually affects the processing of this information, thereby interfering with the ability to maintain balance. Fortunately, there is some evidence that balance training may be helpful (Hu & Hines, 1994).

Exercise in the Early Stages   The term *exercise* may conjure up images of rowing machines, stationary cycles, and sweaty joggers huffing and puffing after a run through the park. However, dancing, swimming, cycling, and hiking are also good exercise and a great deal of fun besides.

There is no known reason that a person in the early stages of Alzheimer's disease cannot do the same exercises as any other person of the same age and physical condition. In fact, those who already exercise should be encouraged to continue, but with some caveats.

First, judgment about the appropriate intensity and duration of any exercise may become impaired and should be monitored closely. A person should be able to carry on a conversation while walking, cycling, or running. If the person is too breathless to do so, the intensity of the exercise should be decreased.

Second, safety is an issue with some forms of exercise. Solitary walking or jogging is no longer appropriate when the individual becomes spatially disoriented and cannot find the way home. The danger is not only the anxiety that this engenders but the possibility that the person may continue walking or running to the point of exhaustion. If becoming lost is a problem, the individual should be accompanied during exercise or should exercise in a gym where supervision is available. As the disease progresses, some of the equipment may present a safety problem—even the stationary cycle, which requires some balance to remain in the seat.

Third, the progression of the disease eventually affects the ability to perform certain types of exercises. When motor ability diminishes, even walking becomes difficult.

Finally, the effects of other chronic conditions must be considered. In particular, degenerative diseases of the heart, blood vessels, lungs, and joints may limit the individual's exercise capacity. Direction regarding modification of exercise routines should be sought from the physician treating these problems because traditional stress tests may not be suitable (May, 1990), and the individual may not cooperate when confronted with the unfamiliar equipment and procedures.

Exercise in the Later Stages   Therapeutic exercise is not simply being lively or remaining active. Instead, it is work on one or more of four aspects of physical activity: strength, flexibility, balance, and endurance. Exercises that affect one of these areas may not affect others: long-distance runners who do little stretching actually may have limited flexibility (Pollock & Wilmore, 1990).

Strength   Decreases in activity, poor circulation, poor nutrition, and other metabolic changes contribute to loss of muscle strength in older adults. Walking and cycling do not increase upper body, especially arm and trunk, strength. To increase upper body strength, stretchy resistance bands (Dynabands or Therabands), water resistance, small weights, or exercise equipment such as a set of pulleys are needed. From 8 to 15 repetitions through the full range of motion of the major muscle groups is suggested for healthy older adults. Special care must be taken to protect the joints when any weights are used (May, 1990; Van Norman, 1995).

Flexibility   Flexibility is an important consideration for older adults because joint pain and stiffness can discourage movement, which further increases stiffness, seriously decreasing function. A good example of diminished function resulting from joint stiffness and inflexibility is the inability to put on one's own socks and shoes. Inactivity; aging changes in the ligaments, tendons, and joint capsules; and joint diseases all contribute to joint stiffness and inflexibility.

Slow, gentle movement through the full range of motion at the shoulder, trunk, and hips is especially useful for older adults. A small towel held behind the back can be used to work on shoulder flexibility. May (1990) suggests combining the following movements:

- Stretch arms to the ceiling, then bend to each side.
- Place hands on shoulders (bend arms at the elbows) and turn from side to side. This can be done from a sitting position.
- Lie on the back, knees bent, arms at side, and roll to the right side, bringing the left knee up and over to the side and the left arm over the head, letting the shoulders follow. Reverse for turning to the left side.

Flexibility work is best done at the end of an exercise session, when the body is warm and pliable (Pollock & Wilmore, 1990).

Balance   As mentioned previously, people with Alzheimer's disease probably have more trouble with balance than do cognitively intact older adults, although all older people require more time to interpret and respond to information about their body position than do younger people. Exercises that involve weight shifting can be helpful. For people with severe balance problems, an individual assessment and prescription of appropriate exercise is recommended.

Endurance   Entirely different activities are used to improve cardiorespiratory endurance, for example, dancing, rowing, walking, cycling, stair stepping, and swimming. High-impact activities such as jogging, rope skipping, and jumping have a much higher rate of injury and are generally not appropriate for older adults.

Walking is probably the easiest and safest of the low-impact activities for the person with Alzheimer's disease from the perspective of limiting cardiovascular and orthopedic risks. Individuals with poor balance, limited lower limb strength, and similar problems may need assistive devices such as a cane or walker or may need to walk behind a wheelchair for support. A gait belt may be needed to prevent falls.

Highly deconditioned people may be able to do these activities for only 5–10 minutes at a time. Rest periods should be allowed if there is evidence of fatigue or increased shortness of breath or if the person requests it. If the individual complains of any pain, its source should be investigated before proceeding. Complaints must never be ignored. Because of the wide variation in physical condition of people in the later stages of Alzheimer's disease, it is recommended that advice about maximum heart rate increases allowable during exercise be obtained from a physician.

Exercise for Nonambulatory Individuals   Often, it is assumed that people who use wheelchairs or who cannot leave their beds can no longer participate in any type of exercise. In fact, there are both active and passive exercises that can be of benefit to nonambulatory individuals. Some exercises use upper body (arms) equivalents of the exercises just described, and others use lower limbs as well or are done with assistance.

A surprising amount of exercise can be done in a sitting position. Some examples are arm ergometry (i.e., a cycle-type mechanism that uses the hands instead of the feet), propelling oneself in a wheelchair, and swimming. Neck, arm, and trunk exercises can be done sitting down, as can leg raises.

In the supine (lying down) position, the arms, trunk, and legs can be moved actively or passively to maintain flexibility. The smaller joints of the hands and fingers also should be kept as flexible as possible to maintain function and prevent contractures. Even cycling can be done in bed if the individual has sufficient energy, as can weight training. The majority of people with Alzheimer's disease who cannot leave their beds, however, are too ill to engage in these strenuous activities.

Additional Guidelines   Misuse of exercise routines and equipment can result in serious accidents. Some general guidelines to promote safety include the following:

- Assess the individual's ability before beginning an exercise regimen. Obtain medical approval and guidance, especially if the individual has other chronic conditions that may affect exercise tolerance.
- Increase the intensity and duration of exercise gradually and stay within the individual's tolerance levels.
- Ensure that the individual is wearing appropriate shoes and clothing for the particular activity.
- Monitor heart rate during aerobic (endurance) exercise.
- Select low-impact, enjoyable activities for the exercise regimen.
- Plan shorter, more frequent sessions for deconditioned individuals.
- Provide supervision of any exercise activity.
- Include a warm-up and a cool-down period in any exercise plan.
- Help the person follow a regular schedule for exercising, at least three times a week if possible.

Animal-Assisted (Pet) Therapy

Companion animals are experts in the nonverbal communication of unconditional love. Use of companion animals can bring about many positive changes: reduced loneliness, stimulation, mild exercise, relaxation, increased self-esteem, and a renewed purpose in living. One study found that healthy older adults felt joy in caring for another living being and took care of themselves in order to be able to care for their companion animals (Yukl, 1997). Older adults with cognitive impairment may find few other situations in which they can be the giver rather than the receiver of care. Their use goes beyond entertainment to therapy when a bond between animal and human develops (Gammonley & Yates, 1991). Brief weekly or monthly visits from a troupe of dressed-up dogs, cats, and birds, no matter how pleasant, do not lend themselves to the formation of such bonds. Resident pets and pets assigned to longer visit times with specific individuals are more therapeutic. Some considerations in providing a companion animal program include the following:

- Check local and state public health regulations.
- Select healthy, even-tempered animals. This may require a veterinary examination and familiarity with the particular animal's personality.
- Supervision is necessary. Some individuals may become possessive or may handle animals roughly, endangering both resident and animal.
- Some exotic animals (lizards, rats, snakes) may frighten some people.

Dowling (1995) observed that dogs especially may become depressed in residential situations. Lethargy, withdrawal, loss of appetite, and development of skin conditions are indicators that the animal is having difficulty adjusting. He notes that, in residential situations, the companion animals need to be able to leave their "work" in the evening just like staff do.

Like many of the other activities described in this chapter, animal-assisted therapy is not appropriate for everyone with Alzheimer's disease. Some people are simply unable to relate to animals in the manner described. Others dislike animals or are afraid of them. Still others have allergic reactions that preclude close contact. Careful assessment of the individual and observation of the effect of the companion animal are essential for human and animal alike.

Purposeful Activities

Engagement in purposeful activity, as opposed to purposeless activity, is emphasized throughout this book. In particular, participation in the basic (ADLs) and independent activities of daily living (IADLs) is considered essential to maximum well-being. However, as these activities become too complex for the individual to perform alone, many are taken over by caregivers. Losing responsibility for these activities is a loss of a portion of one's purpose in life and of a connection to the ebbs and flows of everyday life. It is easier to help the person with Alzheimer's disease reconnect to these ordinary activities at home, but long-term care facilities willing to shed their traditional rules and job definitions can do the same.

The principles behind provision of opportunities to engage in purposeful activities are much the same as those already described in relation to the basic ADLs and IADLs: assistance should be provided in accord with the individual's capability and tolerance for frustration, and the activity should be meaningful in some way. Pretending that a task is necessary when it is not is demeaning and risks driving the person into further withdrawal if he or she suspects this is being done. Some additional guidelines for engaging the person in purposeful activities follow:

- Purposefulness, not perfection, is the goal (Hellen, 1992). A crooked stamp, a few leaves left on the ground, or a small smear on the window are all acceptable. Overcorrection is discouraging to almost anyone.
- To the extent possible, select familiar activities that provide some satisfaction to the individual.
- Express appreciation of whatever the person has accomplished.
- Provide sufficient supervision to maintain safety.

As to the variety of purposeful activities in which the person may engage, the possibilities are almost endless. They are limited primarily by the capabilities and interests of the individual and the imagination of the caregiver. The following are just a few examples (Hellen, 1992; Vecchione, 1994):

Baking cookies	Washing and drying dishes	Arranging flowers
Raking leaves	Sorting and folding laundry	Clipping coupons
Watering plants	Sweeping floors	Shining shoes
Stamping letters	Dusting books	Putting photos in an album
Taking out garbage	Setting and clearing the table	Planting seeds
Bringing in mail and newspapers	Feeding pets	Sorting buttons
	Feeding wild birds	Washing fruits and
Picking fruit	Washing the car	vegetables
Painting	Sanding	Making beds

Spiritual Practices

Belief in a higher power is important to many older adults. The higher power is a source of love, comfort, hope, strength, well-being, and inner harmony (Young, 1993). Although their impairments limit their ability to take the lead in religious practices and ceremonies, people with Alzheimer's disease can continue to participate in religious activities, especially religious services, song, prayer, and meditation, and to consult with their spiritual advisors.

Formal caregivers need to determine how important spiritual practices are to the individual and his or her religious affiliation. They can encourage participation in formal services and the discussion of beliefs. In addition, they can provide guidance in the most effective ways to provide counseling, especially in the later stages, to those spiritual advisors who are unfamiliar with the needs and characteristics of people with Alzheimer's disease.

Other Pleasant Activities

Teri and Logsdon (1991) argue that it is important for people with Alzheimer's disease to have the opportunity to engage in some pleasant activities. The positive effects they list include 1) enhancement of care recipient–caregiver relationships, 2) reduction in caregiver feelings of burden and hopelessness, 3) alleviation of depression, 4) reduction in disruptive behaviors, and 5) provision of a sense of accomplishment. The activities mentioned here are just a sample of those in which people with Alzheimer's disease can engage until the latest stages of the disease.

Traditions   One of the most important categories of these other pleasant activities is the continuation of national, cultural, ethnic, religious, and family traditions, including everything from celebrating Cinco de Mayo (Mexican independence day) to eating *hamantaschen* on Purim.

Excursions   Outings are a second category of pleasant activities that most people with Alzheimer's disease enjoy well into the course of the disease. Movies, museums, concerts, parks, zoos, restaurants, picnics, factory tours, sports events (a hot dog tastes twice as good at a ball game), favorite historical sites, and places of natural beauty are short trips that can be enjoyed without placing too high a demand on the individual (Alzheimer's Association, 1990).

Later in the disease, however, new places can be too frightening, even when family members accompany the individual. Behavior may become a problem, sometimes because of the demands of the situation. Other times, family members cannot tolerate the embarrassment of some of the person's behaviors, especially the loss of inhibition that can lead to some direct remarks made to strangers ("Help me! I don't know this man" "My daughter needs a husband, are you married?" "You've got great breasts"). Some family members can see the humor in the honesty and directness of these remarks; others are not able to do so.

Social Events   Undemanding social events are another important category. Celebrating birthdays or holidays, eating popcorn while watching a movie at home or in a long-term facility, making ice cream sundaes, joining a sing-along, or listening to a good guitar player all have considerable appeal.

SCHEDULING ACTIVITIES FOR PEOPLE WITH ALZHEIMER'S DISEASE

Boredom is seldom mentioned by experts as a serious problem for people with Alzheimer's disease, but it may well be one that requires more attention. It is often mentioned by family members of people in the middle stages of the disease, when capabilities are considerably diminished but energies are still high.

Often, people with Alzheimer's disease are faced with large amounts of time once filled by employment, household responsibilities, or hobbies that can no longer be pursued. How does one fill the time? It is not necessary to fill every minute of every day, but a schedule of activities that suit the individual and lend a regular rhythm to the day may be therapeutic.

The following are some points to consider when planning a program of activities ("Activity considerations," 1994; Kovach & Henschel, 1996):

- Alternate active and passive, quiet and stimulating activities.
- Include mealtimes in the activity plan.
- Allow time for breaks to stretch, walk, toilet, and rest.
- Schedule cognitively demanding activities in the morning.
- Provide options, especially alternatives with differing levels and types of demand.
- Avoid too much naptime during the day so that the person can fall asleep more easily at night. Keep naps scheduled and time-limited.
- Alternate individual and group (solitary and companion at-home) activities.
- Schedule some of the activities at the same time every day for consistency and predictability.

The consistency and predictability of a routine seem to provide some comfort to people with Alzheimer's disease, whose diminished intellectual capacities are strained by too much variety and unpredictability. This is not a recommendation for dull, flat, monotonous days but rather for familiar, recognizable patterns in the activities of a day.

REFERENCES

Activity considerations for a full day. (1994, Winter). *Respite Report,* pp. 5–10.

Alzheimer's Association. (1990). *Activities.* Chicago: Author.

American Psychiatric Association. (1994). *Diagnostic and statistical manual of mental disorders (DSM-IV)* (4th ed.). Washington, DC: American Psychiatric Press.

Berg, L. (1984). Clinical dementia rating scale. *British Journal of Psychiatry, 145,* 339.

Cohen, U., & Day, K. (1993). *Contemporary environments for people with dementia.* Baltimore: The Johns Hopkins University Press.

Connolly, P., & Gabarini, A. (1995). Certified therapeutic recreation specialists in geriatric rehab. *Vital Signs, 10,* 25.

Dowling, J.R. (1995). *Keeping busy: A handbook of activities for person with dementia.* Baltimore: The Johns Hopkins University Press.

Gammonley, J., & Yates, J. (1991). Pet projects: Animal assisted therapy in nursing homes. *Journal of Gerontological Nursing, 17*(1), 12–15.

Hellen, C.R. (1992). *Alzheimer's disease: Activity-focused care.* Boston: Andover Medical Publishers.

Holloszy, J.O. (1983). Exercise, health, and aging: A need for more information. *Medicine and Science in Sports and Exercise, 15*(1), 1–5.

Hu, M., & Hines, M.H. (1994). Multisensory training of standing balance in older adults. I. Postural stability and one-leg stance balance. *Journal of Gerontology, 49,* M52–M61.

Kovach, C.R., & Henschel, H. (1996). Planning activities for patients with dementia. *Journal of Gerontological Nursing, 22*(9), 33–38.

May, B. (1990). Principles of exercise for the elderly. In J.V. Basmajian & S.L. Wolf (Eds.), *Therapeutic exercise*. Baltimore: Williams & Wilkins.

Omnibus Budget Reconciliation Act of 1993, PL 103–66, 42 U.S.C. § 629 *et seq.*

Pollock, M.L., & Wilmore, J.H. (1990). *Exercise in health and disease*. Philadelphia: W.B. Saunders.

Sclan, S.G., & Reisberg, B. (1992). Functional assessment staging (FAST) in Alzheimer's disease: Reliability, validity and ordinality. *International Psychogeriatrics, 4*(Suppl.), 55–69.

Shepherd, G.M. (1988). *Neurobiology*. New York: Oxford University Press.

Tabloski, P.A., McKinnon-Howe, L., & Remington, R. (1995). Effects of calming music on the level of agitation in cognitively impaired nursing home residents. *American Journal of Alzheimer's Care and Related Disorders and Research, 10*(1), 10–15.

Teri, L., & Logsdon, R.C. (1991). Identifying pleasant activities for Alzheimer's patients: The Pleasant Events Schedule–AD. *Gerontologist, 31*(1), 124–127.

Traber, J., & Gispen, W.H. (1985). *Senile dementia of the Alzheimer type*. New York: Springer-Verlag.

Van Norman, K.A. (1995). *Exercise programming for older adults*. Champaign, IL: Human Kinetics.

Vecchione, K.M. (1994). A recreational therapist's perspective. In I. Burnside & M.G. Schmidt (Eds.), *Working with older adults: Group process and techniques*. Boston: Jones & Bartlett.

Voelkl, J.E., Fries, B.E., & Galecki, A.T. (1995). Predictions of nursing home residents' participation in activity programs. *Gerontologist, 35*(1), 44–51.

Whipple, R.H., Wolfson, L., Derby, C., Singh, D., & Tobin, J. (1993). Altered sensory function and balance in older persons. *Journal of Gerontology, 48* (Special Issue), 71–76.

Whitcomb, J.B. (1993). The way to go home: Creating comfort through therapeutic music and milieu. *Journal of Gerontological Nursing, 8*(6), 1–10.

Young, C. (1993). Spirituality and the chronically ill Christian elderly. *Geriatric Nursing, 14*(6), 298–303.

Yukl, T. (1997, January). *An interspecies kinship: Persons and companion animals in later life*. Paper presented at the Dimensions of Caring and Spirituality in Health Care: Practice, Research and Theory conference, Gainesville, Florida.

Zgola, J. (1987). *Doing things: A guide to programming activities for persons with Alzheimer's disease and related disorders*. Baltimore: The Johns Hopkins University Press.

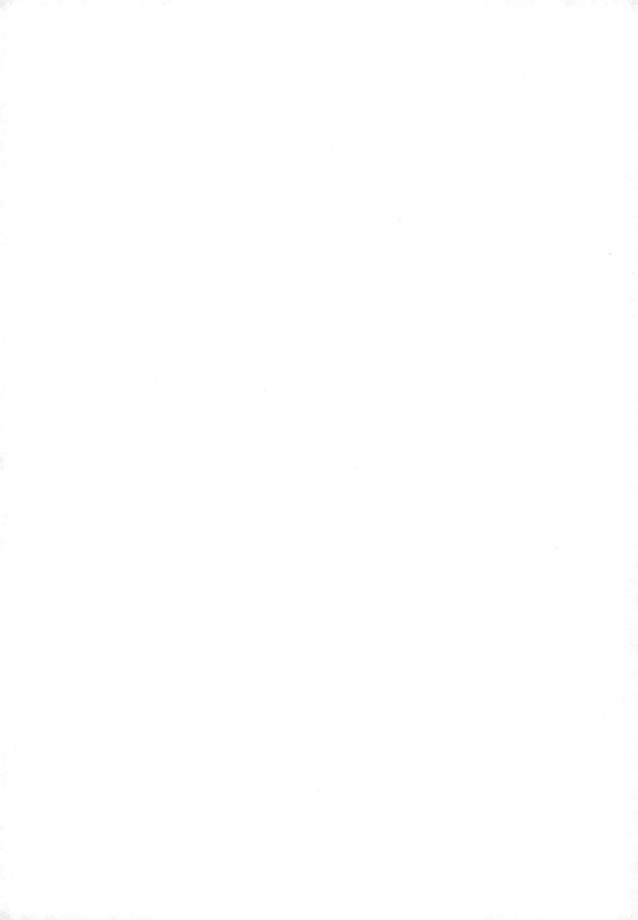

Chapter 11

Environmental Modifications

If they have not spent a day in a wheelchair, tell your architect and designer to do so, and not to cheat. . . . It will open your eyes and sensitize you.

Margaret Calkins (1994)

Before very much had been learned about the effects of Alzheimer's disease on people, family members consoled themselves that "mother doesn't know what is happening to her so it doesn't matter if we take turns having her live with us," or that "my husband no longer knows where he is so it's okay to put him in a nursing home." The assumption was that, because the person could no longer act on the environment, the characteristics of that environment no longer mattered. In fact, the opposite appears to be true. Because the person with Alzheimer's disease has a diminished capacity to adapt to the demands of any particular environment, the characteristics of the environment are even more important than they are to a person who is cognitively intact. Some characteristics of the environment may even determine how functional the person can be. This idea can be taken one step farther: A well-designed environment can be an important element in the treatment of Alzheimer's disease (Hiatt, 1991).

One of the most dramatic examples of the effect of the environment on people with Alzheimer's disease is the response to relocating. Both family members and formal caregivers comment frequently on the impact of moving to a new home, into a long-term care facility, and even from one unit to another in the same facility.

> For years, my husband talked about moving out of the city. When his Alzheimer's was diagnosed, he begged me to agree to a move. So we bought a townhouse 30 miles outside the city. It was so pretty. The problem was that all the townhouses looked alike. Dimitri could never remember which one was ours. He kept ringing neighbors' doorbells, asking for directions.
>
> One evening, he demanded to be let in someone else's townhouse. In fact, he ordered the woman to leave—he said she was in the wrong house and to get out before he called the police. She was very upset. Fortunately, our condominium in the city hadn't been sold yet so we moved back here. Dimitri is much better here, although I don't know how long it will last. I know that eventually he won't be able to find our old apartment either, but for now, he can find his way home.
>
> My mother went downhill so fast when we moved her to Denver. She had been doing okay in her own apartment but was really afraid to be alone anymore. She was getting lost on the way to the supermarket, forgot doctors' appointments, that kind of thing. When she came here, she couldn't even find the

> bathroom. She woke us up one night, screaming in the dark. A moonlit shadow from a tree outside made her think that there was a man leaning over her. She thought he had a knife in his hand.
>
> Our Alzheimer's unit was scheduled for major renovation last summer. We had to move all of the patients out while they replastered walls and carpeted the floors. We put them in the dayrooms and lounges and empty patient rooms on other units temporarily. We tried to reorient them but were not particularly successful. Patients who ordinarily went to the dining room on their own had to be helped with their trays. Our more agitated patients were really upset. One patient socked another one. He had a black eye for a week. Three died. We knew they were very frail but we hadn't expected them to die.

The more subtle effects of the environment are, of course, much more difficult to detect but have been documented in various types of research on people without dementia. Jet lag, for example, is a form of environmental dislocation. Seasonal affective disorder is thought to be a reaction to short, dark winter days that can be countered by exposure to certain wavelengths of light. The arrangement of chairs in a room has been the subject of numerous group dynamics studies. Placing chairs in a row, as is often done in airports and train stations, discourages conversation, whereas placing the chairs so people can see each other ("conversational grouping") encourages conversation.

Although research on this aspect of caring for people with Alzheimer's disease is still relatively sparse, what has been done seems to confirm the idea that the environment does make a difference (Zeisel, Hyde, & Levkoff, 1994). The following is an example of a minor environmental change that affected the person's function, in this case the ability to maintain social graces:

> In celebration of a winning lottery ticket, Ben's wife, Sylvia, recarpeted their entire house. Although she chose soft colors for the bedroom, she put a wildly patterned rug in their living room. Within a week, she noticed a urine odor in the living room. She began to watch Ben, who was in the middle stages of Alzheimer's disease by that time, to see what he was doing. Sylvia finally saw Ben urinating in the middle of the new rug. Dismayed by his action, she cried, "Ben! Why are you doing that?" "I'm just taking a warm whiz in the new urinal," Ben explained. Sylvia walked up behind Ben and looked at the center of the new rug from his viewpoint. She saw a white rectangle the size and shape of an old porcelain urinal. Sylvia rearranged the living room furniture so that the coffee table stood over the white rectangle. Ben stopped urinating in the living room.

In this chapter, a number of goals and principles for modifying environments to better suit people with Alzheimer's disease are examined, followed by more specific suggestions for resolving particular problems such as leaving the house unnoticed or having problems finding the bathroom. Differences between early and late stages and between home and institutional environments are pointed out where they are important considerations.

GOALS OF ENVIRONMENTAL MODIFICATION

Treatment

In environmental modification for people with Alzheimer's disease, the therapeutic effect is given priority over the aesthetic effect of any change in the environment. Aesthetics are not ignored but are given a therapeutic orientation. For example, the location of a fish tank would be chosen for maximum visibility by people who use wheelchairs as well as walkers rather than for being the prettiest spot in a room. A wall hanging would be selected not only for its artistic value but for its interest and lack of disturbing elements. Sometimes it is necessary to use trial and error to determine the effect of these decorative elements of design, as it is with many environmental modifications.

Dignity and Privacy

Every individual, no matter his or her degree of impairment, has a right to as much dignity and privacy as possible. For example, a person with severe impairment will need help taking a shower or using the toilet. The result is that he or she cannot do these things in private with the bathroom door closed to other people. It is still possible, however, to provide some privacy. Although another person must help, the door can be closed to others.

The design of the shower room in many long-term care facilities probably contributes to the agitation and resistance that occurs so frequently there: large, warehouse-like rooms with cold, tiled floors, walls, and even ceilings that echo every sound. Simply adding shower curtains that can be pulled around each shower head would reduce the exposure of the person being showered, cut the echoes, and reduce the cavernous appearance of these rooms.

Childish decorations and furnishings are another affront to the dignity of the adult with Alzheimer's disease. Overuse of primary colors, cartoon figures, and cutesy decorations is common, especially around holidays. Adult designs and themes can be used just as effectively to celebrate holidays, increase visual interest, and provide directional signs.

Normalization

In any setting, a major goal is to treat the person with Alzheimer's disease as much like any other person as possible, which includes providing as normal an environment as possible. It is much more difficult to do this in any but the smallest residential facility than it is at home, but it is possible. Many of the improvisations used by family members at home lend normality to the situation: a rolling, nontippable desk chair instead of a wheelchair, a lawn chair in the shower instead of a special chair, a large dinner napkin tucked under the chin at mealtimes instead of a clothing protector (bib).

The organization of adult day centers, retirement homes, and long-term care facilities works against creating a homelike atmosphere. It is a challenge to provide people with such small pleasures as staying up half the night playing cards, watching a favorite movie (one's own favorite, not everybody's favorite or the activity director's favorite), reading the Sunday comics, or rummaging around in the refrigerator for a snack late at night. None of these options is available in most facilities.

Several innovative facilities are trying to provide these small, homey pleasures for their residents. For example, hospital-like corridors and nursing stations can be broken up into smaller pods or into a wheel-and-spoke design with small clusters (instead of rows) of residents' rooms on each spoke. This design resembles that of a large home or bed-and-breakfast establishment more than it does a hospital. Residential-size living rooms and kitchens instead of large, bare dayrooms and dining rooms also contribute to a homelike atmosphere (Cohen & Day, 1993). These changes also allow smaller, quieter spaces and nooks to explore (Joint Commission on Accreditation of Healthcare Organizations, 1994), areas missing from the typical long, sterile corridors. A Swedish study of 18 small (6–8 residents) group living units for individuals with dementia found less disorientation and restlessness in units with L- or H-shaped designs than in those with one long, straight corridor, the most commonly used design in institutions (Elmstahl, Annerstadt, & Ahlund, 1997). No differences related to noise, lighting, and visual stimulation or attempts to create a more homelike atmosphere were found. These results may be more applicable to home and assisted living settings than to large long-term care facilities, given the small size of the units studied.

Allowance for Individual Differences

No matter how much is learned about modifying the environment to better suit people with Alzheimer's disease, there always will be a need to consider individual preferences and tolerances (Cohen & Day, 1993). Some people like small, cozy corners; others prefer large, open spaces. Either of these may be preferred empty or filled with people. Classical music is relaxing for some people, boring to others. Bright colors versus subdued colors, outdoors versus indoors, active versus quiet—these choices are all affected by our individual preferences. Some people also tolerate noise, change, interruptions, and distractions much better than do other people.

There is no reason to believe that these individual differences in preference and tolerance disappear with the onset of Alzheimer's disease. Thus, careful observation of each person as he or she responds to a new or adapted environment is necessary to determine which modifications are successful and which are not.

Tolerable Stimulation

The amount of stimulation that is best for people with Alzheimer's disease is the subject of some debate. On the one hand, people with Alzheimer's disease need to continue to be as active as possible. Some stimulation is necessary to encourage them to be active. On the other hand, they seem to be quite sensitive to noise and distractions. Quiet, tranquil settings allow the person to concentrate and to remain calm rather than become upset or agitated. Bombardment of disturbing environmental stimuli may contribute to resident agitation. In an observational study of disruptive episodes in the dayroom and hallways of a skilled nursing facility Nelson (1995) noted that the presence of more than 20 people in the room and movement of people or equipment through the area were related to outbursts from the residents. Minor collisions of residents using wheelchairs were also noted, a good reason for wide hallways. Turning down the volume on the television, keeping the level of voices and traffic down, even removing the television or pictures on the wall may keep environmental stimulation at a tolerable level.

Which is best, a high- or a low-stimulation environment? Probably neither high nor low, but whatever amount of stimulation is tolerated well by the individual, is best. In other words, enough stimulation should be provided to encourage activity and maintain function but not to place more demands on the person than he or she can handle comfortably (Cohen & Day, 1993).

Facilitation of Function

Perhaps the most challenging goal of environmental modification is facilitation of remaining functional capacity. In order to assist the person to function at the highest level possible, he or she must be able to find whatever it is he or she needs, recognize it for what it is, and then use it safely.

Some interesting work at the Corinne Dolan Alzheimer Center in Ohio illustrates the application of these principles. Toilets there are located in a corner of each residents' room. Partitions resembling those used in business offices form the remaining two walls, but the doorway is extra wide so that the toilet itself can be seen from the rest of the room. A curtain resembling a shower curtain can be pulled across this wide doorway for more privacy. The visual barriers seem to reduce distractions while the visibility of the toilet from the bedroom when the curtain is open makes it easier to find and use (Cohen & Day, 1993). Use of an ordinary-looking toilet also makes it easier to recognize.

Several additional features of these bathrooms further facilitate function. Grab bars alongside the toilet help the person with impaired perception or limited lower limb strength to sit down on the toilet and then pull him- or herself up again safely and independently. A brighter color is used for the toilet seat in order to attract attention away from the sink or wastebasket, sometimes selected as alternatives to the toilet by people with Alzheimer's disease. A sign for the toilet was placed on a rubber mat on the floor outside the toilet instead of on the wall for a resident who walked head down all the time. Plasticized covers or fabric protectors can be used on chairs or sofas for easier cleaning when accidents occur (Cohen & Day, 1993). Using breathable vinyl that can stand up to spills, accidents, and their cleanup but does not feel hard or stick to the skin may be helpful (DeBauge, 1996).

Another example from the same facility is a good reminder of the trial-and-error nature of some of these modifications. A refrigerator with a glass door seemed to be the perfect solution to reminding residents where snacks could be found. However, it did not increase residents' food intake, either because they could not recognize this appliance with a glass door as a refrigerator or because they did not recognize the food inside its commercial packaging ("Research results document," 1992).

Safety

Many of the cautions observed automatically by cognitively intact adults (e.g., looking before crossing a street, testing a pot to see if it is too hot to touch) may be forgotten by the person with Alzheimer's disease. Common examples are eating or drinking something out of an unknown container without checking the label, leaving the stove on, letting a burning cigarette drop to the floor, or being careless with sharp knives or guns. Adults ordinarily avoid these dangers, but people with Alzheimer's disease gradually lose their ability to make such judgments.

One approach to ensuring safety is to remove as many potential dangers as possible: lock away sharp knives, guns, car keys, toxic or flammable liquids, insecticides, and so forth. Safety devices and switches can be installed to keep the stove and other potentially dangerous devices off. Additional safety precautions are described in the next section and in Chapter 12.

SPECIFIC MODIFICATIONS

More specific modifications can be made to either the home or long-term care facility environment, from exit control to modifying the sensory inputs.

Exit Control

Ensuring that the person with Alzheimer's disease does not wander away from home and become lost or hurt is one of the greatest concerns of caregivers both at home and in residential facilities. Stories of people with Alzheimer's disease wandering away from home or leaving a facility unnoticed are common. Those that make the news are usually the ones in which the person is struck by a car or found dead in a remote area days later.

Exit control and provision of the least-restrictive environment possible are difficult goals to achieve simultaneously, but a number of devices have been produced to help meet this goal. Unobtrusive but immediately accessible exits are desirable (Hyde, 1996).

Simple Methods Several simple methods can prevent *elopement* (i.e., when people with Alzheimer's disease leave without supervision or the capability of finding their own way back). Some families find that all they need to do is move the door locks from their normal placement near the doorknob to either the top or bottom of the doorway. However, even guests will have trouble finding the locks in these out-of-the-way places. Hiding a key nearby is another approach, but it is important not to create a fire hazard by making the key too hard to find when the building must be evacuated.

An identification band similar to those used in hospitals or a metal "ID" bracelet is another simple safety measure for people who elope. Although most family caregivers are safety conscious, many do not think of an ID band or bracelet unless it is suggested to them (Lach, Reed, Smith, & Carr, 1995). Including an address and telephone number provides added safety. Some day centers place clip-on name tags of the sort used in industry and hospitals on the *back* of the collar so people with Alzheimer's disease will not remove and lose them. Individuals in the earlier stages of the disease are aware of these tags and their purpose should be explained to them. If presented with sensitivity to the person's feelings the tag will represent a helpful reminder for added security "in case you forget," not a means for tracking or controlling the person. For a small fee family caregivers can register their loved one with the Alzheimer's Association Safe Return program. This program offers an ID bracelet or necklace, wallet card, toll-free number to report when a loved one is lost, and guidance on the search process. (Additional information is available from the Alzheimer's Association, phone 800-272-3900, Internet home page www.alz.org, e-mail address webmaster@alz.org.)

Entrances and exits that must remain unlocked for some reason (e.g., fire codes) can be concealed. A wall or screen can be placed across an entrance to conceal it. Dickinson, McLain-Kark, and Marshall-Baker (1995) tested three types of visual barriers to prevent potentially unsafe exiting through a door with glass panels on an Alzheimer's unit: closed horizontal mini-blinds the same color as the door; a lightweight cotton covering also the same color as the door, with the blinds left open; and closed blinds with the cloth barrier. Although the blinds reduced exiting by 44%, the cloth alone was even more effective, reducing exiting by 96%. The researchers observed that residents were attracted to the protrusion and shininess of the door's panic bar, which was effectively camouflaged by the cloth covering, and some eventually breached the cloth barrier. They caution that any plans to place visual barriers on exits should be reviewed by a fire marshal before use (Dickinson et al., 1995). An additional benefit to this approach is that it reduces the visibility of traffic in and out of a unit. Doors also can be cleverly camouflaged with paint or wallpaper ("Research brief," 1994). Dutch doors serve a somewhat different purpose. When left half open, they provide some privacy to the person in the room and discourage other residents from wandering in uninvited, yet caregivers can still see and hear if the resident needs some help.

Secure Systems Outdoors   Outdoor areas also must be secure. Stockade fences were once the favorite material for closing in an outdoor area, but their resemblance to an old military prison (especially the pointed tops) was not aesthetically pleasing. Actually, any kind of outdoor wall can be softened with appropriate plantings. Plants that can be reached by anyone with Alzheimer's disease should not be toxic. (A list of toxic plants common in your area can be obtained from state agricultural services.)

Automatically locking gates are also essential in outdoor areas. Most of the locks are complex enough to require some thought before figuring out how to open them. They may not be sufficient, however, if people with Alzheimer's disease are unsupervised when they are outside.

Electronic Systems   A more secure (and unfortunately more expensive) system utilizes either codes or alarms to prevent elopement. Gates and elevators can be secured electronically by simple codes such as 4-3-2-1. However, if the codes are too simple, some residents will figure them out, sometimes by watching what visitors do when they leave. Others may discover them accidentally. Another common code system requires that several buttons be pressed at once to unlock the door or gate.

Visitors and staff also should know that they should not allow a resident to pass through these doors or gates, no matter how insistent the resident is. If a resident pushes through the door anyway, the visitor should alert staff immediately. Locked doors with buzzers to summon the staff are inefficient because they require staff attendance, taking staff away from therapeutic activities.

Alarm systems of varying degrees of sophistication are also available. Electronic eyes can sense when a person crosses a barrier and moves too close to the street or other hazards. However, these "eyes" cannot detect whether the person is a resident or a visitor, so false alarms will occur. Other systems are activated by ankle or wrist bracelets worn by the residents so that staff and visitors can pass undetected but a resident with the bracelet on will trigger the alarm (Sloane & Matthew, 1991). These systems can control elevators as well as doors and gates. They are generally effective in detecting possible elopers, but the loud alarms are disconcerting. Those systems that lock the doors or elevators when the alarm is triggered also create an inconvenience to staff and visitors and must be evaluated thoroughly for potential danger in the event of a fire.

All of these devices, from the simplest to the most complex, are restrictive to some degree. However, it is not only impossible but wearying for any caregiver to be eternally vigilant. These systems can prevent serious accidents and deaths, so their judicious and sensitive use is warranted in most cases.

Spaces for Wandering and Pacing

Why some people with Alzheimer's disease pace half the day or night and the potential harm or benefits of this pacing are examined in Chapter 6. Whatever the reasons, it is clear that some people with Alzheimer's disease seem to need to pace and should be allowed to do so within reason.

Pacing is one instance in which it may be easier to accommodate the person in a long-term care facility than at home, especially if home is a small apartment in a locale with much inclement weather. Local shopping malls offer long, flat surfaces suitable for pacing with a companion. The problem may be finding a willing partner. Simple exercise equipment may also provide a satisfying substitute that does not require as much space as a wandering path.

Outdoor Spaces   In good weather outdoor spaces for walking and wandering are easier to find, but a companion may still be needed. Fenced-in backyards at home and outdoor parks at long-term care facilities are ideal for outdoor wandering. In either case flat surfaces and secure gates are needed so that the person can wander or pace at will without constant supervision. Many Alzheimer's day centers and residential facilities have fenced-in outdoor areas that the person can access at will. For some residents, this seems to be a favorite pastime and source of great satisfaction.

Curved paths add to the attractiveness of outdoor settings and create some visual interest as the person follows the twists and turns of the path. Of course, keeping the exit in sight is also important for people who are easily disoriented. The way back to the house or facility should be visible from all corners of this outside area.

Indoor Spaces   Indoors, long hallways and large day areas are often chosen by residents for pacing and wandering. Whether or not these spaces encourage pacing is not clear. Obstacles of all types may present a problem: people moving slowly in their wheelchairs impede forward motion; laundry carts and other paraphernalia frequently block halls, especially in the morning. Wide hallways that are clear of clutter and equipped with sturdy handrails for unsteady walkers are essential. Glare and overly long halls may exacerbate perceptual problems and disorient some residents.

Places to Gather

Almost every home and long-term care facility has places to gather, but not all are pleasant, comfortable, or conducive to social interaction. Huge, bare dayrooms seem to repel visitors and promote institutional behavior in residents. More homelike living areas are preferable for conversation and small group interaction. The large areas, however, do lend themselves to other recreational activities, such as parties, dancing, and entertainment. Moveable partitions allow the same space to be used for multiple purposes.

Furniture Arrangement   As mentioned in the introduction, chairs lined up against a wall do not encourage people to sit facing each other and, therefore, discourage conversation. Even worse are stationary furnishings that cannot be moved to accommodate different size groupings. Soft (although not too soft, or people will have difficulty rising out of them), comfortable chairs and small sofas in "conversational groupings" do encourage conversation.

Use of carpet in places where spills and toileting accidents are common is still somewhat controversial, but carpet in "living room" areas reduces the cold, institutional feel of a residential facility and adds to personal comfort. Properly installed low-pile carpeting is preferable because shuffling feet, walkers, and wheelchairs become caught in or are slowed down by deep-pile carpeting (Hughes, 1995).

Televisions A television, sometimes called "the electronic hearth" for its ability to draw family members into a circle around it, can be placed in some, but not all, of these gathering places. Too often, televisions in residential facilities present green faces and loud static, not exactly what a person with impaired perception needs.

As Alzheimer's disease advances, people seem to experience increasing difficulty comprehending television programs. Some facilities have found that eliminating the ubiquitous television from the lounges used by people in advanced stages of the disease has decreased the amount of disruptive behavior. However, because televisions are an important source of information and entertainment, judicious use would seem to be the best policy for all but the most impaired residents.

Places to Get Away

Places to get away from the crowd, to be quiet or private outside of one's bedroom, are rare in most long-term care facilities. Ironically, perhaps, special Alzheimer's units may be the noisiest, most conflict-filled places in such facilities. Resident rooms are often the only small, quiet space to which a person can retire for peace and quiet. It is usually easier to provide such spaces in a private residence, although crowded living quarters can present almost as much of a challenge as a busy Alzheimer's care unit.

How important are these places to get away? The Joint Commission (1993) encourages provision of irregular spaces and nooks to explore in its standards for special care units. These spaces may be small porches or patios outdoors or small rooms or alcoves indoors. Some spaces are created by the use of plants or furniture arrangements, and others are designated "quiet areas," rooms set aside for this purpose.

It is often forgotten that a person with Alzheimer's disease can be as distressed as are staff and visitors by the sometimes bizarre behavior and unexpected outbursts of fellow residents. Because he or she does not understand clearly why other residents are acting the way they do, the person frequently concludes, not entirely illogically, that the other residents are "crazy" and will advise his or her family not to visit "this crazy house I'm in" because it will upset family members too much. Clearly, the small and irregular spaces are important not only for exploration but also for getting away from the sometimes distressing behaviors of fellow residents.

Allowing these small private spaces means that staff cannot observe all residents at all times. Some staff may find this restriction difficult to accept, especially those who are accustomed to a hospital type of environment. It also requires that extra attention be devoted to the safety issues examined earlier in this chapter.

Natural Areas

The provision of access to outdoor areas is probably more of a quality-of-life than a necessity-of-life issue. However, outdoor sounds and sights have long been used to promote relaxation and provide enjoyment. Outdoor areas are also important sources of healthy recreational activities. For people with Alzheimer's disease, these may be one of the few sources of enjoyment left. Some comments from family caregivers illustrate this well:

> I try to take my wife out every evening to see the sunset. She can't say much anymore, but her "oohs" and "aahs" at the colors in the sky are clear enough to me.

Raul always loved to fish. He's not very good at it anymore, but he will sit in the boat for hours, as content as he ever gets nowadays.

Gardens, terraces, patios, courtyards, and gazebos are magnets for the eye as well as places for visitors and residents to gather. Safe, pleasant places with both sun and shade, sheltered spaces, screened spaces, and spaces open to catch the breeze should be available outside of every long-term care facility (Cohen & Day, 1993). In cold locales or high-rise facilities an indoor atrium or screened-in rooftop garden or terrace is also attractive, although expensive to build and maintain.

Of course, safety must still be a concern. When people with moderate or severe Alzheimer's disease are outside alone, the area must be secure so they cannot wander away. The area also must be safe (e.g., no obstacles or irregular walkways to trip on, no toxic plants within reach, no sharp gardening implements or chemicals left untended).

Sensory Input

The modification of sensory inputs may be the most complex aspect of environmental modification. Sounds, sights, and smells abound in most long-term care facilities. Some may be essential, others helpful, but a number may be disturbing or confusing to people with Alzheimer's disease. For example, staff rushing from one task to another may inadvertently raise the tension level on a special care unit. Moving more slowly and keeping voices low may help residents (Cohen & Day, 1993).

Visual Input   Color coding to distinguish important objects (e.g., "your room has a green door, his is blue") may be too abstract for people late in the disease and not useful for people with color blindness. More concrete cues using representative symbols (e.g., the outline of a toilet for the bathroom, forks and spoons for the dining area) may be more helpful (Hiatt, 1991). However, if the individual needs glasses to see these signs clearly, then they will only be helpful when glasses are being worn. (This is a problem in some facilities where hearing aids, dentures, and glasses are not carefully guarded and residents are therefore rendered incapable of interpreting or acting upon their sensory environments. Prevention measures include careful labeling of these valuable items, checking food trays before they are returned to the kitchen, and checking laundry before it is sent out.)

Other visual elements can cause confusion. Too many directional arrows in one area leave the person sorting through a jumble of abstract symbols, a task many people with Alzheimer's disease are no longer capable of accomplishing. However, simple, direct, readable word signs can be helpful. A sign with the resident's name on it can help distinguish his or her room from others' rooms until relatively late in the disease. Elaborate lettering or decoration on the sign may defeat the purpose, however. Use the simplest, most direct words possible: *toilet* is easier to understand than *restroom*, for example ("Research brief," 1995).

Colors can be chosen for their tranquilizing effect. Peach, pink, beige, ivory, light blue, green, and lavender are all believed to be relaxing colors. White, yellow, orange, and red are considered livelier, more stimulating colors. Flat paint is preferable to enamel, which may add to problems residents have with glare.

Small prints on wallpaper can be mistaken for insects crawling on the wall or for snakes slithering in a window (Alzheimer's Association, 1990). Alternating light and dark tiles on the floor can cause it to appear to have holes (the dark tiles) that need to be avoided. A dark stripe across a floor can cause a person with Alzheimer's disease to stop in his or her tracks and refuse to proceed past the "chasm" ahead (called *visual cliffing*). Contrast in colors can be helpful in other places where they help the individual distinguish architectural features such as stairways or doorways.

Mirrors also can be confusing, especially when used for decorative purposes. Imagine walking into a room for the first time and trying to judge its length where the far wall is covered with mirrors. Smaller mirrors in expected places (bathroom, dressing areas, bedrooms) do not seem to contribute to confusion for most people.

Olfactory Inputs   It is harder to evaluate the effects of odors on people with Alzheimer's disease. The smell of strong cleaning fluids and disinfectants, urine, feces, and insecticides are unpleasant and likely to be distressing. In contrast, the scents of a garden or a kitchen are usually welcome and may evoke pleasant associations (Cohen & Day, 1991). Good ventilation is essential in any setting.

Aural Inputs   Many noises—loud televisions, alarms, call bells, paging systems, staff shouting down the hall to each other—may be disturbing. In general, soft, muted tones are considered more calming than loud, harsh tones. Quiet time with the lights dimmed and noises diminished may reduce sundowning syndrome, which occurs late in the afternoon or early evening. "Sundowners," as they are called, are people who are usually calm and reasonable during the day but become restless and agitated when the sun goes down.

Individual Assessment

The importance of assessing individual differences in tolerance and preference should be emphasized once more. Observation of the individual's response to any modification of the environment is a major part of the assessment. However, many caregivers sometimes forget that the most straightforward way to assess these effects is to *ask* the person, as in the following example from a recreational therapy aide:

> I brought Mrs. Silver a compact disc player to listen to. I thought she might like to hear some Jewish folk songs but wasn't sure. After I turned it on, she started to say something but I couldn't understand her. She had such a strange look on her face that I nearly took the CD player away. She kept struggling to say something and finally got the word out. She said, "beautiful." I'd never heard her speak before.

Imagination, flexibility, and a willingness to test and discard ideas that do not work are important ingredients when creating a therapeutic environment for people with Alzheimer's disease.

REFERENCES

Alzheimer's Association. (1990). *Environment.* Chicago: Author.
Calkins, M. (1994). Quoted in "How to create a therapeutic environment." *Respite Report,* 6(2), 3–10.

Cohen, U., & Day, K. (1993). *Contemporary environments for people with dementia*. Baltimore: The Johns Hopkins University Press.

DeBauge, L.K. (1996). Interior design/renovation of the special care unit. In S.B. Hoffman & M. Kaplan (Eds.), *Special care programs for people with dementia* (pp. 139–148). Baltimore: Health Professions Press.

Dickinson, J.I., McLain-Kark, J., & Marshall-Baker, A. (1995). The effects of visual barriers on exiting behavior in a dementia care unit. *Gerontologist, 35*(1), 127–130.

Elmstahl, S., Annerstedt, L., & Ahlund, O. (1997). How should a group living unit for demented elderly be designed to decrease psychiatric symptoms? *Alzheimer Disease and Associative Disorders, 11*(1), 47–52.

Hiatt, L.G. (1991). Designing specialized institutional environments for people with dementia. In P.D. Sloane & L.J. Matthew (Eds.), *Dementia units in long-term care*. Baltimore: The Johns Hopkins University Press.

Hughes, E.M. (1995). Creating functional environments for elder care facilities. *Geriatric Nursing, 16*(4), 172–176.

Hyde, J. (1996). Alzheimer-friendly assisted living regulation. *American Journal of Alzheimer's Disease, 11*(2), 2–9.

Joint Commission on Accreditation of Healthcare Organizations. (1993). *1994 Standards and survey protocol for dementia special care units*. Oak Brook Terrace, IL: Author.

Lach, H.W., Reed, T., Smith L.J., & Carr, D.B. (1995). Alzheimer's disease: Assessing safety problems in the home. *Geriatric Nursing, 16*(4), 160–164.

Nelson, J. (1995). The influence of environmental factors in incidents of disruptive behavior. *Journal of Gerontological Nursing, 21*(5), 19–24.

Research brief: Supportive cues. (1995). *Respite Report, 7*(1), 6.

Research results document ways to help Alzheimer's patients. (1992, Fall). *Advances: Newsletter of the Robert Wood Johnson Foundation*, p. 10.

Sloane, P.D., & Matthew, L.J. (1991). *Dementia units in long-term care*. Baltimore: The Johns Hopkins University Press.

Zeisel, J., Hyde, J., & Levkoff, S. (1994). Best practices: An environment-behavior (E-B) model for Alzheimer special care units. *American Journal of Alzheimer's Care and Related Disorders and Research, 9*(2), 4–21.

Chapter 12

Promotion and Maintenance of Health and Function

Theris Touhy

Couldn't it be said that as long as he could appreciate the magnolia he was still very much alive?

S. Ariyoshi (1987)

The widespread belief that nothing can be done to improve the lives of people with Alzheimer's disease reduces the individual to a nonperson status, devoid of treatment options. Because these people are viewed as unable to benefit from treatments, they are often excluded from services. Perhaps even more distressing than this exclusion, human services professionals often overlook treatable problems or dismiss them as untreatable solely on the basis of the Alzheimer's diagnosis and, in doing so, fail to plan for appropriate goals for these people. In fact, the expectation that people with Alzheimer's disease face imminent and irreversible decline is so ingrained that professionals often view any setbacks, both subtle and dramatic, as inevitable consequences of the disease progression and therefore do little to counteract these setbacks or rehabilitate the individual. The following vignette illustrates this:

> I received a report on the nursing unit one Monday morning and was told that they felt Marta had progressed to the last stage of the disease. Thinking that this was a bit unusual because Marta had been her usual self when I left on Friday, I began asking a few more questions of the nursing staff. Marta's normal pattern for the 3 years I had known her was to constantly walk all over the facility. She rarely spoke, but always had a smile when she stopped long enough to be with one of us. The staff went on to report that Marta was eating well, showed no evidence of pain, fever, or other symptoms, and still had her sunny disposition and ready smile. What was very different was that Marta had spent the entire weekend on the unit, mostly sitting in a chair, and most definitely not walking around the facility as usual. Narrowing the problem down to one of mobility, rather than a progression to the nonambulatory stages of Alzheimer's, X rays were taken and confirmed a fractured hip. The fracture was

subsequently repaired and, after several weeks of therapy, Marta was up and walking again—still, I might add, in the same "stage" of her disease.

Caregivers and service providers must remember that the maintenance of good health can help to ensure that the experience of the disease is not compounded by untreated illness.

This chapter examines strategies to promote and maintain the physical health of people with Alzheimer's disease in order to prevent excess disability and maintain the highest quality of life possible.

DETECTION OF SIGNS AND SYMPTOMS OF PHYSICAL ILLNESS

Maintaining physiological balance in the frail older adult with multisystem problems has been likened to walking a tightrope because these individuals live very close to the outer limits of normal physiological function. Stress on their systems often disrupts their fragile conditions, leading to illness. Yet, because of the nature of Alzheimer's disease, illness in these individuals is difficult to detect and easily ignored. By the time dramatic presentations surface, these adults can be *very* sick.

Delineating Barriers to Adequate Treatment

The subtle influence of age-discriminant health care practices has been documented in the literature (Binder & Robins, 1990; Foreman, 1986; Levine, 1989; Mentes, 1995; Tappen & Beckerman, 1993; Weddington, 1982). Older adults with Alzheimer's disease experience this age discrimination even more acutely, which ultimately affects their ability to obtain adequate care for the following reasons:

- Adults with Alzheimer's disease often cannot tell health care professionals how they are feeling.
- Aggression and other behavior disturbances that accompany the illness are frequently misunderstood and incorrectly treated with psychoactive medications.
- Adults with Alzheimer's disease cannot advocate for themselves or fight for the treatment they need.
- Because adults with Alzheimer's disease are often seen as hopeless, practitioners frequently see no point in providing treatment.

Older people frequently present symptoms of acute illnesses in subtle ways that are missed by practitioners. Exacerbations of chronic illnesses or new disease processes, infections, drug toxicity, elimination problems, sensory deprivation, or overstimulation are commonly manifested in unconventional symptoms in frail older adults (Mentes, 1995).

> Colby, an ambulatory man with Alzheimer's disease, was quite prone to urinary tract infections. The only indication that an infection was developing was his gait, which became more unsteady, causing him to lean to one side while he was walking. The staff knew they should report his condition and assess him for a possible urinary tract infection when Colby started leaning.

In fact, the cognitive and behavioral changes are often the first signs of physical alterations. In a person who already demonstrates cognitive impairment, further decline in mental status, changes in behavior, or both often go unnoticed and untreated. These important cues to the development of health problems are overlooked and simply assumed to be a result of the existing disease process. Even worse than being dismissed, the behaviors may be seen as psychiatric problems and treated with psychoactive medications, while their underlying cause goes undetected, leading to further morbidity (Lyness, 1990; Weddington, 1982).

In addition, pain is often unrecognized or inadequately treated in older adults (Ferrell & Ferrell, 1993; Haley & Dolce, 1986; Herr & Mobily, 1991; Sengstaken & King, 1993), especially among older people with Alzheimer's disease, who often have many other chronic health concerns that predispose them to pain. Osteoarthritis and osteoporosis, for example, can make any movement or touch painful. Unable to explain their hurt or to even recognize their pain, behavior changes such as increased withdrawal, screaming, aggression, and combativeness may be the only available way for these individuals to communicate their illness (Marzinski, 1991).

> An older lady with Alzheimer's disease spent most of her waking hours self-propelling her wheelchair down the hall of the long-term care facility calling out: "Miss, Miss, please help me, my back, my back." At the same time, she grabbed and pinched whomever came within her reach. Her behavior was distressing to the staff, visitors, and other residents. She was placed on Haldol, which had no effect on her behavior. Her back was extremely kyphotic (curved), and she had a history of osteoporosis and several old fractures. Fortunately, her primary care provider was reluctant to increase the Haldol and requested an orthopedic consultation. After the initiation of around-the-clock pain medication, placement in a comfortable padded recliner chair when out of bed, and frequent rest periods in bed during the day, her distress-related behaviors stopped completely.

A more unusual mode of communicating pain is the following:

> Having lost the ability to express herself in words, one woman used numbers. During the morning care routine, she would call out a series of numbers. The staff were intrigued; they even began playing the lottery with the numbers, thinking she might be psychic. After some time, the staff finally figured out what the numbers meant. When she was comfortable, she repeated 578, but when she was in pain, the number 64 was used. Once the staff decoded her messages, they were able to meet her comfort needs.

Improving Assessment

Recognizing, diagnosing, and treating illness in adults with Alzheimer's disease is comparable to fitting hundreds of small pieces of a jigsaw puzzle into a meaningful whole.

Changes in Behavior It is important to be acutely aware of subtle changes in behavior and daily life patterns that may herald the onset of acute illness. To recognize these subtle changes and diagnose them correctly, the care provider must know the person and his or her own unique patterns of behavior. Wolanin and Phillips (1981) cautioned against misunderstanding an older person's behavior and suggested three simple questions to ask when assessing behavior: "1) Does the behavior make sense to the person? 2) How does the present behavioral response compare to past responses the person has made under similar circumstances? 3) Does the behavior make sense to you within his framework?" (p. 90). Structured assessment protocols such as those developed by Foreman (1986) and

Mentes (1995) should be utilized in any setting to assist the practitioner in recognizing and diagnosing delirium (see Table 12.1). It is also important to gather information on past history from family, caregivers, and any others who know the person well. So-called "problem" behaviors should not be dismissed as disruptive or a characteristic of Alzheimer's disease, but rather viewed as a possible mode of communicating needs when words fail and people cannot communicate their pain.

> Jacques, a resident of a long-term care facility, was diagnosed with Alzheimer's disease, which was compounded by an additional diagnosis of paranoia and aggressive behavior. Prior to admission to the nursing facility, Jacques suffered sepsis (disseminated infection) related to a urinary tract infection and spent 5 days in an intensive care unit of a local hospital. His aggressive behavior, according to his wife, began during this hospitalization. She reported that he cursed and hit any caregiver who attempted to perform invasive treatments such as catheterization and intravenous therapy, necessitating the use of bilateral wrist restraints and antipsychotic medications.
>
> These behaviors had not been evident at home or in the long-term care setting, where Jacques did well without psychoactive medications. He lived in a private room and had a set routine, and the staff knew that he needed his personal space. Activities related to toileting or incontinence care were approached gently and with much explanation because these were areas of potential stress for this man.
>
> All seemed to be going well since his admission to the nursing facility. Then, on one of her frequent visits, Jacques's wife told him her shoulder was sore and asked him to rub it for her. He began rubbing gently and then very roughly pinched her and would not let go. This frightened her and she reported it to the staff, wondering if his aggression was escalating again. The next day, staff reported that Jacques had struck out at one of his favorite caregivers while she was assisting him to the toilet. It was also reported that he had moved his bowels in the sink. Much discussion followed as to the advisability of a psychi-

Table 12.1.   Examples of causes of delirium in frail older adults[a]

Systemic	Exacerbation of chronic illness or new disease process (e.g., diabetes, chronic obstructive pulmonary disease, thyroid disease, gastrointestinal bleeding, electrolyte imbalance)
	Infections (e.g., respiratory, urinary)
	Drug toxicity/interactions
	Elimination problems (e.g., fecal impaction, urinary retention)
Mechanical	Exacerbation of chronic illness or new disease process (e.g., cardiovascular accident, cardiac dysfunction, cancer, brain trauma)
Psychosocial/environmental	Losses (e.g., death of loved one, loss of possessions)
	Sensory deprivation/overstimulation
	Level of personal control

From Mentes, J. (1995). A nursing protocol to assess causes of delirium. *Journal of Gerontological Nursing, 21*(2), 26–30; reprinted by permission.

[a]This list of causal factors is not exhaustive, and multiple factors are possible.

atric consult and the need for medication to stop these behaviors. His wife expressed concern that his disease had progressed and was saddened at this possibility because he had been doing so well.

Looking at his past history of sepsis related to a urinary tract infection, and knowing the experiences this gentleman underwent in his last hospitalization, an astute practitioner ordered a urinalysis, which showed red blood cells and bacteria. A culture followed, treatment was given, and Jacques returned to his stable state with no recurrence of aggression or inappropriate behavior. While focused on his behavior, the staff found an additional reason for it: On occasion, the door to his bathroom had been shut. Unable to see the visual cue of the toilet and unable to work through the process of locating another toilet, Jacques had utilized the next best option—the sink in his room. His care plan now clearly reflects the importance of always leaving the door to his bathroom open, and his "inappropriate behaviors" have subsided.

Hanson's story further illustrates the importance of interpreting any and all forms of verbal and nonverbal communication as potentially indicative of some need.

Hanson was transferred to the Alzheimer's unit from another facility. He had a malignant melanoma on his face and was disfigured. His eyes were shut tightly and he was not able to verbalize except for almost constant loud, grunting moans. Thorazine (a major tranquilizer) was given whenever he became particularly loud. When asked why this man was moaning, his physician said that he also had dementia and the loud, grunting moans were a result. However, after observing the ineffectiveness of the thorazine, the nursing staff concluded that the moans were related to pain. After much lobbying to convince the doctor, pain medication was ordered. With each dose of pain medication, the moaning became quieter. Within 3 days, it was heard only rarely. Hanson appeared less restless and much more comfortable.

Now the pattern of his moans is recognized by staff members who can interpret his needs by the characteristics of the sounds. The moan of pain is easily differentiated from the moan related to constipation or hunger. Hanson communicates his needs the only way available to him, and the nursing staff listens and responds. This is the intimate knowing that must be brought to full awareness in caring for the person with Alzheimer's disease.

Changes in Vital Signs   Baseline patterns of vital signs should be obtained in order to detect change and identify abnormalities. Unless professionals know what is normal (or at least customary) for the person, they will be unable to detect subtle changes and may even initiate unnecessary treatment. For example, a temperature of 98.6° F may indicate impending infection in a frail older adult with a baseline temperature of 96° F.

In older people, hyperthermia (overheating) can occur with temperatures as low as 100° F and can be accompanied by shaking and tremors. The absence of other abnormal findings, however, does not reliably rule out serious illness when there is fever. A 1995 study of older people admitted to an emergency room with fevers of 100° F or higher showed that 76% of them were seriously ill. Half of this 76% showed no other indications of serious illness, yet 13% of those discharged were later admitted with serious ailments, primarily pneumonia, urinary tract infection, or sepsis. The presence of fever is significant in older people and requires careful investigation. Parenthetically, the researchers noted that emergency room physicians consider evaluation and treatment of older patients to be more time consuming and difficult because they usually need more extensive evaluation of physical, immunological, social, and psychological conditions (Marco et al., 1995).

Hypothermia (lower than normal temperature) is also a significant risk in the frail older person. Inactivity, inability to communicate feeling cold or to cover up or dress more warmly, thermoregulatory changes, thin skin, and the effect of medications predispose frail older people to hypothermia. Careful attention must be paid to maintaining a comfortable room temperature, providing warmth and adequate covering during bathing, and providing lap robes and sweaters to people unable to move from chairs.

> A new staff nurse received a report that an older person was very confused. He sat all day in a chair in his room with a blanket on his head, the staff reported. She had just finished a class on delirium in the older adult and was sure that she could find out what was going on with this gentleman. She was determined to show the rest of the nursing staff that there were probably reversible causes for his confusion that they had missed, not having the advantage of her recent learning. She provided his morning care and came to learn that he was only mildly forgetful. In fact, he was a retired professor of English.
>
> The nurse saw little indication of confused behavior and was quite pleased with her skills. She got him out of bed and settled comfortably into the chair. Then, as she was leaving, he asked her for a blanket. She gave it to him, and he promptly placed it on his head, just as had been reported to her. She asked him why he had a blanket on his head, to which he replied, "Everyday they put me in this chair next to the air conditioner and it's cold. I am accustomed to wearing a hat and, since I do not have one here, the blanket will have to do."

Changes in Biorhythms   Changes in sleep, rest, and activity patterns may also herald the onset of illnesses and require close observation. Not only are these patterns unique for each individual but they typically change with age and may be affected by Alzheimer's disease. Close observation of these patterns is useful in detecting change and in helping individuals maintain their usual patterns. For example, some people usually nap several times a day, whereas others remain alert and active all day. It is also important to note that people with Alzheimer's disease may have difficulty sleeping through the night. Often, it is unrealistic to expect them to stay in bed or to sleep soundly all night. The use of hypnotics for sleep induction should be avoided, and sleep disturbances should be treated as problems only if they interfere with the function of the person.

PREVENTION OF HEALTH PROBLEMS

Many health problems can be avoided with simple preventive measures. Immunizations, dental examinations, influenza vaccines, tuberculosis screenings, routine mammograms, Pap smears, and prostate examinations should be available to all older adults, including those with Alzheimer's disease. In addition, care providers should be cognizant of the health benefits of maintaining mobility and fitness in the older adult and ensuring adequate intake of food and liquids.

Maintaining Mobility and Fitness

The positive effects of activity for people of all ages are well documented (Spirduso, 1995). Increased muscle tone and strength, joint flexibility, peripheral circulation, and lung vital capacity; improved perfusion of nutrients into body tissues, sleeping and eating patterns, and self-esteem and mood; and decreased blood pressure, stress, and anxiety are just some of the benefits of exercise (Clarkson-Smith & Hartley, 1989; Miziniak, 1994; Parent & Whall, 1984; Roberts & Wykle, 1993; Simpson, 1986). For the older adult, even the frail long-term care facility resident, an increase in muscle strength and mobility, which can reduce the use of assistive devices, is a potential benefit (Fiatarone et al., 1990, 1994; Mulrow et al., 1994; Walker, 1986). Inactivity, in contrast, predisposes the person to falls, fractures, depression, incontinence, and pressure ulcers.

Several researchers have noted that the health of people with Alzheimer's disease seems to improve with exercise. Exercise maintains or increases functional abilities, improves appetite and quality of sleep, reduces stress and disruptive behaviors, helps alleviate depression, enhances self-esteem, and improves the person's ability to communicate (Friedman & Tappen, 1991; Miziniak, 1994; Posner & Ronthall, 1991; Teri & Logsdon, 1991). For example, Friedman and Tappen (1991) studied walking and conversation with a group of 30 individuals with moderate to severe cognitive impairments resulting from Alzheimer's disease. Individuals who walked and engaged in conversation with the investigator for 30 minutes three times a week improved on two tests of communication skills. The researchers noted that this intervention can be accomplished easily in any setting because it involves walking at the individual's pace and engaging in conversation on topics of relevance to the person.

It is distressing to note the continued resistance to inclusion of people with Alzheimer's disease in rehabilitation and exercise programs because of their supposed "zero rehabilitation potential." Their failure to comprehend and retain instructions for rehabilitation therapies are viewed as evidence of their inability to achieve program goals. A 1995 study of falls and gait training, for example, noted that cognitive impairment was a major risk factor for falls, yet indicated that individuals with dementia are not good candidates for physical therapy (Galindo-Ciocon, Ciocon, & Galindo, 1995).

Perhaps it is the goal of rehabilitation that ought to be reconsidered when applied to the person with Alzheimer's disease. Rehabilitation efforts focus primarily on restoring function after an acute event such as stroke or hip fracture, rather than maintaining or improving strength and function (Rubenstein, Josephson, & Robbins, 1994). In contrast, improvement and maintenance of function and prevention of unnecessary decline are appropriate goals for the person with Alzheimer's disease. As Monicken (1991) reported, "regardless of functional potential, few patients should be eliminated from rehabilitation programs. Any goals, no matter how limited, that could possibly enhance a patient's discharge status, quality of life, or level of independence should be given at least a short term trial" (p. 241). Everyone has potential and goals, although they are sometimes harder to identify in people with Alzheimer's disease. Being able to move on one's own and participate in social situations contributes to as high a level of functioning as possible, thereby enhancing an individual's quality of life. Keeping people moving—any way possible, for as long as possible—often demands creativity and patience on the part of caregivers. Performing tasks for the person, although easier and more efficient for the caregiver, robs people of control and dignity and increases excess disability.

Designing Interventions to Promote Mobility and Fitness
Interventions to promote mobility and fitness must be individualized for each person and based on a functional assessment of their abilities and physical capabilities, knowledge of their past

interests and life patterns, and their response to the activity. Activities should be within their physical and cognitive capabilities and should be enjoyable. Rubenstein et al. (1994) noted that simple walking programs can improve strength and function, indicating that older adults "should be encouraged to be as physically active as possible, even if that only consists of walking with assistance a few minutes each day, as long as it can be done with reasonable safety" (p. 448).

Interventions range from formalized gait training and therapist-directed progressive ambulation to kicking a ball or raising arms to reach for the stars in a small group activity. One person may enjoy throwing a bean bag into a basket on the floor, another may prefer folding towels or dusting. Activities should be as varied as the individuals participating in them.

> A tall, portly gentleman in the late middle stage of Alzheimer's disease was admitted to a long-term care facility. He was essentially nonverbal, making only grunting noises. He kept his eyes shut and required a great deal of stimulation to respond to staff. Occasionally, they saw a smile or a glimmer of understanding but his primary strength was his ability to ambulate. His wife reported that she and a home health aide had established a toileting routine in which they would use a rolling walker and assist him to the bathroom every morning at home. Looking at the man's size, the staff questioned the advisability of this routine and instead suggested the use of diapers for the management of toileting needs and the use of a mechanical lift for out-of-bed transfers. They cited staff time, efficiency, and their backs as reasons for the suggestion. His wife was adamant in her belief that he could and should be walked, and that the toileting regimen she had established had eliminated the need for enemas and disimpactions related to his constipation problems.
>
> After several strenuous sessions of enemas in bed, combined with pushing and pulling this large man back and forth to provide incontinence care, ambulation to the bathroom was seen as worth a try. To the amazement of the staff, once he got up and moving he was clearly capable of pushing the walker and moved at a slow pace to the bathroom. After 3 months, his morning toileting routine had not only restored normal bowel patterns without the use of enemas but had also improved his ambulatory abilities so that he could walk 60 feet.

One long-term care facility introduced twice-daily "rock and roll" times. When the upbeat music started, residents were to grab a partner and start moving. People who needed assistance were paired with partners. Those who could move their wheelchairs independently started rolling; others may have needed a push. Staff members and residents alike enjoyed watching the parade move through the halls and outside the facility, with visitors and office staff often joining in to help. Everyone exercised at their own pace in a joyful and enthusiastic manner. Another Alzheimer's day center located in an elementary school coordinated its outdoor walking time with the children's recess hour. Children often came by to walk outdoors with their older friends.

Another way to promote and maintain function in people with Alzheimer's disease is to incorporate exercise and fitness activities into small group work. The SERVE (*self-esteem*, *relaxation*, *vitality*, and *exercise*) model described by Schwab, Rader, and Doan (1985) is a good example. The program combines music, exercise, touch, and relaxation into a small group activity in which individuals with Alzheimer's disease interact for 1 hour three times a week. Using these and other creative activities, staff and residents can experience a renewed sense of vitality and enthusiasm. Staff members should remember to plan activities that are failure-free, in which everyone experiences success and abundant praise.

Ensuring Adequate Intake of Food and Fluids

Ensuring the adequate intake of food and fluids to prevent malnutrition and dehydration should be a priority for caregivers of people with Alzheimer's disease. Clinical reports indicate that weight loss and malnutrition are typical, particularly among people with cognitive impairment who live in long-term care facilities (Hall, 1994; Sandman, Adolfsson, Nygren, Hallmans, & Windblad, 1987). Although few concrete data are available for people with Alzheimer's disease who live at home, caregivers frequently report concerns in this area. Older adults are increasingly diagnosed with "failure to thrive" in hospital and long-term care facility admissions, primarily as a result of unexplained weight loss and resultant malnutrition (Newbern, 1992). The weight loss associated with Alzheimer's disease, still unexplained, may even be present in people with adequate caloric intake (Sandman et al., 1987; Singh, Mulley, & Losowsky, 1988). However, this should not be assumed to be an inevitable consequence of the disease. Caregivers should thoroughly investigate changes in weight and eating patterns, which may herald pathological conditions. Possible explanations for weight loss include physiological consequences of the disease process itself, functional losses affecting eating ability, behavioral manifestations of the disease that interfere with adequate intake, ineffective feeding approaches, and inadequate assessment of eating abilities (Bonnel, 1995; Hall, 1994; Osborn & Marshall, 1993; Sandman et al., 1987; Van Ort & Phillips, 1992). Increased energy consumption (possibly related to pacing or wandering), less lean body mass, less body fat, low fasting blood sugar levels, hyperinsulinism (a generalized impaired metabolism syndrome), and dysphagia (swallowing problems) are also possible explanations for weight loss and malnutrition among people with Alzheimer's disease (Hall, 1994; Sandman et al., 1987; Singh et al., 1988). Hall (1994) noted that choking on foods and fluids may be caused by forgetting how to swallow or stuffing their mouth with food.

Designing Interventions to Ensure Adequate Intake   Interventions to assist in providing adequate nutrition and fluid intake must be based on accurate assessments. Observation of eating abilities, dining environments, feeding techniques and time allotments, and dysphagia should help to determine which components of the activity are problematic. In residential settings, nursing staff, dietitians, speech-language pathologists, and occupational therapists may be involved in the assessment. Enlisting family or friends to determine the cause of eating problems is also helpful.

Encouraging good oral hygiene, repairing diseased teeth, and obtaining properly fitting dentures are also essential to adequate intake. Because people with Alzheimer's disease may not recognize their thirst or may exhibit apraxia (i.e., not understand what to do with a glass or cup), water and other liquids should be easily accessible and frequently offered. Food should be available around the clock for those who are awake at night or may be receptive to eating outside of scheduled mealtimes.

Large meals and the provision of many dishes and utensils may be confusing. Not knowing what to do, the person may play with the food or simply not eat. Offering only one food at a time may be more effective than serving a full tray of food at each meal.

Older adults also may experience dysphagia. The practice of syringe feeding should be avoided because it may force foods and fluids into the person's mouth without allowing for the swallowing reflex to take place, increasing the risk for aspiration. Careful assessment of potential dysphagia is important to prevent choking and aspiration pneumonia, a leading cause of death among people with Alzheimer's disease (Hall, 1994).

The symptoms of abnormal swallowing are difficulty initiating the swallow, packing of food into the cheeks, drooling, coughing or throat clearing, an absent or weak coughing reflex, and fluid leaking from the nose after swallowing (Donahue, 1990). Interventions may include the following (Donahue, 1990; Gauwitz, 1995; Hall, 1994):

- Thickening liquids with nonfat dry milk or a commercially prepared thickener
- Using semisolid foods rather than puree
- Observing or feeling for the swallow after each bite
- Offering small quantities of food at a time
- Allowing adequate time for eating and limiting distractions
- Offering solids and liquids at different times
- Checking the mouth for lodged or pocketed food
- Avoiding the use of straws
- Keeping the drinking glass three-quarters full or using a partially covered cup to prevent tipping the head too far back
- Keeping the person in an upright position during eating and for 45–60 minutes after eating
- Sitting the person up straight and slightly forward, with the head slightly flexed during meals
- Maintaining close observation and having assistance and suction equipment available
- Training staff in cardiopulmonary resuscitation (CPR) and Heimlich manuever
- Providing precut meats and avoiding foods easy to choke on, such as crackers, popcorn, or hot dogs
- Developing an extensive finger-food menu

Initiating Enteral Feeding and End-of-Life Decisions Caregivers should be certain that all available interventions have been instituted before initiating long-term enteral (tube) feeding. If enteral feeding is begun, ongoing assessment of eating abilities and the need for continued use of the tube should be conducted. Hall (1994) reported comparable mortality rates between individuals with dementia who were fed by nasogastric tube and those who were fed naturally. Some individuals who required short-term nasogastric feeding during periods of acute illness were able to have the tube removed once the episode resolved.

Issues related to the use of enteral feeding to sustain the lives of people in the end stage of Alzheimer's disease should be discussed with the patient and family early in the disease process. Ideally, the person chooses his or her own preference in this regard before losing the ability to communicate such complex ideas. If the person cannot do so, it is important to provide caregivers with adequate information regarding available treatment options and the consequences related to nutritional intake. The question of whether the burdens of medical hydration and nutrition outweigh the benefits in treatment of those with terminal illness is a matter of considerable discussion and concern (Taylor, 1995).

SPECIAL HEALTH CARE ISSUES

Caregivers should be aware of several special health care issues such as incontinence. Also, older adults with Alzheimer's disease frequently require extra help in caring for their skin and maintaining their dental hygiene.

Skin Integrity

Age-related factors and the sequelae of superimposed illnesses place older people at great risk for skin breakdown and pressure ulcers. Additional risk factors related to Alzheimer's disease include the inability to recognize pressure-related discomfort or to reposition oneself because of mobility-related problems or the use of restraints, poor nutritional and fluid intake, and injuries to the skin as a result of bumping into things or falling. Skin should be inspected daily for any redness, irritation, or open areas. The liberal use of lubricants to keep skin supple and observance of adequate fluid intake to maintain hydration are also important.

Dental Care

In the late stages of the disease people with Alzheimer's disease lose the ability to routinely care for their teeth or dentures. Unfortunately, provision of dental care for older people in long-term care facilities is frequently less than adequate. It is often difficult for caregivers to provide dental care or even to examine the teeth and gums because the person does not comprehend commands to open the mouth or resists allowing others access to the mouth. As a result, dental problems are common. Caregivers should seek guidance from dental professionals when designing interventions for dental care. Nighttime applications of solutions to prevent decay, soft sponge applicators, ingestible toothpaste, and the appropriate use of suction or electric toothbrushes may help prevent tooth decay and keep the mouths of the older adults clean and fresh.

Incontinence

People with Alzheimer's disease are at high risk for developing incontinence because of impaired mobility and cognition (Jirovec & Wells, 1990). It is estimated that 30%–40% of people who enter residential facilities become incontinent while in the facility (Newman, 1996; Newman, Steidle, & Wallace, 1995). Incontinence may be overlooked or untreated because it is considered inevitable. Additional contributing factors are the apraxia associated with the disease, the use of medications that dull the senses or increase perfusion and output, the effects of relocation to an unfamiliar facility, lack of clearly marked signs combined with appropriate verbal reminders, lack of easy-to-manage clothing, and inadequate staffing patterns (Jeter, 1990). Functional incontinence, usually the result of restricted mobility, cognitive impairment, apraxia, or lack of assistance to toilet, is most common among persons with Alzheimer's disease (Newman et al., 1995).

Designing Interventions for Incontinence   Before designing interventions, a thorough assessment of the reasons for incontinence should be conducted. Assessment should include a continence history, medication review, physical examination, functional assessment of ability to use the toilet or toilet substitute, environmental assessment, bladder diaries (tracking frequency, timing, and amount of continent and incontinent episodes), and additional tests such as urinalyses, cultures, and postvoiding residual measurements. Many tools are available to assist in the assessment of types and causes of incontinence (Penn, Lekan-Rutledge, Joers, Stolley, & Amhof, 1996; Urinary Incontinence Guidelines Panel, 1996). Treatable conditions such as urinary tract infections, constipation, or fecal impaction should be corrected.

For individuals unable to express their need to evacuate, toileting routines should be developed using such cues as increased restlessness, wandering, pulling at clothing, or attempting to get out of bed or a chair. Establishing individualized toileting regimens in long-term care facilities has been shown to require less nursing time and cost less than care provided for an incontinent episode (Creason, Burgener, & Farrand, 1992).

> One gentleman with cognitive impairment spent most of his day singing lovely operatic tunes. When his singing became quite loud and was interspersed with "Oh, God," caregivers knew to take him to the bathroom.

Loose-fitting clothing, Velcro fly closures on pants, and wearing minimal or no undergarments may make toileting easier (Jeter, 1990).

If incontinence episodes occur, the person's skin requires meticulous care to prevent fungal infections and skin damage, which predispose to pressure ulcers. Frequent changing of wet bedding and clothing; adequate cleansing of the skin, with limited use of drying soaps or powder; and implementing pressure ulcer prevention programs can help to alleviate skin complications.

External Urinary Devices   If interventions to lessen incontinence are unsuccessful or if a person is unable to participate in interventions, the use of adult briefs or external urinary devices should be considered. For some older adults, these products and devices can restore social continence and allow for more participation in activities (Jeter, 1990; Newman, 1996). For others, these devices may allow continued care at home, especially when relatives are physically or emotionally unable to manage using other alternatives. However, these types of interventions should not be the first choice of treatment. They should be used only for the protection and dignity of the person, never for the convenience of staff (Jeter, 1990).

A wide array of incontinence products are available. Pads, which are placed in the underwear, are preferable to full briefs. If the full brief is required, underwear may be placed over them to promote a more typical feeling and appearance. A fully absorbent and disposable adult brief with an elastic waistband that allows for easy application and removal is most convenient for people who can still toilet themselves. External urinary devices are also helpful, especially for men, but must be used with caution. They should be changed at least every 24 hours and applied correctly to avoid constriction of the penis. The person's skin should be observed frequently for irritation.

PROMOTING HEALTH WITH SAFE ENVIRONMENTS

Aging places people at high risk for injury and fatal accidents. Dementia, even more than age, further increases risk (Van Dijk, Meulenberg, Van DeSande, & Habbema, 1993). The effects of Alzheimer's disease on a person's neurological and cognitive function eventually make him or her completely dependent on caregivers to maintain safety. A study of 35 caregivers of people with Alzheimer's disease living in the community identified wandering, cooking, driving, and displaying antisocial and aggressive behavior as the most commonly occurring safety problems. Common accidents included becoming lost, cuts, and falls (Lach, Reed, Smith, & Carr, 1995). In the long-term care setting the use of physical and chemical restraints to prevent injury also contributes to the risk of injury and accidents (Evans & Strumpf, 1990; Jantti, Pyykko, & Hervonen, 1993; Rubenstein et al., 1994; Sloane et al., 1991; Tinetti, Liu, & Ginter, 1992; Van Dijk, Meulenberg, Van DeSande, & Habbema, 1993).

Incidence and Consequences of Falls

Accidents are the fifth leading cause of death in older adults, accounting for two thirds of accidental deaths (Rubenstein et al., 1994). Statistics indicate that 35% of people 75 years and older living in the community will experience falls (Tinetti & Speechley, 1989). In long-term care settings the incidence of falls is even higher. An estimated 40%–50% of residents fall each year (Ejaz, Jones, & Rose, 1994), of whom half fall repeatedly (Tinetti, 1987).

Older adults living in residential facilities may have more intrinsic risk factors for falls and are more susceptible to falling as a result of even minor hazards in the environment. For the frail older adult with multiple risk factors, the performance of daily activities, such as toileting, can precipitate a fall (Rubenstein et al., 1994; Tinetti & Speechley, 1989).

Although only 5%–10% of falls result in serious injury, the older person may experience postfall syndrome and limit activities because of fear of another fall (Murphy & Isaacs, 1982; Rubenstein et al., 1994; Ruthazer & Lipsitz, 1993; Sloane et al., 1991; Tinetti, Williams, & Mayewski, 1986; Van Dijk, Meulenberg, Van DeSande, & Habbema, 1993), also known as "fallaphobia" (Kemp & Mosqueda, 1997). Caregivers may also limit the activities or mobility of someone afraid of another fall, which may be more hazardous than the fall itself. Caregivers must be alert, though, because falls can herald the onset of acute illness or disease states in the older adult (Granek et al., 1987; Jantti et al., 1993; Kuehn & Sendelweck, 1995; Meddaugh, 1996; Micelli, Waxman, Cavalieri, & Lage, 1994; Tinetti, 1987).

Etiology of Falls

Fall risk increases with the number and severity of chronic illnesses and disabilities. Chronic conditions that impair sensory, cognitive, neurological, and musculoskeletal functioning increase fall risk. Gait abnormalities significantly increase the risk of falls. Foot problems, such as toe deformities, bunions, or calluses, may contribute to gait disorders, instability, and falls. The decline in visual acuity, perception, hearing, vestibular function, and proprioception (i.e., reception of stimuli produced by the organism) that accompany age-related changes or disease processes also contributes to falls. A direct relationship exists between someone's total number of medications and his or her risk of falling (Rubenstein et al., 1994; Tinetti & Speechley, 1989).

It has been suggested that environmental factors play a greater role in falls among community-based older adults (see Table 12.2). Two studies noted that stumbling and slipping in urine accounted for a number of falls in long-term care facility residents with Alzheimer's disease (Meddaugh, 1996; Pieter et al., 1993). Little research exists to explain how the environment may contribute to falls in the long-term care setting (Rubenstein et al., 1994; Tinetti & Speechley, 1989). Speculated causes include the physical and psychosocial adjustment to the communal nature of a long-term care setting; changes in daily living patterns; limitations of activity and independence; new equipment and devices, such as wheelchairs, mechanical lifters, and shower rooms; and the use of physical restraints. Staffing levels, education and training, proper use of equipment, and time of day and location in which most falls occur are also variables that should be analyzed in assessing fall risk factors in the facility (Ejaz et al., 1994; Ginter & Mion, 1992; Jantti et al., 1993; Kuehn & Sendelweck, 1995; Luukinen, Koshi, Laippala, & Kivela, 1995; Rubenstein et al., 1994).

The first few weeks after admission to a hospital or long-term care facility are associated with a high fall risk. Unfamiliarity with the new environment, the aftereffects of a hospital stay, or physical deterioration at home necessitating admission contribute to increasing risks for falls during this period (Van Dijk, Meulenberg, Van DeSande, & Habbema, 1993). It is important to explore past fall events in as much detail as possible

Table 12.2.   Environmental factors affecting the risk of falling in the home

Environment area or factor	Objectives and recommendations
Lighting	Absence of glare and shadows; accessible switches at room entrances; night light in bedroom, hall, or bathroom
Floors	Nonskid backing for throw rugs; carpet edges tacked down; carpets with shallow pile; nonskid wax on floors; cords out of walking path; small objects (e.g., clothes, shoes) off floor
Stairs	Lighting sufficient, with switches at top and bottom of stairs; securely fastened bilateral handrails that stand out from wall; top and bottom steps marked with bright, contrasting tape; stair rises of no more than 6 inches; steps in good repair; no objects stored on steps
Kitchen	Items stored so that reaching up and bending over are not necessary; secure step stool available if climbing is necessary; firm, nonmovable table
Bathroom	Grab bars for tub, shower, and toilet; nonskid decals or rubber mat in tub or shower; shower chair with handheld shower; nonskid rugs; raised toilet seat; door locks removed to ensure access in an emergency
Yard and entrances	Repair of cracks in pavement, holes in lawn; removal of rocks, tools, and other tripping hazards; well-lit walkways, free of ice and wet leaves; stairs and steps as above
Institutions	All the above; bed at proper height (not too high or low); spills on floor cleaned up promptly; appropriate use of walking aids and wheelchairs
Footwear	Shoes with firm, nonskid, nonfriction soles; low heels (unless person is accustomed to high heels); avoidance of walking in stocking feet or loose slippers

upon admission in order to identify those individuals at risk and implement fall prevention interventions as early as possible.

Alzheimer's Disease as a Fall Risk Factor

Although the diagnosis of dementia is consistently mentioned as a risk factor for falls, few studies have been carried out to assist in understanding the unique characteristics of people with dementia in relation to fall risk, fall prevention, and the effectiveness of interventions (Van Dijk, Meulenberg, Van DeSande, & Habbema, 1993). Researchers have found that cognitive impairment increases fall risk by impairing judgment, neurological function, balance control, visuospatial perception, and the ability to orient oneself geographically (Jantti et al., 1993; Roberts & Wykle, 1993; Rubenstein et al., 1994; Van Dijk, Meulenberg, Van DeSande, & Habbema, 1993). Cognitive impairments may also affect a person's capacity to perceive his or her actual abilities, which leads to attempts to perform activities outside of his or her physical capabilities, thus increasing fall risk (Roberts & Wykle, 1993). For example, a person may attempt to get up and walk unassisted, climb over siderails, or wander into unsafe areas. Among those who can ambulate, risk increases when they are unable to recognize increasing fatigue, know when to stop, or recognize hazards in the environment such as people or objects.

> One older man who loved to walk rapidly, unless redirected to the circular path, would keep walking until he ran into the bushes or fell down.

Older people control their postural stability almost entirely by visual input. One study suggested that adults with dementia are at greater risk for falls because of a lack of visual fixation, which may explain why, despite good physical and neurological status, they fall more often (Jantti, Pyykko, & Hervonen, 1993). In addition, dementia is the most consistent predictor for the use of physical and chemical restraints in the long-term care setting, further predisposing those with dementia to increased fall risk (Rubenstein et al., 1994; Sloane et al., 1991; Tinetti et al., 1992; Van Dijk, Meulenberg, Van DeSande, & Habbema, 1993).

Assessment of Fall Risk

Fall risk analysis should be conducted after a fall or whenever a person's condition changes (see Table 12.3). Assessments should include an examination of those physical and psychological conditions that can be treated or modified. For example, simple adjustment of medications, provision of an appropriate assistive device, treatment of a urinary tract infection, or a change in prescription lenses may lessen the risk of falls.

A fall risk assessment should also include an observation of the person performing position changes and gait maneuvers during customary ADLs. Balance and gait assessment can provide valuable information about fall risk, underlying conditions that may predispose one to falls, the hazards associated with certain activities, and the types of rehabilitation and environmental interventions that may facilitate reducing fall risk. Especially helpful is observing the person's ability to get in and out of bed and walk to the bathroom, because a high number of falls occur during these activities.

Finally, a comprehensive review of the person's history of falls, including a description of how the fall occurred, review of medications, the person's activity at the time of the fall, environmental factors that may have had an impact on the fall event, and strategies the person utilizes to prevent and cope with falls should also be assessed (Rubenstein et al., 1994; Tinetti & Speechley, 1989; Van Dijk, Meulenberg, Van DeSande, & Habbema, 1993).

Fall Prevention Interventions

Maintaining dignity, independence, and freedom while preventing injury is a major caregiving dilemma in Alzheimer's disease. Designing safety programs to minimize accidents and injuries without compromising quality of life requires creative intervention. The most challenging aspect of a fall prevention program is the design of appropriate interventions that minimize the risks of falls and injuries while supporting and enhancing functional independence. Interventions must be individualized, taking into consideration intrinsic risk factors, the person's functional level, the impact of the environment, and the effect of the treatment on the person's quality of life (Kiernat, 1991; Rubenstein et al., 1994).

Identifying Patterns   Cohen, Neufeld, Dunbar, Pflug, and Breuer (1996) reported success with the use of a behavior mapping instrument to assist staff in identifying patterns of behavior and choosing appropriate interventions. With careful assessment, staff were able to see that many risky behaviors, such as attempting to stand up unassisted, were related to a specific need such as toileting or comfort (Bradley, Siddique, & Dufton, 1995;

Table 12.3.   Fall risk assessment[a]

Physical appearance	Poorly fitting shoes
	Shoes in poor condition with heels and lasts broken down
	Frail
	Flat affect, suggesting depression
Postural control	Balance Test Results
	Positive Romberg's sign
	Unsteady tandem gait
	Unsteady gait
	Uses wide base of support when standing and ambulating
	Use of an assistive device for ambulation
	Poor muscle strength of trunk and lower extremities
	Unable to rise from a chair without moving toward the edge of the seat or using arms to push off
Skeleton	Severe deformities of the feet
	Severe limited range of motion in the knees, hips, and ankles
	Severe kyphosis
	Severe limitations in the range of motion of the neck
Nervous system	Abnormalities in vibratory sensation of the lower extremities
	Abnormal patellar reflex
	Corrected visual acuity less than 20/50
	Postural hypotension on arising from a chair or bed
Mental status	Cognitive impairment
Psychological status	Depressive symptoms
	"Fallaphobia"
	Perceptions of physical abilities and risk for a fall that are inconsistent with the physical findings
Functional status	Dependency in physical ADLs and instrumental ADLs
	Impaired motor coordination
Environment	Poor lighting
	Cluttered hallways
	Absence of handrails
History	History of a fall, slip, or trip in the past 6 months

Adapted from Roberts, B.L., & Wykle, M.L. (1993).

[a]The risk for a fall increases as the number of abnormal findings increases.

Cohen et al, 1996; Strumpf, Wagner, Evans, & Patterson, 1992; Werner, Cohen-Mansfield, Koroknay, & Braun, 1994).

Reviewing Medication   If possible, caregivers should eliminate medications that may contribute to impaired balance, perception, awareness, and cognitive function. Sedatives, benzothiadiazides, phenothiazines, antidepressants, antiarrhythmics, and diuretics have the most impact on a person's fall risk. Psychoactive medications have been associated with a twofold increase in the rate of recurring falls among ambulatory long-term care facility residents (Granek et al., 1987; Thappa, Gideon, Fought, & Ray, 1995), although it is not clear if the increased fall risk is the result primarily of the medication itself or of the combination of the medication and other inherent conditions in the individual.

The 1987 Omnibus Budget Reconciliation Act (OBRA; PL 100-203) mandates the right of all residents of skilled nursing facilities to be free from any physical or chemical restraint imposed for the purposes of discipline or convenience and not required to treat the resident's physical symptoms. Chemical restraints are generally considered to be in use when psychoactive drugs are given on a regular basis (Sloane et al., 1991). These medications should be prescribed only to treat the symptoms of a specific disease state and must contribute to maintaining or improving the condition for which they are being used, without decreasing the functional abilities of the person. If these medications are used, caregivers must monitor for side effects and reduction of symptoms and explore the effectiveness of nonpharmacological alternatives.

Enhancing Function   Lower extremity weakness, especially ankle dorsiflexion (i.e., flexion toward the back), has been found to be a significant risk factor for falls among older adults (Kiernat, 1991; Luukinen et al., 1995). Balance and gait training programs have been shown to improve ambulation (Galindo-Ciocon et al., 1995; Jantti et al., 1993; Roberts, 1989). Skilled therapists need to be involved in both the assessment of the fall risk of frail residents of long-term care facilities and the design and adaptation of fitness and exercise programs. Simple walking programs, range of motion exercises, and exercise groups should be a part of any fall prevention program. Even walking a few steps with assistance is preferable to immobility and may ameliorate fall risk.

Providing Appropriate Clothing   Proper footwear and footcare can improve mobility and gait and lessen fall risk. Gait and balance assessments should be conducted with the person wearing his or her customary footwear and also without shoes. Shoes that are well fitting with firm, nonskid soles may maximize proprioceptive input (Tinetti & Speechley, 1989). Kiernat (1991) noted that women accustomed to wearing high heels may have shortened Achilles tendons and may benefit from a low-heeled shoe. Podiatric care should be routinely provided for assessment and treatment of conditions such as toe deformities, bunions, calluses, and long nails.

It is recommended that people not wear loose-fitting slippers or slipper socks. However, one study noted a decrease in fall rates among residents of a dementia care unit when nonskid terry slipper socks were worn during the night (Meddaugh, 1996).

People also should be dressed in clothing to which they are accustomed and that they like. Clothing should fit well and be comfortable. Ill-fitting clothing and pants that are too long have been mentioned as possible causes of falls. Jogging suits, which are easily put on, provide warmth, and are easy to launder, are highly recommended. However, many older women refuse to wear them and prefer housedresses.

Utilizing Protective Devices   Some individuals may require assistive ambulation devices. A plastic walker with an attached seat may be useful for some people who can ambulate but need support and protection. It can promote independence, strengthen lower extremities, improve gait and ambulation, and help people to move about without the assistance of a caregiver. Bicycle helmets and hip pads have also been noted as useful in the prevention of injuries related to falls among older adults at high risk (Jantti et al., 1993; Rubenstein et al., 1994).

Making the Environment Safe   Environmental changes useful in fall prevention include grab bars in hallways, bedrooms, and bathrooms; elevated toilet and bathtub seats; nonskid wax on floors; nonslip treads in tubs and showers; handrails on stairs (textured and extending beyond the last step); and kitchen arrangements that allow for convenience without bending over or reaching up. Because older people with vision losses or proprioceptive abnormalities require adequate illumination to assist them in maintaining balance, caregivers should provide optimal lighting in bedrooms and bathrooms, even at night, while reducing glare. In addition, stronger visual stimulation, such as sharp contrasts, bright colors, and vertical stripes on the walls, may help these adults avoid falls.

Bed and chair alarms or wanderer alert systems are also useful to alert caregivers that people are attempting to get up or go into unsafe areas. Widder (1985) reported that bed alarms reduced falls by 20%–30%. One caregiver places a string of Christmas bells on every bedroom door in her house to alert her that her husband is up and about. In addition, customized seating devices such as wedge cushions, positioning pillows, deeply inclined seats, solid seat inserts in wheelchairs, antitipping devices, rocking chairs, recliners, and lap trays can increase comfort in seating, compensate for postural instability, and prevent falling or sliding out of chairs (Kiernat, 1991).

Walking paths should be free from obstacles, especially moveable furniture. Beds should be in a low position and locked, and mattresses can be placed on the floor next to the bed to cushion a fall. Residential facilities should consider the use of double bed–size mattresses instead of the standard single mattresses and should avoid full siderails.

Because many older people use touch to assist in postural stability, it may be helpful to locate rails or nonmovable objects on the path between the bed and bathroom. Wide open spaces with nothing to hold onto or touch may increase fall risk (Kiernat, 1991; Rubenstein et al., 1994). Personal items and call lights should be within easy reach. In the home setting, devices that are worn around the neck and can activate a telephone call are useful. Occupational therapy evaluation and treatment can contribute greatly to the assessment of fall risk and the design of safety interventions.

Restraints   Physical restraints traditionally have been a standard intervention in a fall prevention program. Designing safety programs without restraints requires caregivers to reframe their thinking.

Incidence of Restraints   As a result of mandates in the 1987 OBRA legislation, restraint use in long-term care facilities declined from 41% in 1987 to 22.5% in 1992 (Strumpf & Evans, 1992). Since 1992, several studies have reported even lower rates of restraint use (Cohen, Neufeld, Dunbar, Pflug, & Breuer, 1996; Ejaz et al., 1994; Werner et al., 1994). Although national rates for restraint use in hospitals are not reported, published studies estimate that between 7% and 50% of hospitals use restraints (Ludwig & O'Toole, 1996; Strumpf & Evans, 1992). The Joint Commission on Accreditation of Healthcare Organizations, the national accrediting body for hospitals, has begun closely scrutinizing restraint use in hospitals, which may lead to more accurate data about the appropriate use of restraints and alternatives in the acute care setting, as well as to a decrease in the use of restraints.

Nevertheless, the national restraint rate suggests that thousands of older adults, especially those who are old-old (age 80 and older) or have cognitive impairment, are routinely restrained in health care institutions across the United States (Strumpf & Evans, 1992). It further suggests that many caregivers are still unaware of effective alternatives (Cohen et al., 1996).

Effects of Restraints   Prevention of falls is most frequently cited as the primary reason for using restraints among older adults. However, restraints do not prevent serious injury and may even increase risk of injury (Ginter & Mion, 1992; Tinetti, Liu, & Ginter, 1991,

1992). For example, vest restraints, which have been found to be the cause of several deaths, are still commonly used (Ludwig & O'Toole, 1996; Miles & Irvin, 1992). As noted by Ejaz et al. (1994),

> Allowing previously restrained residents the freedom to fall does not appear to place them at greater risk than other elderly nursing home residents. These findings raise the question of why we restrain only the most physically and cognitively impaired residents in nursing homes, while other residents may enjoy liberty and are allowed to face the consequences of freedom.

Other common reasons offered for the use of restraints include inadequate staffing, wandering, confusion, interference with medical treatment, agitation and aggression, moral duty to protect residents from harm, and fear of legal liability (Cohen et al., 1996; Evans & Strumpf, 1990; Ludwig & O'Toole, 1996).

Some people believe that society's attitudes toward older adults and those with mental illness influence this practice. Physical restraints were originally used to control the behavior of individuals with mental illness considered to be dangerous to themselves or others (Evans & Strumpf, 1990). Using restraints on frail older adults with cognitive impairment reflects society's attitudes and beliefs about the worth of older people and its limited understanding of the meaning of behavior (Cohen et al., 1996; Hall & Buckwalter, 1991; Miller, 1994; Rantz & McShane, 1995; Ripich, Wykle, & Niles, 1995; Taft et al., 1992; Whall, Gillis, Yankou, Booth, & Beel-Bates, 1992).

The inappropriate and indiscriminate use of restraints is a source of great physical and psychological distress to older adults and may intensify agitation or contribute to depression (Strumpf & Evans, 1992, p. 126):

> I felt like a dog and cried all night. It hurt me to have to be tied up. I felt like I was nobody, that I was dirt. It makes me cry to talk about it (tears). The hospital is worse than a jail.

> I don't remember misbehaving, but I may have been deranged from all the pills they gave me. Normally, I am spirited, but I am also good and obedient. Nevertheless, the nurse tied me down, like Jesus on the cross, by bandaging both wrists and ankles. . . . It felt awful, I hurt and I worried, "What if I get leg cramps; what will I do then if I can't move?" It was miserable . . . and an awful shock. . . . Because I am a cooperative person, I felt so resentful. Callers, including men friends, saw me like that and I lost something; I lost a little personal prestige. I was embarrassed, like a child placed in a corner for being bad. I had been important . . . and to be tied down in bed took a big toll. . . . I haven't forgotten the pain and the indignity of being tied.

Alternatives to Using Restraints   The conflict between the legal/professional imperative to protect individuals from harm and the federal mandate to decrease the use of restraints is a source of concern to professional caregivers. Removing restraints without careful attention to safety and the use of effective alternatives can jeopardize an individual's safety. Evans and Strumpf (1990) offer the following guidelines for standards of practice for restraint use with older adults:

1. The use of restraints should trigger further investigation and treatment aimed at elimination of the problem causing the need for restraint.
2. Restraints should be applied only as a result of collaborative decision making between health team members.
3. Restraints should never be used as a substitute for surveillance.
4. The use of restraints should incorporate informed decision making by patients and families.
5. Restraints should be used only on a short-term basis and as a last resort by staff members who are properly trained for their use. (p. 126)

When using restraints to prevent interference with medical treatment, the risks and benefits of both the treatment and the short-term use of restraints should be considered (Evans & Strumpf, 1990). Alternatives include disguising tubes under clothing or binders; limiting the duration of invasive treatments; using volunteer or family assistance in observation; and utilizing headphone radios, therapeutic touch, relaxation, and distraction techniques. If restraint is essential, the least-restrictive restraint should be utilized.

Evans and Strumpf (1990) noted that long-term care facilities in the United Kingdom, which emphasize active rehabilitation, expect falls and accidents to occur. Although falls are common, the rate of serious injury is not high. Scottish nurses, who believe that restraints are unethical, rarely use them, and in a 1987 study were able to identify a significantly higher number of alternatives than nurses in the United States (Evans & Strumpf, 1990). Similar findings related to the limited use of alternatives were reported in a study of hospital nurses on medical-surgical floors (Ludwig & O'Toole, 1996).

WEIGHING TREATMENT OPTIONS

Early detection and prevention efforts with adults with Alzheimer's disease will not always be sufficient to ward off illness, and treatment efforts will need to be instituted. In these instances both the benefits and risks of extensive diagnostic testing and treatment should be carefully considered. It is important to consider the least invasive and least-restrictive treatment option available. The short-lived trauma of having a diseased tooth removed usually is preferable to suffering the long-term consequences of inaction, such as pain related to the infection or inability to take adequate nutrition. These are issues that require careful consideration and discussion between health care providers and those responsible for the person's health care decisions, if he or she is unable to make them. The preparation of advance directives specifying the person's wishes related to these issues can be used as a basis for decision making (see Chapter 15). The role of the health care professional is not to make such decisions or impose beliefs, but rather to assist patients and families by providing information, encouraging discussion and expression of feelings, and respecting the decisions of the person with dementia or of those responsible for making health care decisions for him or her.

If extensive procedures or invasive treatments are undertaken, careful thought must also be given to how best to accomplish them. Scheduling treatments and procedures for the person's best time of day and having familiar caregivers nearby are important. The practitioner providing treatment should be familiar with the issues surrounding individuals with Alzheimer's disease in order to communicate with the person, promote comfort, and prevent behavior disturbances related to fear, pain, or the inability to understand.

A resident of a long-term care facility required sutures in his forehead as a result of a fall. Although a familiar staff member accompanied him, he still managed to terrorize the entire emergency department. Within a few minutes of having been sutured and his forehead covered with a pressure dressing, he had pulled three of the sutures out, while hitting and screaming at everyone within his reach during the procedure. Back in his familiar surroundings, his favorite nurse re-dressed the wound, using Steristrips to close the wound and a clear plastic occlusive dressing that he had difficulty removing. It healed nicely.

· · ·

Can urine specimens be collected utilizing external urinary devices rather than by inserting a straight catheter? Do intravenous lines need to be inserted to provide antibiotic treatment, or can crushed tablets be mixed into the person's favorite flavor of ice cream to accomplish effective treatment of the infection? Should a person in end-stage Alzheimer's disease with a deep pressure ulcer undergo a surgical debridement or skin graft, or should conservative treatment be continued to avoid painful surgery? Physicians, practitioners, and family caregivers must consider many ethical issues when providing treatment for people with Alzheimer's disease.

REFERENCES

Ariyoshi, S. (1987). *The twilight years.* Tokyo: Kodansha International.

Binder, E.F., & Robins, L.N. (1990). Cognitive impairment and length of hospital stay in the older person. *Journal of the American Geriatric Society, 38,* 759–766.

Bonnel, W. (1995). Managing mealtime in the independent group dining room: An educational program for nurse's aides. *Geriatric Nursing, 16*(1), 28–32.

Bradley, L., Siddique, C.M., & Dufton, B. (1995). Reducing the use of physical restraints in long term care facilities. *Journal of Gerontological Nursing, 21*(9), 21–34.

Clarkson-Smith, L., & Hartley, A.A. (1989). Relationship between physical exercise and cognitive ability in older adults. *Psychology of Aging, 4*(2), 183–189.

Cohen, C., Neufeld, R., Dunbar, J., Pflug, L., & Breuer, B. (1996). Old problem, different approach: Alternatives to physical restraints. *Journal of Gerontological Nursing, 22*(2), 23–29.

Creason, N.S., Burgener, S.C., & Farrand, L. (1992). Guidelines for assessment of incontinence in elderly institutionalized women. *Geriatric Nursing, 13*(2), 76–79.

Donahue, P. (1990). When it's hard to swallow: Feeding techniques for dysphagia management. *Journal of Gerontological Nursing, 16*(4), 6–9.

Ejaz, F., Jones, J., & Rose, M. (1994). Falls among nursing home residents: An examination of incident reports before and after restraint reduction programs. *Journal of the American Geriatrics Society, 42*(9), 960–964.

Evans, L., & Strumpf, N. (1990). Myths about elder restraint. *Image, 22*(2), 124–128.

Ferrell, B.R., & Ferrell, B.A. (1993). Pain assessment among cognitively impaired nursing home residents. *Journal of the American Geriatrics Society, 41*(4), 960–964.

Fiatarone, M., Marks, E., Ryan, N., Meredith, C., Lipsitz, L., & Evans, W. (1990). High intensity strength training in nonagenarians: Effects on skeletal muscle. *Journal of the American Medical Association, 262,* 3029–3034.

Fiatarone, M., O'Neill, E., Doyle, N., Clements, K., Solares, G., Nelson, M., Roberts, S., Kehayias, J., Lipsitz, L., & Evans, W. (1994). Exercise training and nutritional supplementation for physical fragility in very elderly people. *New England Journal of Medicine, 330,* 1769–1773.

Foreman, M. (1986). Acute confusional states in hospitalized elderly: A research dilemma. *Nursing Research, 35,* 34–38.

Friedman, R., & Tappen, R.M. (1991). The effects of planned walking on communication in Alzheimer's disease. *Journal of the American Geriatrics Society, 39,* 650–654.

Galindo-Ciocon, D., Ciocon, J., & Galindo, D. (1995). Gait training and falls in the elderly. *Journal of Gerontological Nursing, 21*(6), 10–17.

Gauwitz, D. (1995, August). How to protect the dysphagic stroke patient. *American Journal of Nursing,* pp. 34–38.

Ginter, S., & Mion, L. (1992). Falls in the nursing home: Preventable or inevitable? *Journal of Gerontological Nursing, 18*(11), 43–48.

Granek, E., Baker, S.P., Abbey, H., Robinson, E., Myers, A.H., Samkoff, J., & Klein, L. (1987). Medications and diagnoses in relation to falls in a long-term care facility. *Journal of the American Geriatrics Society, 35,* 503–511.

Haley, W.E., & Dolce, J.J. (1986). Assessment and management of chronic pain in the elderly. *Clinical Gerontologist, 5*(3–4), 435–458.

Hall, G.R. (1994). Chronic dementia: Challenges in feeding a patient. *Journal of Gerontological Nursing, 20*(4), 21–30.

Hall, G.R., & Buckwalter, K. (1991). Whole disease planning: Fitting the program to the client with Alzheimer's disease. *Journal of Gerontological Nursing, 17*(3), 38–41.

Herr, K.A., & Mobily, P.R. (1991). Complexities of pain assessment in the elderly: Clinical considerations. *Journal of Gerontological Nursing, 17*(4), 12–19.

Jantti, P.O., Pyykko, V.I., & Hervonen, A.L. (1993). Falls among elderly nursing home residents. *Public Health, 107,* 89–96.

Jeter, K. (1990). *Nursing for continence.* Philadelphia: W.B. Saunders.

Jirovec, M., & Wells, T.J. (1990). Urinary incontinence in nursing home residents with dementia: The mobility-cognition paradigm. *Applied Nursing Research, 3*(3), 112–117.

Joint Commission on the Accreditation of Healthcare Organizations. (1996). *Comprehensive accreditation manual for hospitals.* Oakbrook Terrace, IL: Author.

Kemp, B., & Mosqueda, L. (1997). Aging-related conditions. In M.J. Fuhrer (Ed.), *Assessing medical rehabilitation practices* (p. 399). Baltimore: Paul H. Brookes Publishing.

Kiernat, J. (1991). *Occupational therapy and the older adult: A clinical manual.* Rockville, MD: Aspen Publishers.

Kuehn, A., & Sendelweck, S. (1995). Acute health status and its relationship to falls in the nursing home. *Journal of Gerontological Nursing, 21*(7), 41–49.

Lach, H., Reed, T., Smith, L., & Carr, D. (1995). Alzheimer's disease: Assessing safety problems in the home. *Geriatric Nursing, 16*(4), 160–164.

Levine, M.E. (1989). Ration or rescue: The elderly patient in critical care. *Critical Care Nursing Quarterly, 12,* 82–89.

Ludwig, R., & O'Toole, A. (1996). The confused patient: Nurses' knowledge and interventions. *Journal of Gerontological Nursing, 22*(1), 44–49.

Luukinen, H., Koshi, K., Laippala, P., & Kivela, S.L. (1995). Risk factors for recurrent falls in the elderly in long term institutionalized care. *Public Health, 109,* 57–65.

Lyness, J. (1990). Delirium: Masquerades and misdiagnosis in elderly inpatients. *Journal of the American Geriatrics Society, 38,* 1231–1238.

Marco, D., Schoenfeld, D., Hansen, K., Hexter, D., Stearns, D., & Kelen, G. (1995). Fever in geriatric emergency patients: Clinical features associated with serious illness. *Annals of Emergency Medicine, 26*(1), 18–24.

Marzinski, L.R. (1991). The tragedy of dementia: Clinically assessing pain in the confused nonverbal elderly. *Journal of Gerontological Nursing, 17*(6), 25–28.

Meddaugh, D. (1996). Special socks for special people: Falls in special care units. *Geriatric Nursing, 17*(1), 24–26.

Mentes, J.C. (1995). A nursing protocol to assess causes of delirium. *Journal of Gerontological Nursing, 21*(2), 26–30.

Micelli, D., Waxman, H., Cavalieri, T., & Lage, S. (1994). Prodromal falls among older nursing home residents. *Applied Nursing Research, 7*(1), 18–27.

Miles, S.H., & Irvin, P. (1992). Deaths caused by physical restraints. *Gerontologist, 32*(6), 762–766.

Miller, R. (1994). Managing disruptive responses to bathing by elderly residents. *Journal of Gerontological Nursing, 20*(11), 35–39.

Miziniak, H. (1994). Persons with Alzheimer's: Effects of nutrition and exercise. *Journal of Gerontological Nursing, 20*(10), 27–32.

Monicken, D. (1991). Immobility and functional mobility in the elderly. In W. Chenitz, J. Stone, & S. Salisbury (Eds.), *Clinical gerontological nursing* (pp. 233–245). Philadelphia: W.B. Saunders.

Mulrow, C.D., Gerety, M., Kanten, D., Cornell, J., De Nino, L., Chiodo, L., et al. (1994). A randomized trial of physical rehabilitation for very frail nursing home residents. *Journal of the American Medical Association, 271*, 519–524.

Murphy, J., & Isaacs, B. (1982). The post-fall syndrome. *Gerontology, 28*, 265–270.

Newbern, V.B. (1992). Failure to thrive: A growing concern in the elderly. *Journal of Gerontological Nursing, 18*(8), 21–25.

Newman, D. (1996, February 6). *Incontinence: Prevalence, evaluation, and intervention.* Paper presented at Convatec 1995–1996 Advanced Practice Lecture Series, Ft. Lauderdale, FL.

Newman, D., Steidle, C., & Wallace, D. (1995). Urinary incontinence: An overview of the diagnosis and management. *American Journal of Managed Care, 1*(2), 68–74.

Omnibus Budget Reconciliation Act of 1987, PL 100-203, 42 U.S.C. § 13951-3 *et seq.*

Osborn, C., & Marshall, M. (1993). Self-feeding performance in nursing home residents. *Journal of Gerontological Nursing, 19*(3), 7–14.

Parent, C.J., & Whall, A.L. (1984). Are physical activity, self-esteem and depression related? *Journal of Gerontological Nursing, 10*(9), 8–11.

Penn, C., Lekan-Rutledge, D., Joers, A., Stolley, J., & Amhof, N. (1996). Assessment of urinary incontinence. *Journal of Gerontological Nursing, 22*(1), 8–19.

Posner, C.M., & Ronthal, M. (1991). Exercise and Alzheimer's disease, Parkinson's disease, and multiple sclerosis. *Physician and Sports Medicine, 19*(2), 85–92.

Rantz, M., & McShane, R. (1995). Nursing interventions for chronically confused nursing home residents. *Geriatric Nursing, 16*(1), 22–27.

Ripich, D., Wykle, M., & Niles, S. (1995). Alzheimer's disease caregivers: The focused program. *Geriatric Nursing, 16*(1), 15–19.

Roberts, B.L. (1989). The effects of walking on balance among elders. *Nursing Research, 38*, 180–182.

Roberts, B.L., & Wykle, M.L. (1993). Pilot study results: Falls among institutionalized elderly. *Journal of Gerontological Nursing, 19*(5), 13–20.

Rubenstein, L., Josephson, K., & Robbins, A. (1994). Falls in the nursing home. *Annals of Internal Medicine, 121*(6), 442–451.

Ruthazer, R., & Lipsitz, L. (1993). Antidepressants and falls among elderly people in long term care. *American Journal of Public Health, 83*(5), 746–749.

Sandman, P., Adolfsson, R., Nygren, C., Hallmans, G., & Windblad, B. (1987). Nutritional status and dietary intake of institutionalized patients with Alzheimer's disease and multi-infarct dementia. *Journal of the American Geriatrics Society, 35*, 31–38.

Schwab, S., Rader, J., & Doan, J. (1985). Relieving the anxiety and fear in dementia. *Journal of Gerontological Nursing, 11*(5), 8–15.

Sengstaken, E.A., & King, S.A. (1993). The problems of pain and its detection among geriatric nursing home residents. *Journal of the American Medical Association, 41*, 541–544.

Simpson, W.M. (1986). Exercise: Prescription for the elderly. *Geriatrics, 41*, 85–97.

Singh, S., Mulley, G., & Losowsky, M. (1988). Why are your Alzheimer's patients thin? *Age and Ageing, 17*(1), 21–28.

Sloane, P., Mathew, L., Scarborough, M., Desai, J., Koch, G., & Tangen, C. (1991). Physical and pharmacological restraint of nursing home patients with dementia. *Journal of the American Medical Association, 265*(10), 1278–1282.

Spirduso, W. (1995). *Physical dimensions of aging.* Champaign, IL: Human Kinetics.

Strumpf, N., & Evans, L. (1992). Alternatives to physical restraints. *Journal of Gerontological Nursing, 18*(11), 4.

Strumpf, N., Wagner, J., Evans, L., & Patterson, J. (1992). *Reducing restraints: Individualized approaches to behavior.* Huntington Valley, PA: The Whitman Group.

Taft, L., Delaney, K., Simon, D., & Stansall, J. (1992). Dementia care: Creating a therapeutic milieu. *Journal of Gerontological Nursing, 19*(11), 38–42.

Tappen, R., & Beckerman, A. (1993). A vulnerable population: Multiproblem older adults in acute care. *Journal of Gerontological Nursing, 19*(11), 38–42.

Taylor, M. (1995). Benefits of dehydration in terminally ill patients. *Geriatric Nursing, 16*(6), 271–272.

Teri, L., & Logsdon, R.G. (1991). Identifying pleasant activities for Alzheimer's disease patients: The Pleasant Events Schedule–AD. *Gerontologist, 31*(1), 124–127.

Thappa, P., Gideon, P., Fought, R., & Ray, W. (1995). Psychotropic drugs and risk of recurrent falls in ambulatory nursing home residents. *American Journal of Epidemiology, 142*(2), 202–211.

Tinetti, M.E. (1987). Factors associated with serious injury during falls by ambulatory nursing home residents. *Journal of the American Geriatrics Society, 35*(7), 644–648.

Tinetti, M.E., Liu, W.L., & Ginter, S.F. (1991). Mechanical restraint use among residents of skilled nursing facilities: Prevalence, patterns, predisposition. *Journal of the American Medical Association, 265*, 468–471.

Tinetti, M.E., Liu, W.L., & Ginter, S.F. (1992). Mechanical restraint use and fall related injuries among residents of skilled nursing facilities. *Annals of Internal Medicine, 116*, 369–374.

Tinetti, M., & Speechley, M. (1989). Prevention of falls among the elderly. *New England Journal of Medicine, 320*(16), 1055–1059.

Tinetti, M.E., Williams, T., & Mayewski, R. (1986). Fall risk index for elderly patients based on number of chronic disabilities. *American Journal of Medicine, 80*, 429–434.

Urinary Incontinence (UI) Guideline Panel. (1996, March). *Urinary incontinence in adults: Acute and chronic management.* AHCPR Publication No. 96-0684. Rockville, MD: Agency for Health Care Policy and Research, U.S. Public Health Service, U.S. Department of Health and Human Services.

Van Dijk, P., Meulenberg, O., Van DeSande, H., & Habbema, J. (1993). Falls in dementia patients. *Gerontologist, 33*(2), 200–204.

Van Ort, S., & Phillips, L. (1992). Feeding nursing home residents with Alzheimer's disease. *Geriatric Nursing, 13*(5), 249–253.

Walker, J.M. (1986). Exercise and aging. *New England Journal of Physiology, 14*(1), 8–12.

Weddington, W. (1982). The mortality of delirium: An underappreciated problem? *Psychogeriatrics, 33*, 1232–1235.

Werner, P., Cohen-Mansfield, J., Koroknay, V., & Braun, J. (1994). The impact of a restraint-reduction program on nursing home residents. *Geriatric Nursing, 15*(1), 142–146.

Whall, A.L., Gillis, G.L., Yankou, D., Booth, D.E., & Beel-Bates, C.A. (1992). Disruptive behavior in elderly nursing home residents: A survey of nursing staff. *Journal of Gerontological Nursing, 18*(10), 13–17.

Widder, B. (1985, September/October). A new device to decrease falls. *Geriatric Nursing,* 287–288.

Wolanin, M., & Phillips, L. (1981). *Confusion: Prevention and care.* St. Louis: C.V. Mosby.

Supporting Mechanisms and Services Related to Alzheimer's Disease

Chapter 13

Care for the Caregiver

No person was ever honored for what he received. Honor has been the reward for what he gave.

C. Coolidge (1992)

Caregiving should be classified as a noble profession.

F. Raymond (1994)

Simply being with a person with Alzheimer's disease can sometimes be discomfiting; providing that person's care can be a daunting task. Those who do so need the guidance and support of professionals well versed in the care of people with Alzheimer's disease and in the psychodynamics of caregiving. Caregivers need to understand what is happening to their loved one and how they can help that person without doing harm to themselves.

The myth that families coldly abandon their older relatives to the formal care system persists despite reams of research data to the contrary. In reality, families are the *sole* source of care for 70% of older adults with disabilities in the community. Another 23% of older adults with disabilities rely on both formal and informal caregivers; only 7% rely entirely on formal caregivers (DeVita, 1994).

These figures are often questioned by health care professionals whose experience tells them otherwise. They see families disappear into the night after dropping an obstreperous older relative off at the emergency room, families who seem to begrudge the older person even a new pair of slippers, families who promise to visit but never reappear. What these professionals forget, in coming to conclusions about families in general from their own experience, is that they simply do not see the families who are providing all the care at home that an older person needs as often.

According to figures from the Alzheimer's Association (1995), 70% of the 4 million Americans with Alzheimer's disease are cared for at home. This fact implies the presence of at least an equal number of caregivers. Unlike most other chapters in this book, in which the focus is primarily on the person with Alzheimer's disease, the focus of this chapter is on the perspective of family caregivers and the various interventions that support their efforts to care for their family members with Alzheimer's disease.

CAREGIVERS' EXPERIENCES

Living with Alzheimer's Disease

How does it feel to see a loved one live through the slow but steady decline of Alzheimer's disease? A number of people have written about their experiences and, for the most part, they do not mince words in their descriptions: Tragic, devastating, exhausting, chaotic, desperate, and a living hell are all terms that have been used in these chronicles of life with a person with Alzheimer's disease. Yet they also find humor in the situation and consistently speak of the person with Alzheimer's disease with deep and lasting affection.

The effects of Alzheimer's disease pose special challenges to family and friends of the person with the disease. The subtle early signs of the disease may be mistaken for carelessness, depression, paranoia, even marital infidelity. Anger and suspicion may lead to shouting matches, exchanges of insults, or worse (Danna, 1995). Overdrawn checking accounts, problems at work, and forgotten chores add to a general atmosphere of discord until the family member realizes that memory loss is responsible for these distressing behaviors.

As the disease progresses, the person with Alzheimer's disease is no longer able to express thoughts, opinions, or feelings very clearly. Many caregivers receive little directly expressed recognition or appreciation from the care receiver, thereby being denied one of the intangible benefits of caregiving for most people. In addition, the person with Alzheimer's disease eventually becomes unable to recognize or fully comprehend the needs of the caregiver—to notice that the caregiver is ill, fatigued, or stressed. Thus, the reciprocal nature of most human relationships becomes severely imbalanced; most of the giving comes from the caregiver and most of the receiving from the care receiver, with little interaction in the reverse direction.

In addition to the lack of reciprocity, there is also the problem of the stigma that is still attached to mental health problems. The seemingly bizarre behavior of people with Alzheimer's disease often makes others uncomfortable. The result is a tendency of most people to flee from the situation, further isolating caregiver and care receiver (Reese, Gross, Smalley, & Messer, 1994).

A comparison of caregivers of family members with Alzheimer's disease and stroke found that the caregivers of people with Alzheimer's disease were more distressed than those caring for a family member who had a stroke (Reese et al., 1994). The difference may be attributable to the more unpredictable nature of problems associated with Alzheimer's disease. In addition, barring additional strokes, many people who have suffered strokes show some improvement over the first few months, followed by a period in which they plateau. For people with Alzheimer's disease the decline is continuous, something that often leaves caregivers feeling helpless in the face of increasing deterioration.

Providing Care to a Person with Alzheimer's Disease

Providing care to a person with Alzheimer's disease has its rewards as well as its problems.

Rewards   Most of the literature on caregiving in Alzheimer's disease emphasizes the problems that occur, probably because it is the problems that bring people to professionals for guidance and assistance. Yet the reward portion of the equation may be more important than is generally recognized: If caregivers can be helped to improve the balance between rewards and problems, they may feel less distressed by their caregiving responsibilities.

Caregiving activities involve engagement in an intimate person-to-person relationship from which both parties can potentially derive satisfaction. The potential for reward from these encounters emerges from the connections between the individuals involved and from the caregiver's concern for the person receiving care (Tagliareni, Mengel, & Sherman, 1993). The rewards a caregiver may derive from the caregiver–care receiver relationship and concomitant activities are many.

Opportunities for Closeness   The increasing dependency of the person with Alzheimer's disease virtually forces caregiver and care receiver to spend more time in close proximity to one another. In addition, the physical intimacy of helping with such tasks as personal grooming and the psychological intimacy of helping the person cope with the fears and insecurity engendered by increased forgetfulness and disorientation may bring a greater understanding and appreciation for one another than had existed before (Lustbader & Hooyman, 1994).

Opportunities for Reconciliation   Although the stresses of coping with Alzheimer's disease may strain already tenuous or conflicted relationships even further, they may also act as a catalyst, accelerating movement toward reconciliation (Lustbader & Hooyman, 1994). Crises often open up previously closed relationships and can accelerate work toward healthier coping styles, if handled appropriately.

New Bonds with Family and Friends   Crises also can bring out the best in people, stimulating them to reach out to the person in need. Family and friends may come to the aid of the overwhelmed caregiver, leaving both feeling closer to one another.

Intrinsic Reward of Helping   For some people, providing care is a way to repay past help and kindness from the person who now has Alzheimer's disease. One often hears, "If I were in this position, I hope someone would help me out as I am doing for so-and-so." For others, simply being able to help is its own reward. It is also a recognition of the importance of mutual aid in maintaining the bonds of family and community.

Moments of Lightheartedness and Humor   Many caregivers find moments of humor, even hilarity, in the sometimes absurd world of Alzheimer's disease. Wirsig (1990), for example, describes a moment of wry amusement when he discovered that his wife, Jane, had suddenly forgotten how to sit down. Laughter defuses tensions and lifts spirits when they are down. Raymond (1994) recounts a story from the daughter of a woman with Alzheimer's disease. Her mother called her into the bedroom in a panicky voice, saying, "Look at how much weight I've gained." The daughter looked again and explained to her size 16 mother that she was trying to get into her daughter's size 6 nightgown. They both laughed at the absurdity of the situation.

Spiritual Renewal   Moral and spiritual bases for helping others in need also exist. Many caregivers find much satisfaction and solace in turning or returning to their faith.

Problems   The types of problems associated with providing care to a person with Alzheimer's disease may be divided into two categories, subjective and objective. The subjective problems include feelings of entrapment, resentment, and grief. The objective problems may include disruption of function in other roles, the financial costs of care needed, or the changes in lifestyle necessitated by the disease (Vitaliano, Young, & Russo, 1991).

The number of problems experienced by a particular caregiver and the resulting feelings of stress and burden depend on many factors, including prior relationship with and commitment to the individual; other demands on the caregiver's time, money, and energy; the care receiver's response to the disease; and the caregiver's own physical and

emotional health and resources. Each caregiver will place his or her own unique inter-
pretations on these factors and their effects. It is important to explore and discuss the
meaning of each of these factors with the caregiver before developing a plan of care.

As indicated earlier, the phenomenon of caring for one's older relation (not necessarily one who has Alzheimer's disease) has been the focus of a substantial amount of
research. One interesting study of daughters and daughters-in-law who were experiencing above-average stress from their caregiving roles found confirmation of many of what
have been reported to be the most frequent concerns of informal caregivers (Smith,
Smith, & Toseland, 1991):

- *Need to improve coping skills.*   This need includes managing time better, sharing
  rather than holding in feelings, and coping with stress. Some caregivers have trouble
  using and organizing their little leisure time. Others suffer tension headaches, back-
  aches, insomnia, muscle tension, and other symptoms of stress.
- *Providing the care needed.*   The most difficult aspect of providing care is meeting
  the emotional/behavioral needs of the care receiver. Physical, safety, legal, and financial needs are additional concerns for some caregivers.
- *Managing family issues.*   Dysfunctional as well as functional families find themselves in the role of caregiving for a person with Alzheimer's disease. When they
  shoulder the burden alone, caregivers may feel unappreciated, used, and resentful
  that other family members are not helping out as well.
- *Relationship with care receiver.*   Conflicts with the care receiver, including difficulty
  communicating, are fairly common. In addition, as the care receiver's world shrinks,
  the caregiver may find him- or herself becoming an important part of the care receiver's social life.
- *Seeking additional help.*   Often, one of the most difficult tasks for health care professionals is to convince caregivers to accept outside help. Simply providing information about these resources is not sufficient: Caregivers need to be persuaded that
  it is reasonable to accept additional help and that this in no way diminishes their
  role or their ability to determine what is best for their older relative.
- *Feeling guilt and inadequacy.*   Many caregivers feel that they are not doing enough
  for the older person. This feeling may occur despite the fact that they are doing
  everything possible for the care receiver.
- *Planning for the future.*   Decisions about continuing to keep the person at home or
  in the caregiver's home or to place the person in a long-term care facility are often
  difficult to make. Feelings of guilt and inadequacy often enter into these decisions
  even when caregivers recognize their need for relief.

Which of these problems is most difficult for caregivers of people with Alzheimer's
disease to face? The person's memory loss, aggression, and wandering were the problems
most often mentioned in one study of rural caregivers (Bowd & Loos, 1996). In another
study, given 11 different situations, 174 caregivers of all ages chose memory problems,
the person's general decline, and difficulty communicating with the person as the 3 most
difficult. The next three were personality changes, the caregiver's loss of freedom, and
the person's inability to recognize familiar people or things. The person's denial of his
or her problems, incontinence, caregiver depression, eating problems, and caregiver guilt
were chosen less often (Williamson & Schulz, 1993). Fatigue was a significant problem
for many of the rural caregivers: Less than half said they were able to get enough sleep
(Bowd & Loos, 1996).

The researchers emphasized that many people manage the responsibilities of caregiving quite well, and that those who are stressed by their caregiving responsibilities are

not all affected by the same factors. In other words, caregiving per se is not a unitary source of stress (Williamson & Schulz, 1993).

The intensity of the emotions experienced by some caregivers is lacking in these lists of problems and concerns. Interviews of caregivers and narratives of caregivers' experiences better reflect the depth and breadth of the feelings generated by the experience. For example, Raymond (1994) wrote a guide for family caregivers following her own experience of caring for her mother. Speaking of guilt and related feelings, Raymond wrote

> Ambivalent feelings occur to everyone caring for an emotionally and physically unstable patient. As you face problems which have no immediate answers, your spirit is tested repeatedly. There is a very thin line between love and hate when difficult circumstances give rise to churning emotions. As the burden of caregiving escalates, resentment grows. Then you suffer the torment of secret shame for allowing such disloyal feelings to surface. (p. 31)

To reassure the caregiver that such feelings are natural, Raymond continued

> Remember that you've got enough on your shoulders without adding the burden of guilt. When you feel overwhelmed and resentful, it is because you are a stressed-out human being, subject to the frailties and weaknesses that beset all of us living under overwhelming pressures. This is a time to be gentle with yourself and find loving ways to replenish. (p. 32)

INTERVENTIONS

General Approach

It is easy to fall into the habit of assuming that all caregivers feel the same way about their responsibilities and about what has happened to their loved one. In reality, both individual circumstances and cultural differences enter into the caregiver's interpretation of his or her situation. Gubrium and Holstein (1994) warned of the tendency to fit different people into the same mold, the "normal" course of caregiving. For example, whereas many caregivers may eventually decide that they can no longer manage their loved one at home, other caregivers may prefer to keep the person at home. This second group needs as much support for their decision as does the first group, rather than being labeled "martyrs" or "in denial" because they insist on doing it their way rather than the prevailing way (Ganzer & England, 1994).

Specific Interventions

The most common interventions offered to caregivers of people with Alzheimer's disease are informational, support group, individual and family counseling, and case management services (Collins, Given, & Given, 1994). These interventions are frequently combined in various packages of services. Much counseling, for example, is provided under the more palatable guise of education, a more acceptable term to those who do not want to be identified as in need of mental health therapy. The same type of treatment, therefore, may be administered in several different formats.

Despite earlier reservations about the effectiveness of these interventions and the continuing need to refine and further test them, there is now a consensus that these interventions can be helpful to caregivers, especially to those who are experiencing some difficulty with their role (Haley, 1991; Whitlach, Zarit, & von Eye, 1991). Preventive programs are probably more appropriate for those who are not experiencing above-average stress or depression as a response to their caregiving responsibilities.

Information   The effects of Alzheimer's disease on a person's behavior can be baffling, dismaying, hurtful, and sometimes even horrifying to a caregiver. When the reasons for that behavior are explained, the caregiver may be able to respond in a more therapeutic manner and to take the behavior less personally—that is, the caregiver may be able to say, "He (or she) is not doing this on purpose" (Gallagher-Thompson & DeVries, 1994).

Over the course of the disease, caregivers need information on a whole range of subjects, including but not limited to the following:

- Diagnosis and treatment
- Effects of the disease at various stages
- Emotional response to Alzheimer's disease
- Care needs at various stages
- Formal services available and how to access them
- Financial and legal implications
- End-of-life decisions

Caregivers also need information about keeping themselves healthy. This may include information on

- Exercise
- Nutrition
- How to balance activity and rest
- Stress reduction
- How to recognize the warning signs for stress, anxiety, and depression

Handling Feelings   Caregivers need opportunities to express the "unacceptable" negative feelings that they may be experiencing (Gallagher-Thompson & DeVries, 1994). They need to learn how to accept these feelings in themselves and how to handle them constructively rather than destructively.

Caregivers also need to understand the risks of allowing stress, anxiety, or depression to build unchecked. At the very least, they should recognize such signs of stress and anxiety as irritability; insomnia; vague aches and pains; rapid heart rate; digestive upsets; and increased drug, alcohol, or tobacco use. They also should be able to recognize depressive symptomatology, including inability to fall asleep or stay asleep, difficulty concentrating, a sense of hopelessness or failure, and crying spells (Danna, 1995). In addition, it is important that caregivers know where they can get help if they are at risk for depression or stress-related illness, and that they feel free to ask for that help. Often, the development of a relationship of trust with a health care provider will make it easier for a caregiver to share these concerns and accept help in dealing with them.

Grieving   As the person with Alzheimer's disease progresses through the stages referred to so often in this book, the caregiver also experiences a parallel series of losses related to the changes occurring in the loved one. These losses may include the abandonment of hopes and plans both had for the future, companionship, emotional support, and a sense of security as well as the obvious financial and physical demands that are placed on the caregiver when the care receiver can no longer assume any responsibility for maintaining home and health.

Caregivers need to be able to grieve for themselves and for the person with Alzheimer's disease. The downward spiral of Alzheimer's disease may lead them to cycle over and over again through the stages of the grieving process. The goal is to eventually achieve acceptance of the inevitable but not to withdraw entirely from the loved one before death occurs (Walker, Pomeroy, McNeil, & Franklin, 1996).

Managing Family Issues   Unresolved family conflicts may resurface when a problem such as the need to provide care for a family member with Alzheimer's disease arises. These conflicts may be acted out in discussions about who is responsible for providing what kind of care. Often, a single family member is given the primary responsibility for caregiving. Offers to help from other family members may not be forthcoming, leading to resentment and feelings of being taken advantage of. Some caregivers find it difficult to confront such issues within their families. They may need help with polishing their communication skills before attempting any confrontation. Individual and family counseling may be necessary in some cases.

Improving Coping Skills   When problems arising from caregiving are solvable, problem-solving approaches are appropriate. However, when the problems are not amenable to change, emotion-focused coping skills may be needed (Williamson & Schulz, 1993). Some coping skills that family caregivers find helpful include the following:

Humor   The ability to laugh at oneself occasionally is often mentioned by family caregivers as one of the ways they cope with their overwhelming responsibilities.

Faith   Although seldom mentioned in the professional literature, many family caregivers report that one of the ways they manage to continue with their responsibilities is to pray.

Relaxation Techniques   Deep breathing, progressive muscle relaxation, and guided imagery may all be helpful in modulating stress responses.

Communication Skills   The ability to share one's feelings is often a safety valve in emotion-laden situations. As mentioned earlier, it is especially important for caregivers to be able to handle their ''unacceptable'' feelings about the care receiver and about their caregiving responsibilities. In addition, many caregivers can benefit from learning how to use assertive, rather than aggressive or passive, communication with family members and formal caregivers.

Help Seeking   Assertive communication skills are also useful in seeking assistance with caregiving tasks. As mentioned earlier, some caregivers need ''permission'' to seek help, that is, to give up feeling that they must handle this task alone. Tebb (1995) developed a well-being scale for caregivers that can be used as a guide in helping them to identify their strengths as well as their limitations and in empowering them to make some constructive changes in their situation. The scale guides caregivers to consider the degree to which their own basic needs (for expression of feelings, physical needs, security, and esteem) are being met and their satisfaction with their daily activities (time for self, household maintenance, leisure activities, functions outside the home, and family support). Asking caregivers these questions helps to validate their need to think of their own welfare as well as the welfare of the care receiver. It can also help them make the decision to seek outside help, find some time to care for themselves, or bring a little more pleasure into their own lives.

Reducing Negative Thinking, Increasing Positive Thinking   Caregivers also may find themselves caught up in a downward spiral of self-defeating thought patterns. Recognizing their strengths and accepting the fact that they cannot reverse the disease process may help to counteract the self-negating thoughts. A realistic appraisal of the kinds of changes and improvements that can be expected at any stage may help to banish self-defeating thoughts.

Flexibility   As with so many things, there are often no right or wrong ways to handle a problem with a person with Alzheimer's disease—simply ways that work and ways that do not. Many of the suggested management techniques were discovered by families as they struggled with their responsibilities. As Raymond suggests, "When the old way of doing things no longer works, try a new way!" (1994, p. 36).

REFERENCES

Alzheimer's Association. (1995). *Caregiver stress.* Chicago: Author.

Bowd, A.D., & Loos, C.H. (1996). Needs, morale and coping strategies of caregivers for persons with Alzheimer's disease in isolated communities in Canada. *American Journal of Alzheimer's Disease, 11*(3), 32–39.

Collins, C.E., Given, B.A., & Given, C.W. (1994). Interventions with family caregivers of persons with Alzheimer's disease. *Nursing Clinics of North America, 29*(1), 195–207.

Coolidge, C. (1992). In *The Forbes scrapbook of thoughts on the business of life* (p. 397). Chicago: Triumph Books.

Danna, J. (1995). *When Alzheimer's hits home.* Briarwood, NY: Palomino Press.

DeVita, C. (1994). Five myths about aging in the United States: Findings from the National Academy of Science's *Demography of Aging,* edited by Linda G. Martin and Samuel H. Preston. *Aging Today, 1,* 1–2.

Gallagher-Thompson, D., & DeVries, H.M. (1994). "Coping with frustration" classes: Development and preliminary outcomes with women who care for relatives with dementia. *Gerontologist, 34*(4), 548–552.

Ganzer, C., & England, S.E. (1994). Alzheimer's care and service utilization: Generating practice concepts from empirical findings and narratives. *Health and Social Work, 19*(3), 174–181.

Gubrium, J.F., & Holstein, J.A. (1994). Analyzing talk and interaction. In J.F. Gubrium & A. Sankar (Eds.), *Qualitative methods in aging research.* Thousand Oaks, CA: Sage Publications.

Haley, W.E. (1991). Caregiver intervention programs: The moral equivalent of free haircuts? *Gerontologist, 31*(1), 7–8.

Lustbader, W., & Hooyman, N.R. (1994). *Taking care of aging family members.* New York: Free Press.

Raymond, F. (1994). *Surviving Alzheimer's: A guide for families.* Forest Knolls, CA: Elder Books.

Reese, D.R., Gross, A.M., Smalley, D.L., & Messer, S.C. (1994). Caregivers of Alzheimer's disease and stroke patients: Immunological and psychological considerations. *Gerontologist, 34*(4), 534–540.

Smith, G.C., Smith, M.F., & Toseland, R.W. (1991). Problems identified by family caregivers in counseling. *Gerontologist, 31*(1), 15–22.

Tagliareni, E., Mengel, A., & Sherman, S. (1993). Parallel worlds of nursing practice. In S. Burke & S. Sherman (Eds.), *Ways of knowing and caring for older adults* (pp. 91–106). New York: National League for Nursing Press.

Tebb, S. (1995). An aid to improvement: A caregiver well-being scale. *Health and Social Work, 20*(2), 87–92.

Vitaliano, P.P., Young, H.M., & Russo, J. (1991). Burden: A review of measures used among caregivers of individuals with dementia. *Gerontologist, 31*(1), 67–75.

Walker, R.J., Pomeroy, E.C., McNeil, J.S., & Franklin, C. (1996). Anticipatory grief and AIDS: Strategies for intervening with caregivers. *Health and Social Work, 21*(1), 49–57.

Whitlach, C.J., Zarit, S.H., & von Eye, A. (1991). Efficacy of interventions with caregivers: A reanalysis. *Gerontologist, 31*(1), 9–14.

Williamson, G.M., & Schulz, R. (1993). Coping with specific stressors in Alzheimer's disease caregiving. *Gerontologist, 33*(6), 747–755.

Wirsig, W. (1990). *"I love you, too!"* New York: Evans & Co.

Chapter 14

Special Services

Let me live and grow old in a place I know. It is enough that my body becomes a stranger and my thoughts unclear.

J. Ossofsky (1993)

If you think I need a day center, please enroll me . . . so I can have some fun while you play tennis and go shopping. If I want to think of it as going to school or to work, humor me.

Burton Reifler (1994)

In an open letter to his wife, Frances, Burton Reifler (1994) expressed his concern for her and his preferences for treatment should he ever develop Alzheimer's disease. The problem with the system of services for people with Alzheimer's disease, he said, is that it too often forces a choice between extremes: the family caregiver trying to handle all of the responsibility at home or placement in a long-term care facility. He continued with a poignant point–counterpoint of two items that he found in the same issue of his local newspaper: a news item about a desperate man caring for his wife with Alzheimer's disease who felt so alone and overwhelmed that he shot her and then himself, and a letter from a husband describing how helpful an Alzheimer's day center had been.

The amount and quality of assistance available to the person with Alzheimer's disease and his or her family caregivers has a considerable impact on the quality of life and health of all involved. In this chapter, a range of services designed especially for the person with Alzheimer's disease, from community-based Alzheimer's disease centers to special care units of long-term care facilities, is examined. Some of the most important points to consider in selecting a particular service are included where appropriate.

COMMUNITY-BASED SERVICES

Alzheimer's Disease Centers

In 1994 there were 28 federally funded Alzheimer's Disease Centers operating within major health care institutions in the United States (Alzheimer's Disease Education and Referral Center [ADEAR], 1994). These centers offer clinical services, information resources for professionals and lay people, and opportunities to participate in research on Alzheimer's disease. Many also have satellite centers that reach out to rural and minority communities.

Although the appropriate procedures for diagnosis and treatment of Alzheimer's disease are rapidly becoming familiar to most health care professionals, there are still some advantages to seeking the assistance of experts associated with the Alzheimer's Disease Centers. Comprehensive diagnostic evaluations are usually available in memory disorder clinics run by these centers. Information, counseling, support groups, access to experimental medications, and nonpharmacological interventions are also generally available at these centers.

Alzheimer's Disease Education and Referral Center

ADEAR[1] is part of the National Institute on Aging's program of research and information dissemination on issues related to the health of older adults. ADEAR was authorized by Congress to "compile, archive, and disseminate information concerning Alzheimer's disease" for professionals, people with Alzheimer's disease, their families, and the public (ADEAR, 1993). The center can provide information on the following topics:

- Research findings
- Clinical trials of new drugs
- Services for patients and families
- Publications and audiovisuals
- General information about Alzheimer's disease

Alzheimer's Association

In 1979 a group of family caregivers of people with Alzheimer's disease representing local support organizations from across the country met with professionals in the field to form a national voluntary organization now called the Alzheimer's Association.[2] This association has been a strong advocate of research on Alzheimer's disease. It is also an excellent source of current information and educational materials about Alzheimer's disease.

Through its network of local chapters, the Alzheimer's Association offers referral services, hotlines, respite services, and support groups for people with Alzheimer's disease and their loved ones. Most of the special services described in this chapter can be located by contacting the nearest chapter of the Alzheimer's Association. The efforts of the local chapters have markedly reduced the isolation of people with Alzheimer's disease and their families, many of whom had felt that they were struggling alone with their problems before the Association came into being (Lombardo, 1988).

Support Groups

Many of the Alzheimer's Disease Centers, Alzheimer's Association chapters, and other organizations offer support groups for both people with the disease and their families.

Support Groups for People with Alzheimer's Disease   Support groups for people with Alzheimer's disease are far less common than family support groups. The groups may emphasize opportunities to talk with other people with similar concerns or they may emphasize recreation, providing opportunities for participation in social activities (see Chapter 7 for further information). The socially oriented groups are often called "clubs" to increase their acceptability to prospective participants. Groups vary in terms of cost, number of participants, and the age and degree of impairment of the participants.

Transportation is often a problem for group members and their families. One solution is to hold group meetings for people with Alzheimer's disease and for caregivers

---

[1]Located in Silver Spring, Maryland, the ADEAR Center's telephone number is 1-800-438-4380.
[2]Located in Chicago, the Alzheimer's Association headquarters' telephone number is 1-800-272-3900.

at the same time. Another consideration is the fit between a person's needs and the group's purposes. For example, groups in which participants openly discuss the problems associated with Alzheimer's disease may not be appropriate for people who are still coming to terms with the idea that they are experiencing memory loss. The level of impairment of group participants is another concern. Individuals with severe impairment cannot manage the higher-level activities and discussions in which people in the early stages can engage.

Group experiences may have a powerful effect, constructive or destructive, on the participants. It is therefore important that a skilled, empathic individual who is knowledgeable about the effects of Alzheimer's disease function as group facilitator.

Family Support Groups   Caregiver support groups have existed for many years. Their sponsorship and requirements for membership have just as many or more variations as the patient support groups.

A support group's emphasis may be social, educational, therapeutic, or a combination of the three. For many caregivers, the educational format is easier to accept because it does not imply a need for "therapy" (Lustbader & Hooyman, 1994). Again, the skill of the facilitator and the match between caregiver needs and group purpose should be the critical elements in selection of an appropriate support group for a given caregiver or family.

Respite Care

Respite care services are designed to provide a break for family caregivers. Their purpose is to relieve caregivers of some small portion of their responsibility, thereby enabling them to continue in their role and delay placement in a long-term care facility (Kosloski & Montgomery, 1995). The manner in which respite is provided spans a wide range of options, from hour-long visits in the home by a volunteer to a temporary stay of a week or two in a residential facility for the person with Alzheimer's disease. Typically, respite is an intermittent service, the use of which is often limited by availability and cost (Danner, 1995). The quality of the help provided to the individual with Alzheimer's disease during a respite also varies from simply custodial supervision (sometimes referred to as "baby-sitting," a term some families and people with Alzheimer's disease find offensive) to a comprehensive therapeutic program of activities and services.

Short-Term Respite   Many organizations train volunteers or paid aides to provide brief (several hours a week or month) respite in the home. For the person with Alzheimer's disease a volunteer's visit can be a source of pleasant company and an opportunity for conversation and quiet activities such as dominoes or a stroll outdoors. Acceptability may be increased if the caregiver allows time for the person to become acquainted with the volunteer or aide before leaving them alone. The respite provider needs to know what the person can and cannot do safely, how much help is needed with activities such as toileting, and how to handle upsets if they occur while the caregiver is away.

For family caregivers this respite time is an interlude in which responsibility is lifted from them and they are free to do whatever they wish: golf, lunch with a friend, shop, or spend a few hours of contemplation by the old fishing hole. If possible, caregivers should be encouraged to use this precious free time for themselves, not for finishing chores or running errands for the care receiver. The choice should be based on an assessment of maximum benefit for the caregiver. It is also important that the caregiver feel confident in the volunteer's or aide's ability to care temporarily for the person with Alzheimer's disease. If this is not the case, the caregiver may feel more anxious than relieved to have respite care.

Extended Respite Care   Longer-term respite is likely to be provided within a facility that has set aside beds for this purpose. Reservations for these beds may need to be made well in advance of the time that respite is needed. Stays of several days to several weeks may be available. This allows family caregivers to take a vacation, to go on a business trip, or even to undergo surgery.

Preparation of the person with Alzheimer's disease for an extended period of respite care is even more important than it is for short-term respite, as is the quality of the respite care. The facility's physical plant, staff, and services should be evaluated as if the person were being placed there permanently. In addition, the person with Alzheimer's disease needs preparation for the stay. A visit ahead of time and careful explanation of what is about to happen are helpful. For some individuals, this respite stay is an enjoyable break in the home routine. For others, it is frightening unless adequate support and reassurance that family members will return are provided. Concerns about missing family members are high on the list of worries of many people with Alzheimer's disease and may be exacerbated by respite care if not handled appropriately by both the family and the respite care provider.

Adult Day Centers

Adult day centers for people with Alzheimer's disease provide daytime care for people at various stages of the disease. Some accept people who are incontinent or display troublesome behavior, including wandering; others do not. Although most day center clients return home at the end of the day, some return to assisted living facilities and a few to nursing facilities. Like most of the other services examined in this chapter, adult day centers may be operated on a for-profit or not-for-profit basis.

Services Offered   Some Alzheimer's day centers are limited operations, such as a church-run center that offers social activities and mid-morning coffee for a group of 10 or 15 people several days a week. Others are full-service operations, such as a center run by a hospital, housing development office, or long-term care facility. These may operate 7 days a week from 7:00 A.M. to 7:00 P.M. to allow employed family members sufficient time to work, serving 50–100 people or more in several locations within a community. Scheduled van transportation from home to the center and back in the evening is usually available.

Social work services and nursing care are common components of these full-service day centers. Thorough assessments may be conducted before an individual is accepted into the center. Family counseling, educational sessions, caregiver support groups, referrals to other sources of assistance, formal care management services, immunizations, blood pressure monitoring, physical examinations, and administration of medications during the day are frequently offered. Psychiatric, podiatric, dental, spiritual, and other specialized care also may be made available through these centers. In addition, center staff often help families through crises and recommend effective management strategies to use at home.

Nutrition is another important component of day care. Breakfast and lunch (a complete hot meal) are usually served, and considerable attention is paid to adequate nutritional intake by each participant.

Programs Offered   Every center seems to have a personality of its own. Its character is shaped by a number of factors:

- Characteristics of the people served (a mid-morning service of Cuban coffee distributed in little plastic medicine cups is a common feature in Miami)
- Amount of resources available (card tables and chairs crowded into a small space versus thick carpets and leather recliners for napping in the more luxurious centers)
- Philosophy of the institution (some are therapeutically oriented, others are primarily custodial; some programs feature dance, exercise, and other lively activities, whereas others emphasize talk and current events)
- Preparation and experience of the staff (some programs employ professional staff who thoroughly understand the special needs of people with Alzheimer's disease)

Although cost, clients, and milieu vary considerably, other elements are common to most full-service day centers. A typical day for a client who attends an Alzheimer's adult day center might proceed as follows:

Ben got up early on Monday, Wednesday, and Friday because these were the days that he went to "work," as he referred to the Alzheimer's day center. His wife watched him from the window to make sure that he got on the van when it arrived, but he did not need any reminders about the purpose of the van or where it would take him.

On arrival, Ben got off the van without help and headed straight for the center door. Carmen, his favorite staff member, usually greeted him and helped him remove his jacket with name tag and address discreetly pinned to the collar. Ben sat down in his usual place at the table and was served coffee, a glass of orange juice, and a toasted bagel. The center nurse circulated, greeting clients and looking for any indications of changes that might be of concern or signs of illness in the participants.

Before the first formal activity of the day, some of the clients read magazines and others did puzzles of varying difficulty. Ben liked to pick up the mail for the director. His friend Isaac fed the birds outside every day at this hour. Current events were the topic of the first activity, led by a retired teacher who knew everyone's name and asked questions that almost everyone could answer. Ben usually leafed through the newspaper during this session. In the break between activities clients were reminded to use the restroom or taken there if necessary. Then Carmen turned on the music and led the exercises. During the exercises, clients were taken one by one to the nurse's office for their flu shots.

At 11:30, the exercise equipment was put away and the big room was rearranged for lunch. Ben liked to help move the tables and chairs. He also led some of the clients with greater impairment to their seats when they returned from the restroom. Ben enjoyed lunch. He had a hearty appetite and usually offered to finish any leftover desserts. Sometimes he just helped himself to someone else's dessert, which usually provoked a cry of protest from its owner. Staff were used to his habits, however, and usually prevented the purloining. They tried to limit Ben to one extra dessert because he had a tendency to be overweight.

After lunch, a volunteer arrived with slides of her visit to Kenya. Most clients were restless during the geography portion but paid attention when she began telling stories about the animals. A half hour of this was enough for Ben. Despite urging from the staff to sit and listen to their guest a while longer, Ben got up and wandered around the center. Then he headed for the refrigerator to check for any leftover desserts. He found his friend Isaac there getting more bread for his beloved birds. "They'll be mad," said Ben. "Who cares?" answered Isaac. "I have to feed my birds."

The staff counted heads regularly to prevent a premature departure, so the absence of Ben and Isaac was quickly noticed. Carmen found them, offered an arm to each of them, and took them outside for a short walk around the garden. They returned in time for the afternoon snack of fruit and crackers. After the snack, each participant settled down to work on a favorite craft until it was time to go home. Ben stamped center newsletters. Isaac colored bird pictures and leafed through bird fancier magazines.

On arrival home, Ben's wife met him at the door. "How was your day, Ben?" "Busy," said Ben. "They had a lot of work for me to do so I couldn't listen to that lady." Ben usually slept soundly after a day at the center.

Selecting a Day Center   A number of factors must be considered when selecting an adult day center for a person with Alzheimer's disease:

- Cost
- Type of activities and services offered
- The individual's preferences in terms of the type of program offered
- Location and availability of transportation
- Qualifications of staff
- Attitude of staff toward each other and the clients
- Safety features
- Center policies (e.g., the type of client accepted)
- Hours of operation (especially for the employed caregiver)

Program–person fit is probably the most important element in this selection process. For example, although the condition of the physical plant is important, some of the most modest centers in terms of resources offer warmth, caring, and pleasant activities, which may be just what an anxious or lonely person with Alzheimer's disease needs.

LONG-TERM CARE FACILITY–BASED SERVICES

The decision to place a person with Alzheimer's disease in a long-term care facility is often a painful one for those involved. In the case of Alzheimer's disease the person's increasing need for supervision, rather than a decline in physical condition, is often the turning point in making the decision (Kane, Saslow, & Brundage, 1991). A combination of troublesome behavior (especially aggressiveness or incontinence), poor health in the caregiver, increased sense of burden, and decline in cognitive function often lead to the decision to place the person in a residential facility (Cohen et al., 1993).

Some evidence exists that intervention can delay facility placement (Mittelman et al., 1993). Many families are unaware of the types of assistance available in their community. Others hesitate to ask for help from either formal or informal sources unless they are encouraged to do so. Education and support can also help them become more effective caregivers, thus reducing their sense of burden. Simply knowing that their efforts are appreciated (people in the advanced stages of Alzheimer's disease generally are not able to recognize the strain on the caregiver or to express much appreciation for the caregiver's efforts) and that help is available when needed may be enough to sustain family caregivers.

When families do decide that they can no longer care for the person with Alzheimer's disease at home, both family members and the individual with Alzheimer's disease need help in making the transition. Families can be encouraged to remain actively involved in the care of the person, relinquishing the 24-hour responsibility but maintaining contact and providing the love and continuity of relationships that formal caregivers cannot provide. The person with Alzheimer's disease also needs to be prepared for the change in residence and to be assisted in adapting to new people and a new environment. Families should be encouraged to discuss the impending move with the person. Such a discussion does not occur as frequently as one might assume: In one research study, it was found that only 22% of the families had done this (Gold, Reis, Markieweicz, & Andres, 1995). All but those individuals with Alzheimer's disease with the most severe impairment are able to participate in the process (Cox, 1996). The disease process itself makes adaptation difficult, so both staff and family members need to offer extra assistance and support during the transition.

Two levels of care are available for people with Alzheimer's disease: assisted living and long-term care.

Assisted Living

As the name implies, assisted living is a semi-independent type of residential care. Some assisted living arrangements work well for people with mild cognitive impairment. Others do not, largely as a result of the amount of supervision an individual needs.

Foster Homes and Board-and-Care Homes   Adult foster homes are individual residences whose owners provide room and board for two or three older people in addition to their own families. Board-and-care homes are usually small residential facilities, often homes converted for this purpose. Residents are provided some help with dressing and bathing if needed in these facilities but are expected to toilet themselves and to be able to move around the facility independently. Some board-and-care homes accept people who use wheelchairs, but generally residents must be able to get out of bed, obtain meals on their own, and be able to exit the facility independently in case of fire.

Some foster homes and board-and-care homes have a familylike environment in which people literally feel as if they were at home. Residents develop good relationships with each other, watching out and providing companionship for one another. Staff members act like family caregivers, providing help willingly and reporting any problems to the individual's family or physician promptly. Home health care nurses and therapists visit to provide supervision and management of any health care problems the person may have. Regular activities appropriate for the level of impairment of the various residents are offered: picnics, shopping, swimming, entertainment, and so forth. Residents keep personal possessions in their rooms and are allowed to bring some of their own furniture so that they can retain some connection with their past. Family members are encouraged to visit whenever they wish and are kept informed of the resident's condition.

Unfortunately, not all foster and board-and-care homes are well run. Even in 1997, there are instances of small residential facilities that are dirty, roach infested, and full of health and fire code violations. In some instances, their residents are afraid to complain for fear of retaliation by the staff. Few have any personal possessions with them because they are quickly lost or stolen. Families may be treated with suspicion by the staff. Sometimes, family members find out that their loved one has been ill only when he or she is transferred to the hospital or emergency room.

Licensing and regular inspections by state and local regulatory agencies help to reduce the incidence of such facilities, but their continued existence makes it essential to personally inspect a facility before placing an individual with Alzheimer's disease, even if assurances of good care are offered.

Congregate Living Facilities　　Larger residential facilities offer Alzheimer's care, some of which are freestanding and some are a part of a continuum of long-term care services. Some of these facilities maintain separate apartments for each resident; others provide only dormitory- or hospital-style sleeping areas. All have common areas for dining and daytime activities. These larger facilities usually offer a wider array of services than do the smaller facilities, from exercise programs to religious services. The quality of the care in these larger facilities is as variable as it is in the smaller facilities and requires equally careful evaluation before placement.

Nursing Facilities

Nursing facilities are transforming from places to house older people who can no longer manage their care alone to health care facilities providing rehabilitative and restorative care. Although residents of all ages may be found in such facilities, the average resident is an 80-year-old or older woman with limited ability to manage the basic activities of daily living. Half or more of the residents of most facilities have cognitive impairments (Levenson, 1993). Before the emptying of state mental health institutions in the 1950s and 1960s, most people with Alzheimer's disease were labeled "senile" or as having "organic brain syndrome" and were housed in the geriatric units of these large institutions. Although the care was enlightened and informed in a few of these facilities, most of the older people with dementia were restrained in wheelchairs or beds. Reality orientation (examined in Chapter 7) was the favored intervention in the most enlightened of these facilities; the remainder made little or no attempt at intervention. The traditional nursing "home" was designed primarily for people with physical, not cognitive or emotional, disabilities. Despite being called "homes," their design has been based more on a hospital model than a residential model.

A number of concerns have been raised about the suitability of traditional nursing care facilities for people with Alzheimer's disease (Office of Technology Assessment, 1992):

- Facility staff tend to encourage dependency in residents.
- Staff often are not knowledgeable about the special needs of people with Alzheimer's disease.
- Most nursing facilities do not have spaces in which people can wander safely or features that promote independent functions.
- Most of the activities offered are inappropriate for people with Alzheimer's disease.

Special Care Units　　In order to provide an environment in which people with Alzheimer's disease can be comfortable and secure, special care units have been established in many nursing facilities. The design of these units is based on a therapeutic approach to the care of people with Alzheimer's disease. The main features of these special care units include the following (Maas, Swanson, Specht, & Buckwalter, 1994):

- All residents have cognitive impairment (some units mix in older people with other people with psychiatric problems, although their needs may be quite different).
- The staff are trained in the care of people with Alzheimer's disease and related disorders.
- Activity programs are designed specifically for people with cognitive impairment.
- Family support services are available.
- Residents are physically and socially separated from the rest of the facility.

Although some nursing facilities contain special care units for other purposes as well, the Alzheimer's special care unit is the most common type. More than 1,500 units are already in existence and many more are in the planning stages (Kaplan, 1996). This number is expected to increase rapidly by the end of the 1990s. The average unit comprises 30 beds. Residents placed on these units are usually ambulatory and have less physical impairment than the average nursing facility resident. Despite the proliferation of these units, however, their effectiveness in terms of improving function or resident quality of life remains unproved (Sloane, Lindeman, Phillips, Moritz, & Koch, 1995).

If a "typical" Alzheimer's special care unit exists, the following would describe it:

> One wing of the first floor of the long-term care facility was set aside for the Alzheimer's special care unit. The unit is locked: A five-digit code, which many visitors are embarrassed to admit they keep forgetting, must be entered on a key pad to open the door. Many residents walk up and down the long hallway from dawn to dusk. Some like to rummage in closets and dresser drawers, often not their own. Others sit quietly unless they are disturbed; some cry out intermittently, but this behavior is less common on the special care unit than it is on other units. Occasional scuffles break out between residents but they are quickly broken up by staff.
>
> Residents take their meals together in the small dining area on the unit. Between mealtimes, the room is used for activities and entertainment: often, music, crafts, small group discussions, or exercise. The television is kept in a smaller room and seems to entertain visitors and staff more than it does the residents. Nursing assistants come and go from these areas, identifying residents who need toileting or cleaning up and leading them back to their rooms for this purpose. Most seem to go willingly.
>
> A second door leads outside to a fenced-in garden. Residents can go in and out at will and many do so regularly. Visitors are common at lunch and dinner time. Most seem to know the staff well and discuss their loved one's condition with the staff whenever they come.
>
> Quiet music is piped into the unit during the day. Lights are dimmed in late afternoon after a snack is served in an attempt to reduce sundowning. Evening shift staff have devised distractions for the residents who become restless as the sun goes down. One lady likes to fold laundry, another wants to help make beds. One gentleman likes to walk other residents, although the other residents are not always amenable to his ministrations.

At night, there are fewer staff and most residents sleep. However, some prefer to doze on the dayroom sofas or visit with the staff, who allow this unless the person seems to be in danger of exhaustion. Usually, one particular staff member has the most success in persuading these individuals to finally go to bed and stay there.

Selecting a Nursing Facility   Many of the criteria for evaluating the appropriateness of a particular nursing facility for a person with Alzheimer's disease are the same as those mentioned earlier for day centers and assisted living facilities. The following list serves as a reminder of the most important points to consider:

- Licensing and ratings by regulatory agencies
- Any violations noted by surveyors and actions taken to correct them
- Level of preparation and attitude (nondefensive, noncondescending, caring, responsive, and able to appreciate the uniqueness of each individual resident) of the staff, from the administrators to the nursing assistants and maintenance personnel
- Physical plant, including comfort; visual, aural, and olfactory appeal; access to outdoor areas; health and safety considerations
- Range of services available, including religious services, occupational and physical therapy, and physician services
- Meal service, particularly the attractiveness of the meals, nutritional value, and ability to cater to individual needs and preferences
- Activity programs, particularly the variety and suitability of activities for people who have severe impairments, whether physical, cognitive, or both
- Cost and other terms of any contractual agreement

Again, the fit between the individual and the particular facility is the primary concern when planning to place a person with Alzheimer's disease in a nursing facility, whether or not that facility has a special care unit.

In some communities the types of special services described in this chapter are well established and are staffed by individuals who understand the needs of people with Alzheimer's disease and the needs of their families. In other communities the services are "special" in name only: special care units that are little more than regular units with a locked door and sign indicating the designation, or board-and-care homes staffed by people who have little knowledge about Alzheimer's disease and little incentive to learn more.

Much is still to be learned about what constitutes the best combination of services for people at various stages of Alzheimer's disease and for their families. As awareness of their special needs increases, it is anticipated that more innovative approaches and services will be developed for these people (Office of Technology Assessment, 1992).

REFERENCES

Alzheimer's Disease Education and Referral Center. (1993). *Alzheimer's disease: A guide to federal programs*. NIH Publication No. 93-3635. Silver Spring, MD: Author.

Alzheimer's Disease Education and Referral Center. (1994). *Alzheimer's Disease Centers program directory*. Silver Spring, MD: Author.

Cohen, C.A., Gold, D.P., Shulman, K.I., Wortley, J.T., McDonald, G., & Wargon, M. (1993). Factors determining the decision to institutionalize dementing individuals: A prospective study. *Gerontologist, 33*(6), 714–720.

Cox, C.B. (1996). Discharge planning for dementia patients: Factors influencing caregiver decisions and satisfaction. *Health and Social Work, 21*(2), 97–103.

Danner, J. (1995). *When Alzheimer's hits home*. Briarwood, NY: Palomino Press.

Gold, D.P., Reis, M.F., Markiewicz, D., & Andres, D. (1995). When home caregiving ends: A longitudinal study of outcomes for caregivers of relatives with dementia. *Journal of the American Geriatrics Society, 43*, 10–16.

Kane, R.L., Saslow, M.G., & Brundage, T. (1991). Using ADLs to establish eligibility for long-term care among the cognitively impaired. *Gerontologist, 31*(1), 60–66.

Kaplan, M. (1996). Special care programs: Challenges to success. In S.B. Hoffman & M. Kaplan (Eds.), *Special care programs for people with dementia* (pp. 1–15). Baltimore: Health Professions Press.

Kosloski, K., & Montgomery, R.J.V. (1995). The impact of respite use on nursing home placement. *Gerontologist, 35*(1), 67–74.

Levenson, S.A. (1993). The changing role of the nursing home medical director. In P.R. Katz, R.L. Kane, & M.D. Mazey (Eds.), *Advances in long-term care* (pp. 152–175). New York: Springer Publishing.

Lombardo, N.E. (1988). Alzheimer's Disease and Related Disorders Association: Birth and evolution of a major voluntary association. In M. Aronson (Ed.), *Understanding Alzheimer's disease*. New York: Charles Scribner's Sons.

Lustbader, W., & Hooyman, M.R. (1994). *Taking care of aging family members: A practical guide*. New York: Free Press.

Maas, M.L., Swanson, E., Specht, J., & Buckwalter, K.C. (1994). Alzheimer's special care units. *Nursing Clinics of North America, 29*(1), 173–194.

Mittelman, M.S., Ferris, S.H., Steinberg, G., Shulman, E., Mackell, J.A., Ambinder, A., & Cohen, J. (1993). An intervention that delays institutionalization of Alzheimer's disease patients: Treatment of spouse-caregivers. *Gerontologist, 33*(6), 730–740.

Office of Technology Assessment. (1992). *Special care units for people with Alzheimer's and other dementias: Consumer education, research, regulatory and reimbursement issues* (OTA-H-543). Washington, DC: Author.

Ossofsky, J. (1993). Quoted in *Gerontologist, 33*, 3.

Reifler, B. (1994, Summer). What I want if I get Alzheimer's disease. *Respite Report*, pp. 5, 7.

Sloane, P.D., Lindeman, D.A., Phillips, C., Moritz, D.J., & Koch, G. (1995). Evaluating Alzheimer's special care units: Reviewing the evidence and identifying potential sources of study bias. *Gerontologist, 35*(1), 35–43.

Chapter 15

Ethical and Legal Issues

[M]y rights had become tenuous and delicate.

Diana McGowin (1993)

He lived, you see, longer than expected.
Long enough to see a son graduate from college.
Long enough to see a wedding.
Long enough to live his dying with dignity.

He had choices.

Susan Ragazzo (1993)

The progressive loss of cognitive abilities that makes the care of a person with Alzheimer's disease a challenge also raises a number of complex ethical and legal issues. When mental capacities are limited but not lost entirely, as would occur if a person were in a coma, the guidelines for protecting a person's safety while safeguarding his or her rights are often fuzzy, confusing, and contradictory.

This chapter examines the ethical and legal issues that arise most frequently in the care of a person with Alzheimer's disease. The ethical issues include the often painful decisions that must be made about restrictions on freedom, fulfillment of family obligations, and end-of-life decisions. The legal issues include patient rights, abuse and neglect, incapacity, and guardianship.

Ethical Issues Related to Alzheimer's Disease

It is easy to say in the abstract that it is important to "foster independence," "maintain safety," or "ensure high-quality care," but it is much more difficult to put these guidelines into practice in real-life situations. Consider the following scenarios from caregivers:

> The family doesn't want us to treat her pneumonia. I tried to explain that she is otherwise physically healthy and has many good years ahead of her. But since she was just recently diagnosed with Alzheimer's disease, they believe that nothing should be done to prolong her life—not even a simple antibiotic. I think she was really enjoying life before she got this pneumonia.

> Walking seems to be her favorite activity. When she can't walk, she becomes restless and calls out "Help me, help me!" incessantly. However, when she walks there is a smile on her face. The problem is that, since her stroke, she is quite unsteady in addition to being cognitively impaired from the Alzheimer's disease. We can prevent a fall by restraining her, but then we'll take away her greatest pleasure in life.

He made his daughter promise never to put him in a nursing facility. He said it would remind him of the concentration camps. Now, his daughter is widowed and has just discovered that she has multiple sclerosis. She wants to "live a little" while she is in remission but to protect her father from his worst fear. No family members can help; his wife died years ago and there are no other children.

Health care–related decisions are usually made based on several principles. The first principle is to do no harm (*nonmaleficence*). The second is to do whatever is in the best interest or welfare of the older person (*beneficence*), as depicted in the first vignette. Fairness (*justice*) is a third. A fourth principle, the right to make decisions for oneself (*autonomy*), is often threatened when the older person has a physical or mental impairment, or both, as in the second vignette. Finally, families have certain rights and responsibilities with regard to providing assistance and in making health care decisions (*familial obligation*) (Wetle, 1995).

Safety and Autonomy

Safety and autonomy issues abound in the care of the person with Alzheimer's disease. Driving a car, using the stove, taking medication, living alone, and going out alone are common safety concerns in the early stages, and many more occur in later stages. Handling finances; making health care decisions; choosing what to eat, how to dress, and when to bathe; and many other decisions raise issues of independence in decision making.

Autonomy is a deeply cherished value in Western cultures. The ideal of autonomy is to know one's preferences and desires and to make decisions independently and rationally based on these preferences and desires (Agich, 1995). Actual autonomy is practiced primarily through the many ordinary activities of everyday life. In addition, there are occasions when conflict arises over two or more of the principles listed earlier, such as preserving independence (autonomy) while maintaining the person's safety (beneficence), as illustrated in the second vignette presented earlier in the chapter.

Safety is an overwhelming concern for both formal and informal caregivers, and thus is a dominant force in their decision making with regard to care recipients with Alzheimer's disease. Although much is said and written about the importance of autonomy, it appears that safety is more often the prevailing value in the care of frail, dependent older people. We know several reasons for this. First, the regulatory environment has long emphasized safety and punished those who did not maintain the highest levels of safety for individuals in their care. The same can be said of the legal environment. In addition, the medical model of care emphasizes physical safety over psychosocial well-being.

A second reason is that there are also the enduring stereotypes of older people, especially frail older people, as generally in need of direction, unable to make wise decisions or take full responsibility for themselves. These stereotypes exacerbate caregiver concerns about safety. These concerns are especially powerful when the individual in question is also a nonconformist or an eccentric in terms of lifestyle or values. Actual ability to take responsibility for oneself can be obscured by the stereotypes and the older person's eccentricities or preferences. Together, they may even stimulate increased efforts to "save" the older person from him- or herself (Collopy, 1995).

Clearly, safety and autonomy issues interact. For example, driving a car and going out alone are not only issues of safety but also of independence. Economic welfare is threatened by mishandling financial matters. Unwise health care decisions may have a serious impact on a person's physical well-being.

To assist caregivers in their efforts to assure the safety of the care recipient while maintaining as much autonomy as possible, Collopy (1995) suggests a reframing of the safety–autonomy issue. Instead of viewing safety and autonomy as polar opposites, they may be understood as different aspects of a larger concern. Much of what is usually termed *safety* is actually physical safety, an important but incomplete perspective on the individual's well-being. If psychological and social safety were added to this picture, then the desires and preferences of the individual, including the need for autonomy, would be considered as well.

Considering psychological and social safety along with physical safety may well make the eccentric behaviors of some older people more comprehensible. For example, when older people experiencing progressive physical or cognitive decline resist relocation or other changes in their lifestyle, they may be defending their psychological safety. In trying to come to terms with their progressive losses, older adults may be "struggling to keep the security of familiar places and patterns, to protect themselves from dislocation and diminishment, to mark off their own areas of control" (Collopy, 1995, p. 144). A real understanding of the individual's personal struggle with his or her cognitive decline requires in-depth knowledge of that person's past and present experiences, his or her own construction of the world and sense of personal order and harmony, and the dissonance with which the person struggles (Collopy, 1995). Use of the assessment guidelines outlined in the later section entitled "Ascertaining Preferences of the Person with Alzheimer's Disease" and of the Values Assessment Interview Guide (Table 15.1) may assist caregivers in their efforts to understand the individual's construction of the world and personal sense of order.

Familial Obligation

Although there is no question in Western cultures that families have some obligation to their individual members, exactly what those obligations are is not clear. For example, it is difficult to say how much help is expected, how much is considered sufficient, and how much would be considered excessive. It is no wonder, then, that caregivers and care recipients are confused and conflicted over these questions. A helpful way to think about familial obligation is in terms of achieving some sort of balance between giving and receiving (Hargrave & Anderson, 1992).

In general, people expect to both give and receive something of value from family relationships. The thing of value may be affection, companionship, intimacy, help, money, or a combination of any of these. Over the years, some balance in the "relationship ledger" between giving and receiving is expected. A relationship between two people may eventually break down if one person continually takes but never gives. The effects of Alzheimer's disease clearly have an impact on a person's ability to give to others. As the disease progresses, the relationship ledger may become severely unbalanced, particularly when family members place more emphasis on tangible returns such as help with household responsibilities or verbal expressions of appreciation than on intangible returns such as affection and companionship. Family members who value the simple companionship of the person with Alzheimer's disease may feel less of an imbalance in the relationship ledger than do family members who value more tangible returns.

When Interests Conflict Because it is so much easier to talk with family members than with a person in the advanced stages of Alzheimer's disease, formal caregivers may be inclined to depend on family members for information about the person's preferences

Table 15.1.   Values assessment interview guide

Overall Health
  Current health
  Perceived effect on ability to function
  Feelings about current health
  Feelings about decreases in physical and/or mental capacities (actual and future possibilities)

Living Situation
  Present living situation (e.g., where, with whom, is it comfortable, affected by health?)
  Comparison with past living situations (Did you live alone or with others? Where did you live? In
    what type of arrangement: home, apartment, or ?)
  Anticipated changes in residence and living arrangement

Financial Situation
  Concerns about having enough money
  Preference (to spend what is available on own care or to save for beneficiaries)

Relationships with Formal Caregivers
  With doctors (Do you like them? Do you trust them? Do you want them to make final decisions
    about treatment?)
  With other caregivers (e.g., nurses, social workers, therapists)

Personal Relationships
  Friends, family available to help make decisions about medical treatment, living arrangements
  Any discussions, documents prepared, formal arrangements made with someone to make health
    care decisions
  Any "unfinished business"—personal, financial, or legal

General Attitude Toward Life
  Activities person enjoys
  Feelings about life (Is it worth living? Are you satisfied with what you have achieved? Are you
    happy to be alive?)
  Sources of pleasure, happiness
  Sources of fear, upset, anxiety
  Importance of independence, self-sufficiency
  Goals for the future

Religious Beliefs
  Religious affiliation
  Strength of religious beliefs
  Amount of guidance, support, comfort from religion
  Use of prayer, sacraments, and rites
  Religious teachings, including strictures that pertain to life-sustaining measures, palliative care,
    withholding treatment, ending life

Attitudes about Serious Illness and Death
  Feelings about using life-sustaining measures (e.g., if in a coma, if terminally ill, if person has
    Alzheimer's disease)
  Wishes regarding specific life-sustaining measures:
    Dialysis
    Fluid
    Food
    Respirator
    Resuscitation
  Wishes about organ donations:
    Any limitations about what organs
    Any documentation of wishes, where documents are located, and so forth

(continued)

Table 15.1.   (continued)

What person anticipates will be important when dying (e.g., physical comfort; pain control; presence of religious advisor, family, friends)
Preference as to where he or she would like to die (home, hospital, hospice)

Funeral Arrangements
Preference about cremation, burial
Type of service preferred
Other arrangements made, documented (Who has been told?)

Adapted from Autonomy and long term care. (1990). *Generations* (Suppl.), pp. 54–58.

and desires. This inclination raises several questions: How accurately can most family members predict the preferences of another family member concerning issues such as placement in a long-term care facility and maintaining life by artificial means? Are family members likely to place their own needs ahead of the needs of the older person? What should be done if family interests conflict with the interests of the older person?

When the interests of the family conflict with the person's wishes, formal caregivers face some difficult decisions. On the one hand, Arras (1995) argues that the person's interests are usually more urgent and significant—often measured in terms of life and death—than are the family's interests. In addition, the person's strength—and mental capacity in the case of people with Alzheimer's disease—and ability to fight for his or her own interests are diminished. On the other hand, the family may have legitimate concerns as well. For example, a spouse may be truly incapable of providing the extensive and often exhausting care required by a person in the late stages of Alzheimer's disease. The emotional strain may be equally difficult for some caregivers to manage.

Often, some balance can be found between the two apparently conflicting sets of interests, the person's and the family's. For example, what may initially appear to be in the best interests of the person—being cared for by a spouse at home—may over the long term be harmful if it deprives the person of the companionship of a close family member felled by overwhelming caregiving responsibilities. When this is a real danger, both the person with the disease and the caregiver will ultimately benefit if an alternative plan, such as live-in help, is found.

Ascertaining Preferences of the Person with Alzheimer's Disease   Kane (1995) cautions against "cookie cutter care plans" that show little variation from one person to another. An antidote to this inappropriate uniformity is a comprehensive assessment of the person's preferences and desires. When dealing with a person with Alzheimer's disease, it is preferable to conduct this assessment in the early stages. However, it can be done with a person in the later stages through skillful and sensitive communication and use of the insights of family and friends to supplement information obtained from the older adult. It has been recommended that all people but those who are comatose or with very advanced dementia should be given an opportunity to discuss these matters and select a health care proxy (Mezey, Bottrell, Ramsey, & the NICHE Faculty, 1996).

The elements of the assessment vary with the individual situation, but the following points (adapted from McCullough, Wilson, Rhymes, & Teasdale, 1995) may serve as a guide:

- Who should be involved in the decision-making process? Although older people in general believe that they should make their own decisions when they are able to do so, there is some evidence that they do trust family members to make decisions for them when they become incapacitated (Bailly & DePoy, 1995).

- What is the person's present condition and living situation? The person's satisfaction with his or her current situation should be considered, as well as his or her physical safety in that situation. In addition, the degree to which the person is able to take responsibility for decisions about his or her own health and welfare should be assessed.
- What is most important to this individual? It is necessary to thoroughly explore the values of the individual with Alzheimer's disease and the people who are involved in his or her care. A list of items that can be used to guide this exploration may be found in Table 15.1.
- What alternative treatments, arrangements, or both are available? Creativity and open-mindedness are critical. The interests of the people providing the care as well as those of the person with Alzheimer's disease must be considered.

End-of-Life Decisions

Advance Directives   The purpose of an advance directive is to make known ahead of time the amount or kind of medical treatment one wants to receive in the future in case one cannot express these wishes at that time. It is also possible to designate a person who can act as a substitute or *surrogate* to make decisions on one's behalf (Bresnahan, 1994).

The Patient Self-Determination Act of 1991 (PL 101-508) defines advance directives as "written instruction, such as a living will or durable power of attorney for health care, recognized under State law and relating to the provision of such care when the individual is incapacitated" (Osman & Perlin, 1994, p. 246). Under the act, health care institutions that receive federal health care dollars must provide patients with written information about their right to refuse treatment and to prepare advance directives and document these directives.

Given the effects of Alzheimer's disease, it is unlikely that the individual in the advanced stages will be able to assume direct responsibility for deciding such issues as withholding life-sustaining food and fluids or ceasing aggressive treatment in the face of a terminal illness. However, it is possible to take some steps to ensure that the person's wishes are carried out by others. This requires either clear, detailed instructions given before incapacitation (i.e., advance directives) or appointment of someone to act as a surrogate to make these decisions for the person, or both.

Whichever route is chosen by the individual with Alzheimer's disease and his or her family, it is important that preparations be made in the earliest stages of the disease, when the person can articulate his or her wishes as clearly as possible. Great sensitivity must be exercised in introducing this subject because the discussion of end-of-life issues requires confronting the difficult road that lies ahead.

Researchers who have studied the subject of individual wishes regarding the use of life-sustaining measures have generally found that family members and very close friends are not particularly accurate in their prediction of a person's preferences (Klepac, Coppola, Ditto, & Danks, 1995). Some evidence also exists that older people do want their families to be involved in these important decisions and that they expect their families to make decisions jointly (i.e., to discuss the matter with each other and to try to resolve any differences of opinion) (Bailly & DePoy, 1995; Stern & Hayley, 1995).

Proxy Advance Planning   Many individuals reach the advanced stages of Alzheimer's disease without having prepared advance directives. An alternative approach, proxy advance planning, has been used at the Edith Nourse Rogers Memorial Veterans Hospital in Bedford, Massachusetts (Hurley, Mahoney, & Volicer, 1995). In this approach the patient's surrogate meets with the health care team (including the physician, nurse, social worker, and chaplain) to discuss any indications of the individual's wishes regarding end-of-life medical treatment and decide what the appropriate level of response to a life-threatening illness would be from among the following options:

- Aggressive diagnosis and treatment of illness or other life-threatening event including transfer to an acute care facility, resuscitation, and/or tube feeding as needed.
- All of the above except resuscitation. This would require a Do Not Resuscitate (DNR) order on the chart.
- No resuscitation or transfer to an acute care facility but provision of treatment such as an oral antibiotic if it will increase the person's comfort and enteral feedings if needed.
- Supportive care only; food and fluid will be given only if they can be taken by mouth (no tube feedings).

Changing the Decision   Neither advance directives nor proxy advance planning can cover every eventuality. Callahan (1995) offers an example of the kind of question that can still arise when the time comes to make a termination-of-treatment decision. If, in the past, the individual with advanced Alzheimer's disease expressed a preference for receiving only supportive care but now expresses a wish to live or appears to be content with his or present situation, which preference should be honored? This question has no easy answer, but one of the features of most advance directive guidelines may offer some direction: The emphasis on the fact that the decisions made in either the advance directive or proxy advance planning processes can be changed by the patient or surrogate at any time.

LEGAL ISSUES RELATED TO ALZHEIMER'S DISEASE

Some of the issues raised in the previous section have been addressed by state and federal legislation as well as by medical ethicists. The Patient Self-Determination Act, for example, put legislative force behind the idea that advance directives could spare both patient and caregivers some of the agonizing decisions that sometimes must be made as life nears its end. Patient rights, abuse, neglect, and incapacity also have been legally defined, and certain protections have been put in place to prevent exploitation and other types of wrongdoing directed to vulnerable older individuals.

Patient Rights

Because long-term care facilities often become a person's last "home," the person's rights to a "dignified existence, self-determination, and communication with and access to persons and services inside and outside the facility" (Agency for Health Care Administration, n.d.; National Citizens' Coalition for Nursing Home Reform, 1987), and the enforcement of these rights, are important to the physical and psychological well-being of every resident of an assisted living or nursing facility. If the person has been judged to be incapacitated, his or her rights can be exercised by the court-appointed representative or guardian.

Long-term care facilities that participate in Medicare or Medicaid reimbursement for health care are required to inform each new resident of his or her rights both orally and in writing in language that the new resident can understand on admission. These rights include the following:

- To have access to his or her medical records on request
- To purchase a copy of these records at reasonable cost
- To be provided complete information about his or her health status in language he or she can understand
- To refuse treatment and to refuse to participate in experimental research
- To formulate advance directives
- To be provided with itemized explanations of services covered by Medicare and Medicaid and services that are not covered
- To protect personal funds, to establish eligibility for Medicaid, to have access to advocacy groups (including ombudsmen and state protective agencies), and to file complaints with state regulators about problems such as abuse, neglect, or misappropriation of property
- To be provided with information about the physician in charge of his or her care
- To be notified of any incident involving injury, change in room assignment, change in status, significant change in treatment, transfer, or discharge (resident's physician, legal representative, and/or family members are also notified)

It cannot be assumed that every facility will automatically protect and preserve all of these rights for the person with Alzheimer's disease. Oversight by health care professionals as well as legal authorities can increase the degree to which these rights are respected for individuals with significant impairments.

Abuse and Neglect

The physical and emotional strains of caring for an individual with Alzheimer's disease are sometimes too great for caregivers, both family and paid, to bear. In addition, nonprofessional (i.e., both paid and family) caregivers often lack understanding of the basis of the disturbing behaviors that occur and have little idea as to how to respond to them effectively. The caregiver's own physical or emotional problems may also contribute to incidents of abuse and neglect.

Abuse is incidents of actual physical or psychological harm, or the failure to prevent this physical or psychological harm. Some "punishments" administered by poorly prepared or overstressed caregivers for disturbing behavior fall into this category: ridicule, threats, hair pulling, pushing, scratching, shoving, hitting, excessive seclusion (including locking the older person in a room or closet), and forcing the person to ingest large amounts of inappropriate food or medicine. Forcing an unwilling person to undergo sterilization or experimentation is also defined as abuse.

Neglect is the failure to provide the care needed by the person with Alzheimer's disease. It is an act of omission rather than of commission. Neglect may include the failure to adequately shelter, clothe, or feed the individual. Failure to adequately supervise the person is another type of neglect that may occur with people with Alzheimer's disease. Failure to provide medical care, medication, or other indicated treatments may also be termed neglect (State of Florida, 1988).

The signs of abuse and neglect are related to the type of abuse or neglect that has occurred. The signs of physical abuse and neglect are unexplained bruises, lesions, fractures, or burns; emaciation; and obvious untreated illness. Clues to psychological abuse and neglect include avoidance of eye contact, evident fear, suspicion, or withdrawal when approached by others. The environmental signs of abuse and neglect are usually obvious: filthy kitchens, careless handling of garbage, vermin, missing or broken equipment, overcrowding, inadequate heating or cooling, intermittent or insufficient running water, and fire hazards.

The individual with Alzheimer's disease is especially vulnerable to abuse, neglect, or both because of his or her reduced capacity to object to or to report the problem to others. Even if the problem is reported, the utterances of people with Alzheimer's disease are so often discounted or ignored entirely that action is rarely taken in cases that would ordinarily be swiftly and thoroughly investigated.

Prevention, in the form of counseling, education, and assistance in caregiving (e.g., respite), is preferable to violations and enforcement of the laws. However, the professional involved in the care of people with Alzheimer's disease is obligated to report suspected abuse and neglect to the appropriate authorities if signs of it are observed.

Incapacity and Guardianship

Incompetence or incapacity has both medical and legal definitions. Neuropsychological testing (discussed in Chapter 3) is used to determine decisional capacity medically. However, interviews also should be conducted to determine a person's judgment and insight, because these are not easily assessed via standardized tests (Broward Community College, 1995).

An *incapacitated* person is someone who has been judged by the court to be unable to manage his or her property (e.g., income, real estate) or to meet his or her own health and safety needs (e.g., food, shelter, hygiene, medicine). Clearly, people with Alzheimer's disease eventually meet the criteria for incapacity as the disease progresses, although many are never declared legally incapacitated.

The procedure for determining incapacity begins with filing of a petition to determine incapacity and to appoint a guardian. Attorneys are then appointed and an examination of the individual is conducted. The results of the examination are reported to the court. This report includes the person's diagnosis, prognosis, and assessment of physical and mental function and evaluation of the person's ability to exercise his or her rights to marry, vote, manage property, drive, travel, work, determine place of residence, choose associates, and consent to medical treatment. A hearing is then held and a judgment is rendered (Broward Community College, 1995). These rights can be restored by the court through a similar procedure that is initiated by filing a petition.

Guardianship   When a person is judged to be incapacitated and in need of a guardian, the form of guardianship (known as conservatorship in some states) assigned should be the least restrictive possible given the individual's capabilities so that as much autonomy can be preserved as possible. The court can specify certain areas (e.g., financial management) to be placed under the control of the guardian, or the court can allow the guardian to assume full control of the rights listed earlier. Certain activities, such as commitment to a mental health facility or dissolution of a marriage, must be approved individually by the court. Guardians are also required to report their activities to the court regularly and can be removed for malfeasance (wrongdoing). The reader should be aware that this action does happen and that fraud has been a problem in some jurisdictions. In some instances the person has been left destitute as a result of malfeasance.

Once an individual has been found incapacitated, he or she cannot execute legal documents (e.g., a will), so it is important that the person diagnosed with early-stage Alzheimer's disease take care of such legal and financial matters as soon as possible. Also, while still competent, the person may be able to designate someone to serve as his or her guardian in the future (State of Florida, 1993), avoiding an inappropriate selection by an outside party later. Family members can be designated as guardians.

Alternatives to Guardianship   It is not always necessary for the person to move from a fully autonomous, decision-making status to the complete dependency on another that guardianship implies. Several intermediate steps can be taken instead.

Probably the best known of these intermediate steps is the execution of a *power of attorney*. A power of attorney document authorizes an attorney or other individual to make decisions for the person but does not negate the individual's right to make his or her own decisions. This authorization ends if the person becomes incapacitated unless it is a *durable power of attorney*, in which case it remains after incapacitation (Alzheimer's Disease and Related Disorders Association, Metro Denver Chapter, n.d.).

Another intermediate action would be the use of a private bill-paying service or assistance from a daily money management service, if one is available in the community. These services can ensure that the person's bills are paid on time, reducing concerns about mismanagement of finances (Wilber & Reynolds, 1995).

Two other alternatives are useful in some situations. Under state family consent laws, a family member may be designated as the person who can make health care decisions for the individual with Alzheimer's disease. State statutes may specify the order of preference, beginning with the spouse, then an adult child, another relative, and so forth. It is also possible to designate a representative who can receive an individual's Social Security or Department of Veterans Affairs pension payment on the basis of a physician's assessment that the person is unable to manage the funds alone (Wilber & Reynolds, 1995).

This chapter began with a brief explanation of the principles of beneficence, nonmaleficence, autonomy, and familial obligation. All of the legal measures described were instituted for the purpose of supporting these principles, however imperfectly they have accomplished this for individual older people. Our challenge is to continue to critically evaluate the extent to which these efforts on behalf of people with Alzheimer's disease accomplish these high purposes and to continue to search for better ways to do so in the future.

REFERENCES

Agency for Health Care Administration. (Undated). *Federal Code 42 CFR 483.10. Requirements for Long Term Care Facilities.* Washington, DC: Author.

Agich, G.J. (1995). Actual autonomy and long-term care decision making. In L.B. McCullough & N.L. Wilson (Eds.), *Long-term care decisions: Ethical and conceptual dimensions.* Baltimore: The Johns Hopkins University Press.

Alzheimer's Disease and Related Disorders Association, Metro Denver Chapter. (n.d.). *Legal considerations with Alzheimer's disease*. Denver: Author.

Arras, J.D. (1995). Conflicting interests in long-term care decision making: Acknowledging, dissolving and resolving conflicts. In L.B. McCullough & N.L. Wilson (Eds.), *Long-term care decisions: Ethical and conceptual dimensions*. Baltimore: The Johns Hopkins University Press.

Bailly, D.J., & DePoy, E. (1995). Older people's responses to education about advance directives. *Health and Social Work, 20*(3), 223–228.

Bresnahan, J.F. (1994). Advance directives in the 1990s: Medical care of the dying and the myth of Sisyphus. In J.F. Monagle & D.C. Thomasme (Eds.), *Health care ethics: Critical issues*. Gaithersburg, MD: Aspen Publishers.

Broward Community College. (1995). *Professional guardian training course*. Fort Lauderdale, FL: Author.

Callahan, D. (1995). Treating people with dementia: When is it okay to stop? In E. Olson, E.R. Chichin, & L.S. Libow (Eds.), *Controversies in ethics in long-term care*. New York: Springer Publishing.

Collopy, B.J. (1995). Safety and independence: Rethinking some basic concepts in long-term care. In L.B. McCullough & N.L. Wilson (Eds.), *Long-term care decisions: Ethical and conceptual dimensions*. Baltimore: The Johns Hopkins University Press.

Hargrave, T.D., & Anderson, W.T. (1992). *Finishing well: Aging and reparation in the intergenerational family*. New York: Brunner/Mazel.

Hunt, S., & Burger, S. (1992). *Using resident assessment and care planning as advocacy tools: A guide for ombudsmen and other advocates*. Washington, DC: National Citizens' Coalition for Nursing Home Reform.

Hurley, A.C., Mahoney, M.A., & Volicer, L. (1995). Comfort care in end-stage dementia: What to do after deciding to do no more. In E. Olson, E.R. Chichin, & L.S. Lebow (Eds.), *Controversies in ethics in long-term care* (pp. 73–90). New York: Springer Publishing.

Kane, R.A. (1995). Decision making, care plans, and life plans in long-term care: Can case managers take account of clients' values and preferences? In L.B. McCullough & N.L. Wilson (Eds.), *Long-term care decisions: Ethical and conceptual dimensions*. Baltimore: The Johns Hopkins University Press.

Klepac, L.M., Coppola, K.M., Ditto, P.H., & Danks, J.H. (1995). *Characteristics of the patient-surrogate relationship and the accuracy of substituted judgment*. Paper presented at the 48th Annual Scientific Meeting of the Gerontological Society of America, Los Angeles.

McCullough, L.B., Wilson, N.L., Rhymes, J.A., & Teasdale, T.A. (1995). Managing the conceptual and ethical dimensions of long-term care decision making: A preventive ethics approach. In L.B. McCullough & N.L. Wilson (Eds.), *Long-term care decisions: Ethical and conceptual dimensions*. Baltimore: The Johns Hopkins University Press.

McGowin, D.F. (1993). *Living in the labyrinth: A personal journey through the maze of Alzheimer's*. San Francisco: Elder Books.

Mezey, M., Bottrell, M.M., Ramsey, G., & the NICHE Faculty. (1996). Advance directives protocol: Nurses helping to protect patient's [sic] rights. *Geriatric Nursing, 17*, 204–210.

National Citizens' Coalition for Nursing Home Reform. (1987). *The rights of nursing home residents*. Washington, DC: Author.

Osman, H., & Perlin, T.M. (1994). Patient self-determination and the artificial prolongation of life. *Health and Social Work, 19*(4), 245–252.

Patient Self-Determination Act of 1991, PL 101-508, 42 U.S.C. § 4206, 4751 *et seq.*

Ragazzo, S. (1993). I have choices [Poem]. *Nightingale Songs, 2*(3), 3.

Requirements for Long Term Care Facilities, 42 C.F.R. § 483.10 (1991).

State of Florida. (1988). Statute 415.102; Statute 825.101 Abuse, Neglect and Exploitation of Elderly Persons and Disabled Adults. Tallahassee: Author.

State of Florida. (1993). Statute 744.3045. Tallahassee: Author.

Stern, R.W., & Hayley, D.C. (1995). *Preferences in surrogate decision-making*. Paper presented at the 48th Annual Scientific Meeting of the Gerontological Society of America, Los Angeles.

Wetle, T. (1995). Ethical issues and value conflicts facing case managers of frail elderly people living at home. In L.B. McCullough & N.L. Wilson (Eds.), *Long-term care decisions: Ethical and conceptual dimensions.* Baltimore: The Johns Hopkins University Press.

Wilber, K.H., & Reynolds, S.L. (1995). Rethinking alternatives to guardianship. *Gerontologist, 35*(2), 248–257.

Index

Long-term memory, 9–10, 64
Loss of Self, The, 78
Lost, becoming, 124–125

Magnetic resonance imaging (MRI), 43–44
  testing difficulty of, 45
Magnetic resonance spectroscopy (MRSI), 44
Malnutrition, 181
MAO, *see* Monoamine oxidase inhibitors
Maps, 69, 124
Mattis Dementia Rating Scale, 67–68
McGowin, Diana, 60, 79
Meaning, memory and, 64–65
Medications, 107–116
  cognitive impairment, 107–110
  falls and, 188–189
  noncognitive symptoms, 110–113
  safe use in Alzheimer's disease, 113–116
Mellaril, 112
Memory
  changes in, 9–13, 66–67
  enhance coding and retrieval processes of, 68, 73–74
  external aids, 69
  music as stimulus for, 150–151
  place, 70
  tapes, question-and-answer, 73
  wallets, 69–70, 72–73
Memory Enhancement and General Awareness Training (MEGA), 72
Memory impairment
  AAMI, 7
  covering up, 79
Metal ions, 109
Metamemory, 66
Mini-Mental State Examination (MMSE), 40, 42–43f
  driving and, 125
Mirrors, 171
Misidentification, 86
Misperception, 80
MMSE, *see* Mini-Mental State Examination
Mnemonics, 74
Mobility
  designing interventions, 179–181
  maintaining, 132, 179
Monoamine oxidase inhibitors (MAO), 109, 112
Mood
  disturbances, 82–83
  legibility of, 81
Motor processes, 20, 152

Movement
  alternating hand, 14
  diminished spontaneous, 14
MRI, *see* Magnetic resonance imaging
MRSI, *see* Magnetic resonance spectroscopy
Multitasking, 121
Muscle tone, increased, 14
Music, therapeutic uses of, 149–151

Napkin, using a, 146
National Institute of Neurological and Communicative Disorders and Stroke (NINCDS), 36
Nature, as relaxation device, 169–170
Negative thinking, 206
Neglect, 228–229
Nerve growth factor, 109
Neurofibrillary tangles, 22–24
Neuroleptics, 112–113
Neurological changes, 13–14
  mood disturbances and, 82
Neurons, structural changes in, 22, 23f
Neurotransmitter, 24–25
  enhancers, 108–109
NINCDS, *see* National Institute of Neurological and Communicative Disorders and Stroke
NINCDS-ADRDA criteria for Alzheimer's disease, 36, 37t
Nonverbal communication, 81
Nootropic agents, as memory aids, 110
Norepinephrine, 25
Normalization, 163–164
Nursing facilities, 216–218
Nutrition, 181–182, 212

Objectification, patient, 55–56
Odors, Alzheimer's disease and, 171
Olfaction, 14
Omnibus Budget Reconciliation Act
  of 1987, PL 100-203, 188–189
  of 1993, PL 103-66, 147
On Golden Pond, 63
Oral hygiene, 140, 141, 181, 183
Outdoor spaces, 168
  safety in, 167
Overmedication, 54, 110–111, 112

Pacing, 88
  spaces for, 168
Pain, assessing, 175–177
Parkinson's disease, 4